Out of the Dead House

OUT OF THE DEAD HOUSE

Nineteenth-Century Women Physicians
and the Writing of Medicine

Susan Wells

THE UNIVERSITY OF WISCONSIN PRESS

The University of Wisconsin Press
2537 Daniels Street
Madison, Wisconsin 53718

3 Henrietta Street
London WC2E 8LU, England

1   3   5   4   2

Printed in the United States of America

Library of Congress Cataloging-in-Publication Data
Wells, Susan.
Out of the dead house : nineteenth-century women physicians
and the writing of medicine / Susan Wells.
324 pp.   cm.
Includes bibliographical references and index.
ISBN 0-299-17170-1 (cloth: alk. paper)
ISBN 0-299-17174-4 (pbk.: alk. paper)
1. Women physicians—United States. 2. Preston, Ann, 1813–1872.
3. Jacobi, Mary Putnam, 1842–1906. 4. Longshore, Hannah, 1819–1901.
5. Women in medicine—United States—History—19th century. I. Title.
R692 .W45   2001
610′.82′097309034—dc21   00-010614

for
Laura Rose Grady
and
Constance Claire Grady

Darling,
stand still at your door,
sure of yourself, a white stone, a good stone—
as exceptional as laughter, you will strike fire,
that new thing!

Anne Sexton

Contents

Illustrations

Acknowledgments

Nineteenth-century women physicians could be a sociable group; working on their writing put me in touch with new and hospitable worlds of medical history and medical archives and confirmed my connections with rhetoricians and compositionists. Karyn Hollis's chance remark that she would love to see the materials at the Medical College of Pennsylvania's archives prompted me to visit there; Theresa Taylor, most patient of archivists, gave me a list of basic historical books and put Hannah Longshore's papers into my hands. I owe immense debts to her and her successors at the Archives and Special Collections on Women in Medicine, especially Barbara Williams, who sustained the archive through a chaotic period in the history of the college and who supplied me richly from its immense resources. This book has also benefited from the help of archivists and librarians at the Friends Historical Library, the Center for the Study of the History of Nursing, the Historic Library of the Pennsylvania Hospital, the Thomas Jefferson University Archives, the Quaker Collection of the Haverford College Library, the Rare Book and Manuscript Library at the University of Pennsylvania, the Schlesinger Library at Radcliffe College, the Historical Library at the National Library of Medicine in Washington, D.C., the Library of the College of Physicians of Philadelphia, the Temple University Urban Archives, and the Charles L. Blockson Afro-American Collection at Temple University. In using these archival materials, I preserved original spelling, grammar, and punctuation.

Participants at academic conferences asked especially useful questions about this project. I am grateful to the College Composition and Communication Conference, the Pennsylvania State University Conference on Composition and Rhetoric, the Wayne State University American Studies Colloquium, the Wood Seminars in the History of Medicine at the College of Physicians of Philadelphia, the American Association for the History of Medicine, the Modern Language Association, the Kent State English Graduate Organization, and the Partial Bodies Conference sponsored by graduate students in comparative literature at the University of Pennsylvania. The questions and comments of James Bono and Gretchen Worden have been especially memorable and welcome. The University of Pennsylvania Workshop in the History and Sociology of Science and Technology offered me a benchmark for rigorous reflection on the aims of science studies. And I owe a more sustained debt to the students and auditors in my seminar Feminist Rhetorics of Science and to Robert Caserio, who complied with my unreasonable request for a late change of seminar topic. My colleagues in rhetoric and composition at Temple University—Eli Goldblatt, Dennis Lebofsky, Arabella Lyon, Frank Sullivan, and Steve Parks—tolerated my urgent requests to look at the latest gruesome pictures. Sally Mitchell and Miles Orvell told me things about archival work that I should have learned in graduate school. Maurice Vogel and Gretchen Condon, scholars in the history and sociology of medicine at Temple, helped me locate my work in relation to those challenging and fascinating fields. Steven Peitzman, author of *A New and Untried Course: Woman's Medical College and the Medical College of Pennsylvania* (Rutgers University Press, 2000), a critically important history of the Woman's Medical College, and Michael Sappol, author of *A Traffic of Dead Bodies: Anatomy and Embodied Social Identity in Nineteenth Century America*, a compelling account of dissection and the formation of American medicine (Princeton University Press, 2001), have been generous and helpful colleagues; I have gained immeasurably from dialogue with them. All errors are my own.

I am grateful for support from Temple University, especially a Summer Research Grant, two Grants-in-Aid of Research, and a Research and Study Leave, without which I would not have finished this book. I owe special thanks to Mary Elizabeth Braun and to the University of Wisconsin Press referees, whose advice has been invaluable, and to Rachel Bright, who did final proofreading.

The lines on the dedication page are from Anne Sexton's "Little Girl, My String Bean, My Lovely Woman."

Finally, I am grateful to Hugh Grady, and to Laura Rose Grady and Constance Claire Grady, for their love and support, and for the "large liberty" that sustained this book.

Out of the Dead House

1

Out of the Dead House

In 1840, the ten-year-old Marie Zakrzewska was living at La Charité, the Berlin midwifery school. Her mother had obtained special permission to enter the school, usually closed to married women, and Marie was permitted to join her when the girl's weak eyes needed treatment. (Marie's father, a man of "liberal opinions," "impetuous temperament," and "revolutionary tendencies," had been dismissed from his military officer's commission with an insufficient pension; Marie's mother needed to help support the family.) Marie made rounds, her eyes bandaged, with her physician, Dr. Müller, who called her his "little blind doctor."[1] She listened to what he said with great concentration.

When the bandages were removed, Dr. Müller told Marie that the corpse of a young man who had been poisoned and turned green was in the dead house, the building that was the hospital's morgue and pathology laboratory. Marie went there to look for herself, and while relatives were busy with the young man's body, she toured the nearby rooms: "These were all freshly painted. The dissecting tables, with the necessary apparatus, stood in the center, while the bodies, clad in white gowns, were ranged on boards along the walls. I examined everything, came back, and looked to my heart's content at the poisoned young man." Then she noticed that both the relatives and the caretaker were gone and that the building was locked. Marie looked through all the rooms again, knocked on the door for half an hour, gave up, and went to sleep. Well after dark, Marie's mother found her, "sitting close by [the door] on the floor fast asleep."[2] A few days later, Dr. Müller gave Marie the *History of Midwifery* and the *History of Surgery*, which she read through the six weeks of her summer vacation.

This story rehearses one of the narratives of nineteenth-century women's entry into medicine. The protagonist comes to us as a little girl, curious, unafraid, strangely concentrated, usually accompanied by her mother and almost always by someone who acts as her father. She learns what she can,

3

but then faces an obstacle. She has wandered far from her place, but she has not yet arrived where she wants to be. She is, as far as she knows, fearless. Zakrzewska, in her version of this story, comes to a place that is actively forbidden, the dead house. She comes in search of a magical sight—a man who has changed color, like a victim of enchantment. The dead house is not for her a place of loss or mourning but a domain of almost festive order. There, the girl who has spent weeks only listening can now also look. And so she looks, for as long as she wants. She would rather not sleep all night there by herself, but if she must, she will.

Rescued, she sees clearly and claims medical knowledge for herself. She takes up her books and reads, beginning a medical education that will bring her to the United States, to a long collaboration with Elizabeth Blackwell, to an honored place as "Dr. Zak" in the histories of the New England Hospital for Women and Children and the New England Female Medical College.

Before beginning her education as a physician, Zakrzewska did a lifetime's work: she kept house for her large family, nursed relatives, and assisted in her mother's midwifery practice until she was twenty. Admitted to midwifery school, she was soon assistant to the teacher—her own Dr. Müller. She lectured to the class and then took examinations on her lectures, and she was appointed chief of the school on her graduation. When she heard that a woman had become a doctor in the United States, she immigrated, supporting herself with a small worsted business, and finally contacted Elizabeth Blackwell. When she entered medical school in Cleveland, her father wrote that if she had been a young man, "I could not find words in which to express my satisfaction and pride in respect to your acts; for I know that all you accomplish you owe to yourself: but you are a woman, a weak woman; and all that I can do for you now is to grieve and weep." At one point, Zakrzewska was so dismayed by her father's disapproval that she decided to go as a missionary to "civilize the squaws."[3] But she persevered, graduated, and eventually prospered.

Zakrzewska tells her story in a singular but representative voice—rational, humorous, willing to indulge in sentimentality but not to forgo satire. For Dr. Zak, that voice was grounded in the study and practice of science, a practice that "has no sex."[4] Knowing as we do that medicine not only deals with gendered bodies but also in some ways genders the bodies it treats, we would not make such a statement today. But we might also recover, in an act of historical imagination, the force of such a statement, for Zakrzewska and women like her. Medicine offered them not only the possibility of a wider sphere but the possibility of a world without spheres, where the house of the dead had been set in order, and there was nothing to be afraid of. Like many other women physicians, Zakrzewska was cured by medical knowledge: Ann Preston, Mary Putnam Jacobi, and Hannah Longshore, three early graduates of the Woman's Medical College of Pennsylvania, all felt sure that by becoming physicians they had saved their lives, delivered themselves from confinement and uselessness, permitted themselves to use their strength and talents. The letters of nineteenth-century women physicians include both complaints of overwork or poor health and professions of a singular joy in the work they were able to do, the lives they had imagined into existence.

The work of medicine included reading and writing, beginning for Zakrzewska with those two fat histories. Later, she would become a writer herself: with the help of a loose association of Cleveland feminists, Zakrzewska wrote her thesis in English and went on to produce proposals, articles, letters to official bodies, lectures, and magazine and publicity pieces.[5] In fact, every woman physician wrote a thesis; many continued to write on scientific topics. Women physicians did the writing that characterized the emerging profession: case histories, faculty minutes, public lectures, commencement speeches, scientific papers, political arguments, memoirs, and testimonies to investigative bodies. Their work is perhaps the largest corpus of scientific writing by women before the contemporary period. As medical practice emerged and organized itself in the United States, women physicians constructed a textual representation of medicine, developing the emerging norms of the medical interview, testing the limits of internal criticism of the profession, inventing new forms of medical research. Sometimes celebrated and sometimes marginalized, they participated in the early production of professional medical writing. I am tempted to speculate that these women wrote an alternate medicine, that their texts are sketches for a possible science that never came into being. Instead, I advance a more modest claim: that women physicians did the work of medicine as it was understood in the last half of the nineteenth century, and that their writing can historicize and complicate our understanding of the relations among women and science, gender and knowledge.

Women physicians developed distinctive strategies for speaking and writing in a hostile profession. Many wrote as if they were men of the received order: they insisted on the regularity of their medical views and the rigor of their education. These women sometimes argued for a wider sphere for women or claimed that their gender gave them a special understanding of some neglected (and usually undervalued) aspect of medicine, such as hygiene, public health, or prevention. Theirs was a strategy of masquerade: the woman physician wrote as male but did not present herself as "a man." Instead, she was "a doctor as good as any man"; her disguise is foregrounded as a performance, rendered memorable by the special skill she brought to it.[6]

Other women were quite willing to foreground their gender, to use it as a tool for transforming medicine. Such women were often interested in irregular therapies, such as the water cure, mesmerism, and magnetism; they were active in radical causes, including abolition, women's rights, dress reform, and temperance movements. Rather than writing conventional medicine, women who adopted this strategy sought to transform the nature of medical writing; they often wrote for a broad audience, popularizing medical knowledge as they saw it, lectured, and wrote in radical journals. Their performance of the discourse of medicine was, in a broad sense, travesty—a performance of subversion dressed as compliance.

Women physicians at the end of the century expanded the range of possible gender performances: the woman physician offered herself as a scientist, able to discourse about the body like a philosopher, accountable to the highest standards of rigor. She could fulfill, as much as it was ever to be fulfilled, the promise of Zakrzewska's motto, "Science has no sex." But of course, such a relentless female performance of a discourse configured as male was not uninflected: the woman physician who wrote "normal medicine" was in some sense cross-dressing as male.[7] Individual women physicians adopted various combinations of these strategies at different times during their careers and hoped for a variety of responses from their profession—from transformation to benign neglect. Seeing gender as a performance helps us to appreciate the rhetorical skill of these women physicians and their uses of the slender rhetorical resources available to them.

THE CONTEXT: NINETEENTH-CENTURY MEDICINE AND WOMEN PHYSICIANS

Late nineteenth-century medicine is paradigmatic of successful professionalization: doctors gained control of licensing, training, and disciplining procedures and also expanded exponentially the range of conditions and diseases they could treat successfully.[8] In 1800, only two hospitals were operating in the United States. The range of conditions for which no effective treatment was available could supply several seasons of television medical series plots: typhoid fever, yellow fever, typhus, influenza, appendicitis, most cancers, many forms of heart disease, diabetes, tuberculosis. Surgery concentrated on the treatment of wounds and the repair of fractures; textbooks in surgery devoted more space to amputations than to any other operation. Medicine included a wide range of therapeutic disciplines: regular (or, for homeopaths, "allopathic") medicine, homeopathy, magnetic and electrical treatments (including mesmerism), the water cure, steam treatments, botanicals, hybrid disciplines such as Eclecticism, and self-treatment systems such as Thompsonianism. Some of these disciplines still survive; others, like magnetic appliances, the Thompsonian recipe books for herbal medicines that allowed every man to be his own doctor, and the apparatus for

6

steam treatments, clutter the backrooms of medical archives. But in the mid-nineteenth century, these disciplines were plausible competitors with regular medicine: Eclecticism, which drew on both the allopathic and homeopathic pharmacopeias, sponsored several medical schools and was powerful within a number of midwestern medical societies. Medical practice had been deregulated at the beginning of the century: licenses were not required to practice medicine; charters were freely given to proprietary medical schools. From its formation in 1846, the American Medical Association struggled to establish the hegemony of regular medicine over these disparate schools and to bring hospitals and medical schools under the control of the profession. So dazzling was the association's success that it is difficult for us to imagine the contingency and openness of nineteenth-century medicine, let alone to maintain the relativism that informs contemporary work in the rhetoric of science.

We think of medical education as proverbially grueling, but in the middle of the nineteenth century, a physician enjoyed an easier professional preparation than, say, a minister, who in some congregations was expected to master demanding ancient languages and perplexing questions of theology. The aspiring medical student needed no prior formal education, although he was expected to know enough Latin to write prescriptions. Before reforms established entrance standards in the third quarter of the century, the sole requirement for entry into medical school was a year's preceptorship with an established physician. The medical student heard seven courses of lectures given over a four-month term by practicing physicians who lectured as a sideline. The student repeated the same course a second year, wrote a thesis, and passed an oral examination. It is not surprising that the standard history of nineteenth-century medical education begins with the sentence, "A century ago, being a medical student in America was easy."[9]

The ease of medical school was not necessarily good news for patients, but it was certainly good news for women who wanted a medical education. Opening a proprietary medical school—and, at midcentury, most American schools were proprietary—required only classrooms, a rudimentary library, and the part-time services of seven physicians; after applying for a state charter, the school could enroll students and grant medical degrees. At midcentury, a number of women's schools were founded, usually with scanty initial support. In 1848, in order to protect women's modesty by training female midwives, Samuel Gregory founded the school that would become the New England Female Medical College. The Woman's (originally Female) Medical College of Pennsylvania, founded by a group of Philadelphia Quakers, graduated eight women in its first class in 1851. (The name was changed in 1867; the school is referred to consistently as the Woman's Medical College in this book.) A handful of women, such as Elizabeth Blackwell, graduated from male medical schools or, like her sister Emily, found a medical education abroad. Coeducation, the goal of many women physicians, came slowly; the University of Michigan became coeducational in 1870, and forty-eight women graduated from the Howard University medical department between 1869 and 1900.[10] But women's main point of entry into the medical profession was the women's proprietary school, including, besides the schools in Boston, New York, and Philadelphia, women's medical colleges in Chicago and Baltimore and smaller schools in Atlanta, St. Louis, Cincinnati, and Toronto. By 1898, these colleges enrolled 377 students. Over five thousand women were practicing as regular physicians in the United States, most of them in New York, Pennsylvania, Massachusetts, Maryland, Illinois, and California—they constituted about 5 percent of the medical profession, a percentage that was not surpassed until the 1970s.[11] These women formed a cadre of scientific workers. They met in women's medical societies, corresponded through their school's alumnae associations, and carried out active careers as clinicians, teachers, and researchers.

Women medical students, like male medical students, came from the middle and upper-middle classes,[12] but they faced financial challenges that differed from those of male medical students. Although many enjoyed the support of their families, especially of physician fathers, others battled familial hostility. Many came late to medical school—in 1880, the average graduate at the Woman's Medical College of Pennsylvania was twenty-seven.[13] Women might enter medical school after a sojourn in teaching or nursing or after fulfilling family obligations to care for sick relatives. And women medical students often worked during medical school or interrupted their education to earn money.

Women doctors, their supporters, their opponents, and their patients were all convinced that women physicians practiced a different kind of medicine from that offered by male physicians at the middle of the nineteenth century. Usually, this difference is described in quietist terms: women doctors were less interventionist, less likely to prescribe harsh drugs or surgery, and more empathetic. But Regina Markell Morantz-Sanchez's study comparing the woman-run New England Hospital with the male-run Boston Lying-In during the 1880s and 1890s revealed "no significant divergence between the two hospitals regarding infant mortality or maternal outcome."[14] There were minor differences in treatment. Patients at New England Hospital were always given a systemic fortifying prescription, such as "beef tea," while such prescriptions were less frequent at Boston Lying-In. New England Hospital kept much more detailed records of its patients. But every other significant variable, including the rate of forceps deliveries and success in controlling sepsis, shows no difference between treatment at the two hospitals. At the last quarter of the nineteenth century, women doctors were practicing a quite conventional style of medicine, with no more and no less success than male doctors. But it was, paradoxically, quite common for all sorts of nineteenth-century physicians to feel that their practices were distinct and innovative, even if their therapies were well within common practice.[15] Contemporaneous accounts of women physicians, quite logically, emphasized what was distinct in their practice; why write about what was unremarkable? Women physicians, therefore, worked in a social context in which their practice was seen as distinctly feminine but in which their therapeutic choices were very similar to those of men.

The period during which women physicians formed a distinct and cohesive group came to an end with the rise of coeducation and the professionalization of medical schools following the Flexner report in 1910.[16] The Johns Hopkins Medical School was planned, during its development in the 1880s, on the German model: it would have a full-time faculty, its own teaching hospital, and an orientation to both research and clinical training. Such a school was both unprecedented and extremely expensive, and its opening was delayed from year to year. The Woman's Fund Committee raised the final five hundred thousand dollars needed to open the school and offered these funds to the trustees if they would admit women on the same terms as men. Hopkins opened with a coeducational class in 1893; within five years, most medical schools were open to women. Enrollments at the women's colleges fell from 459 in 1893 to 183 in 1904, and many schools closed.[17] The Flexner report (1910), sponsored by the AMA Committee on Medical Education, proposed a general reform of medical education, including more clinical and laboratory work, the development of a professional faculty, and institutional connections with teaching hospitals. The weakened women's schools were unable to implement these reforms. In Keith Ludmerer's words, "Of all the oppressed groups, women suffered the most ironic setback. In the wake of the Flexner report, all but one women's medical college [the Woman's Medical College of Pennsylvania] closed."[18]

The success of coeducation as a strategy for training women physicians was uncertain. Some schools discontinued the admission of women; very few admitted women at rates higher than 5 percent. Very few of the women who had taught at women's medical colleges joined the faculties of co-ed schools; the intellectual infrastructure that women physicians had enjoyed lost important institutional supports. The number of women medical students actually declined from 1,280 in 1902 to 992 in 1926. The proportion of women in the profession reached 6 percent in 1910 and then shrank steadily until 1950; it did not rise dramatically until the 1970s.[19]

Women's participation in nineteenth-century medicine, then, was uneven and contradictory: women entered a large, loose profession in relatively ample numbers, participated in its work as it developed scientifically, formed their own institutions, were accepted into the male institutions as scientific medicine achieved its greatest triumphs, and then were both marginalized and dispersed. Advances for women physicians were not necessarily significant for women patients; advances for women patients could be setbacks for women physicians. Early women physicians told quite diverse stories about themselves; they saw themselves as pioneers of medicine of material care and placed their own work in a context we can recover only in fragments. One of the imaginative possibilities that nineteenth-century women physicians can suggest to us is that of a less absolute triumph of regular medicine, of multiple and intersecting medical practices.

WOMEN PHYSICIANS AND SCIENCE STUDIES

This book is not a medical history but an intervention into the rhetoric of science. Rhetoric of science analyzes how scientific texts, including the discourses of medicine, constitute social practices and knowledges. A rhetorical study of the discourses of medicine shows that ways of writing and talking about the body supported doctors' and patients' understandings of gender, of race, indeed of embodiment in general.[20] And the relation between those understandings and the material practices they supported, practices studied by feminist historians, can tell us how texts shape other kinds of scientific work. In the case of nineteenth-century medicine, women physicians participated in both scientific discourses and scientific practices. As medicine became professionalized, it portrayed itself as masculine, as an uncompromising search for truth and certainty rather than a project of feminine comfort or care; we need not ourselves participate in that ideology, although we, unlike Zakrzewska, have good reason to think of science as male. In both its subject matter and its institutional practices, medicine has been a gendered science, and the first wave of feminist scholarship passionately dismantled its claim to neutral objectivity, analyzing how medicine constructed gender and how the masculine bias of the profession compromised both its ability to treat women patients and its claim to impartiality.[21] At the same time, feminist scholarship in education and psychology, especially Carol Gilligan's *In a Different Voice* and Mary Belenky and her associates' *Women's Ways of Knowing,* suggested that the continued underrepresentation of women in the sciences was connected to the masculine bias of science education.[22] In the conventional science class, these studies claim, the student is evoked as an isolated, rather than a connected, knower. Belenky and her associates characterized such isolation as more comfortable for men than for women students. Further challenges were mounted by feminist philosophers of science who examined the rhetoric of early scientific programs and the practices of contemporary women scientists. For Evelyn Fox Keller, in *Reflections on Science and Gender,* the rejection of the feminine urged by Francis Bacon suggested that science was in fact a masculine project; in her examination of the work of geneticist Barbara McClintock, Keller suggests that the work of this woman scientist was shaped by a "feeling for the organism" that was at odds with conventional (and therefore masculine) ways of doing science.[23]

These challenges to the authority of science joined the critical analyses of scientific practices undertaken by Latour and Woolgar, the close reading of Darwin's evolutionary theory within the context of nineteenth-century plot structures by Gillian Beer, and the analysis of experiment as spectacle by Shapin and Schaffer.[24] Science studies have emerged as an interdisciplinary examination of the discursive practices of the sciences, including both historical research and ongoing analyses of the daily work of contemporary scientists, undertaken from a variety of political perspectives. The work of Donna Haraway, for example, has evolved from rather conventional studies in the history of anthropology to remarkably inventive texts used by cultural theorists to study how bodies and their pleasures are constructed in a cybernetic culture.[25] Studies in the rhetoric of science consider such topics as persuasion, credibility or *ethos,* the discursive construction of presence, and scientific uses of metaphor, of narrative structure, and of personification.[26] This work is often carried out in a critical dialogue with practicing scientists.[27] Feminist studies of science, in particular, have been strengthened by the participation of feminist scientists, beginning with the early interventions of molecular biologist Evelyn Fox Keller and continuing through the work of the apprentice scholars in the Biology and Gender Study Group.[28] *Out of the Dead House* brings to bear on this work the feminist studies of nineteenth-century women's reading and writing practices.[29] Women's medical writing can be contextualized in the genre of disciplinary medicine, and it can also be read in relation to what women read and wrote; both perspectives help us attend to what nineteenth-century women physicians tell us about professional authority and textual power.

Feminist rhetoricians of science are only beginning to produce historical studies of the rhetorical practices of early women scientists. Much of the work on women scientists before the twentieth century has focused on accumulating records of their bare existence rather than on analyzing the specificity of their scientific practice. It is not surprising, therefore, that the ideological characterization of science as a particularly male activity has not been contested in either feminist or cultural studies of science, except by redefining science to include traditionally feminine activities such as gardening or midwifery.

This book examines the women physicians of the last half of the nine-

11

teenth century as writers, especially as writers of science. If science is understood as constructed by, among other things, certain practices of language, then it is worthwhile to study how women performed those practices. I am encouraged in this study by the rich context within which these early physicians undertook scientific work. They wrote and practiced in company with other women; unlike such isolated eighteenth-century figures as the anatomist Thiroux d'Arconville or the entomologist Maria Sibylla Merian, nineteenth-century women physicians met with other women, wrote for them, and consulted with them, simultaneously taking part, as they were able, in the work of the male profession. Moreover, because their work as physicians was continuous with the traditionally feminine task of caring for the sick, women physicians could draw upon a rich array of textualizations, including practices of correspondence, popular advice, journalism, and fiction, especially the domestic novel.

WOMEN PHYSICIANS, RHETORIC, AND THE WRITING OF MEDICINE

My own approach to nineteenth-century women physicians is mediated by my training as a literary scholar and my commitments as a rhetorician. Although the texts written by nineteenth-century women do not tell us the whole story of their professional lives, such texts are rich sources of information about how they understood themselves, how they constructed the body, how they made sense of their anomalous gender position. These writings also contest the idea that scientific work is alien to women or that women scientists write in a unitary, distinctly feminine voice. The idea of a distinctly feminine scientific voice assumes that science is something produced almost entirely by men, that women have made no contributions to scientific writing, and that science is a unitary and unchanging activity, substantially the same in all fields and during all periods. I argue against all of these assumptions. Women doctors intervened in medical discourse at the very formation of the modern scientific profession. They invented central tropes and strategies for medical research and writing: the use of survey information, methods of taking patient histories, conventions for telling case histories. Women physicians' contributions changed as the profession developed, and individual women physicians produced quite distinct medical texts. This book traces a specific history in its variations, locating women's writing within the changing contours of medicine as a science and as a profession. It also accounts for the pleasure women physicians took in the disciplinary activity of medicine; avid for scientific knowledge, devoted to research and clinical practice, they call into question any notion of scientific discourse as alien to women.

In order to study that work and that pleasure, I have used the terms of my art: rhetoric has long concerned itself with what is probable, what is likely, what is desired differently by different groups; it has been scorned by philosophers since Socrates for attending to the discourses of women, children, slaves, and other rabble.[30] Rhetoric assumes that the speaking self is always presented, always constructed, and that its truths are always provisional; composition studies attend to noncanonical texts, pedagogical settings, students' approximations of achieved texts. My own desire in this work is to question the self-characterization of scientific knowledge as masculine and to recuperate a sense of women's agency in scientific work, a sense of their commitment to their profession and most especially their pleasure in its practices. Overtaken by admiration for these women, I have chosen to repay my filial debt to them by reading them, by seeing their texts as the work of writers handling resistant materials, who made difficult choices and found in the most forbidding situations the available means of persuasion.

In this book, discussions of individual women physicians and their strategies of gender performance alternate with examinations of emerging professional forms. Chapter 2, "Medical Conversations and Medical Histories," reconstructs, from hospital and clinic records and from books of medical advice, how male and female physicians talked to their patients. Many women physicians prided themselves on their ability to speak intimately with their patients; *heart history* was their term for the woman physician's intervention into her patient's personal life. And women physicians do seem to have talked differently to their patients, although the other treatments they offered were completely conventional. But the "heart history" was contradictory: it allowed patients to express themselves and to intervene in their own treatment; it also offered the doctor a clear field for moral instruction of the patient. Women physicians offered financial advice, supervised the patients' reproductive life, and proselytized for their (quite unconventional) religious beliefs; Freud would have called them wild psychoanalysts. All these contradictions became more acute when the physician was an African American woman, as demonstrated by the writing of Rebecca Lee Crumpler.

"Invisible Writing I: Ann Preston Invents an Institution," chapter 3, is an account of the writing of Ann Preston, who was thirty-eight when she graduated with the first class from the Woman's Medical College of Pennsylvania (1850) and was associated with the college for the rest of her life, as professor of physiology and later as dean. Preston wrote a great deal, but much of her writing—school announcements, procedures, minutes of meetings—was anonymous. When she did write under her own name, the occasion was often ceremonial, a commencement or an inaugural lecture. Preston used the available materials, including the doctrine of a separate sphere for women, to construct a rhetoric which supported women physicians. Her gender performance was cross-dressed; Preston presents herself as an entirely regular physician, distinguishable from males only by her interest in the womanly and unglamourous issues of prevention and hygiene. That strategy was replicable, functional in protecting the new Woman's Medical College, and costly, both personally and professionally.

"Learning to Write Medicine," chapter 4, compares theses written by students at the Woman's Medical College with those written at the School of Medicine of the University of Pennsylvania from 1850 to 1852, and examines a group of theses written by African American students at the Woman's Medical College in the 1870s and 1880s. The theses fall into two groups: some offer advice to a lay audience; others are addressed to other physicians. Theses written as advice—those in the register of health—model how the future doctor would perform his duties as family counselor. Those written to other physicians—a register of medicine—show that the student had attended to faculty lectures and was able to reproduce them. While both men and women students wrote in the register of health and the register of medicine, theses from the Woman's Medical College are distinct in two ways: They are sometimes critical of the medical profession—a very exceptional performance for a student suing for professional credentials, then or now. And women's theses are often marked by satire, a distinguishing rhetorical figure for nineteenth-century women physicians. African American women physicians faced additional rhetorical exigencies: they were deeply interested in "race questions," questions which their training did not help them answer, and the issues of authority they negotiated were especially complex.

"Invisible Writing II: Hannah Longshore and the Border of Regularity," discusses a woman physician who was as resistant as Ann Preston was compliant. Hannah Longshore, sister-in-law of a founder of the Woman's Medical College, was associated throughout her life with such irregular medical schools as homeopathy, the water cure, mesmerism, and spiritual healing. Her relationship with the relentlessly regular Woman's Medical College was therefore quite problematic. This chapter analyzes a speech that Longshore gave, in her old age, to the Woman's Medical College Alumnae Association and places Longshore within the context of her extremely eccentric and productive family, a family who adopted strategies of travesty to express both their admiration for and their distance from religious and scientific orthodoxy.

Chapter 6 analyzes the most scientifically engaged of the women physicians I have studied, Mary Putnam Jacobi. With her hundred and fifty medical publications and energetic journalism, Mary Putnam Jacobi helped to change the face of medical writing. In *The Question of Rest for Women during Menstruation*, anonymous winner of Harvard's Boylston Prize for Medical Writing, Putnam Jacobi was the first to use survey research in a medical

14

article. Her work on hysteria mounted a sustained critique of S. Weir Mitchell's rest cure; Putnam Jacobi, in fact, treated C. P. Gilman after the disastrous rest cure recounted in "The Yellow Wall-Paper."[31] Completely unsentimental, resolutely opposed to any separate sphere for women, Putnam Jacobi had come to intellectual maturity in the world of French utopian socialism, where science was seen as an efficacious way of transforming the world. Putnam Jacobi's performance of gender was often remarkably experimental: by turns, she wrote anonymously, collaborated with other physicians, insisted on her gender, denied its relevance, and accepted and rejected membership in the company of women physicians.

The final chapter of *Out of the Dead House* analyzes two medical spectacles: the clinical lecture and dissection. Women physicians managed to contain the potentially transgressive practice of dissection, but their entrance into the more public ceremony of the clinical lecture could provoke riots. These practices can be understood within the context of women's popular and vernacular interest in physiology, demonstrated in the formation of ladies' physiological societies, the vogue for recreational dissection (usually of small animals), and the popularity of public physiological lectures and exhibits. This chapter returns to the issue raised by the young Marie Zakrzewska, delighted in the dead house: How can we understand the pleasures of medical knowledge as women physicians experienced them? How can we locate those pleasures within the political and cultural context that supported them?

2

Medical Conversations and Medical Histories

The medical practice that the first women physicians entered was one which valued talk. The body's story was not read from diagnostic images or test results but composed from information provided by the patient and confirmed, if need be, in direct examination by the physician. Medicine was therefore a heavily discursive practice, worked out patient by patient in a series of conversations. Conversation initiated treatment, and conversations marked its progress. The doctor would inquire about the patient's symptoms, the history of his or her illness, and daily habits and hygiene. The accompanying physical examination might be limited to a cursory glance at the tongue and survey of the pulse or include careful palpation of organs, auscultation of the chest, and rudimentary laboratory work. Treatment almost always included a prescription but possibly also minor surgery or (more and more rarely after midcentury) bleeding or cupping, cautery, or blistering. The doctor's talk to the patient, however, was always a feature of treatment; hygienic counsel, medical information, and calm encouragement were seen as essential to the cure. Since the patient was seen regularly until a cure was certified, the conversation between doctor and patient would be protracted, often over years. Given the uncertain efficacy of so many nineteenth-century treatments and the growing rejection, especially in the middle of the century, of such heroic measures as purging and bleeding in favor of therapies that concentrated on strengthening the system, the medical interview was the central discipline of therapy rather than ancillary to it.

In the later decades of the nineteenth century, when techniques of physical diagnosis developed, these conversations diminished in importance. Diagnostic devices such as x rays and laboratory tests more complex than basic studies of blood and urine became available at the end of the century, and microscopic investigations became common. At midcentury, it was a rare physician who, after medical school, looked through a microscope. Also, although pulse and respiration rates were counted, only the most scientifically advanced physician used thermometers, and stethoscopes were optional.[1]

16

Moreover, there was an extremely close correlation between medical conversations and the most common genre in nineteenth-century medical writing, the patient history. Even today, the patient history is so closely connected with the initial doctor-patient conversation that patients who can accurately narrate the course of their illnesses are called good historians.[2] The case history is a venerable and durable medical genre; from Sigmund Freud's to Oliver Sachs's, case histories have also been read by a lay audience. Contemporary medical histories offer concentrated, formulaic accounts of patients' experiences, sometimes produced by relatively inexperienced physicians, intended to communicate with dispersed professionals and to direct future investigation and treatment. In the nineteenth century, case histories were a staple of medical education but quite diverse in form; standard conventions for collecting and reporting case histories developed, quite unevenly, during the last half of the century. The nineteenth-century case history might orient the attention of students, project a course of treatment, or record a significant therapeutic advance; the form and structure of the history varied with the interests and status of the writer.

Doctor-patient conversations and patient histories are and were important sites for the linguistic performance of gender and so were especially problematic for women. Women patients faced contradictory constraints both to speak frankly and to maintain a decent silence. Many illnesses we see as having nothing to do with gender were, for nineteenth-century physicians and patients, gendered experiences. Women sought treatment during pregnancy, childbirth, or menopause, but conditions such as eye infections and general fatigue could be understood by both doctors and patients as reproductive illnesses. For women patients, the medical interview was a conversation on potentially delicate subjects with a member of the opposite sex, even when her symptoms were located far from her reproductive organs. When the doctor was a woman, gender was even more salient to the conversation: women doctors understood themselves as having conversations with their patients that no male doctor could have had. As physicians and writers of medical histories, women negotiated the cultural expectation that they be empathic; they also developed institutional forms that supported distinct medical conversations and encouraged the writing of distinct texts. At these sites, women's discursive performance of their gender inflected the nondiscursive medical treatment they were likely to provide or receive; an ideology of unorthodox treatment could be combined with the most conservative regular therapy. (But of course, talk was also part of the therapy, so that unconventional talk *was* also unconventional therapy.)

Contemporary studies of medical discourse can inform our investigation of these historical practices. Such studies demonstrate that, while men and women do not use different languages in medical settings, they do use lan-

17

guage differently. Very broadly, sociolinguists have identified no variation in lexicon or syntax that reliably differentiates women's speech from men's. Although some writers have suggested that women use a distinct vocabulary or are more likely to produce certain sentence forms, no empirical study has supported such claims. In speech or in writing, gender difference typically emerges as one of a number of variables, and its significance changes radically depending on class, relations among language communities, and family structures.[3] But sociolinguists have repeatedly identified gender differences in the large rhetorical structures of conversation. In the sites of American culture that have been studied, men talk more than women, and the two genders follow different conversational strategies. They have different expectations of one another and treat one another differently, although those differences are themselves inflected by race, class, and age. These differences were probably more marked in the mid-nineteenth century, when men's and women's economic and social spheres were more distinct, although we should not assume any simple story of progress.

The medical interview was central to clinical care and unavoidably gendered; women participated in the interview as both patients and physicians. The histories based on such interviews form an important body of medical texts. The rich body of contemporary studies of doctor-patient interviews poses questions about nineteenth-century conversations, demonstrating that the work of the medical interview affects patients' understandings of the diagnosis, their emotional attitude toward treatment, and their compliance with it. The interview also affects the doctor's orientation toward the patient and the course of his or her treatment.[4] To study how women participated in, formed, and were themselves constructed by the medical discourse of the nineteenth century, then, I begin by listening to the talk of the consulting room.

IMAGINED CONVERSATIONS I: THE DOCTOR'S HOPE

Any analysis of nineteenth-century medical conversations must rely on indirect evidence; nineteenth-century medical records, including hospital notes and clinic books, rarely quote patients directly but often suggest something of what passed between doctor and patient. Other genres of physicians' writing, including the voluminous popular medical literature, supplement these accounts. In popular medical literature, male and female doctors told exemplary stories, often organized as dialogues with patients. In examining these records, it is not at all my intention to evaluate the medical care that these physicians provided—an evaluation that would be ill-informed and impertinent. After all, these patients and their physicians, even if they had received and given the best conceivable care, would certainly be dead today. Their ways of speaking and hearing have perhaps survived them, if only in the medical imaginary. In the records of these conversations, we can discern how doctors and patients, women and men, constructed bodies that were gendered, articulated into the family and the economy, and treatable in scientific ways, and we can appreciate both the productive, generative possibilities of such constructions and their potential for oppression and control.

Two assumptions salient to contemporary doctor-patient interactions simply did not operate in nineteenth-century medicine: the constraint of universalism, under which all patients suffering from the same ailment should receive the same treatment, and that of functional specificity, which demands that the doctor's intervention be limited to medical matters.[5] While neither of these principles has ever been more than a goal of medical treatment, each does regulate the discourse of medicine; the patient's social class or moral state cannot be explicitly given as a reason for a course of treatment. To a mid-nineteenth-century physician, both assumptions would have seemed wrongheaded. Hospitals routinely offered or denied treatment on the basis of the patients' perceived moral state;[6] doctors prided themselves on their ability to transform patients' personal lives and beliefs. Nor did physicians accept universalism as an axiom of treatment: the Woman's Hospital associated with the Woman's Medical College of Pennsylvania, like other Philadelphia hospitals, refused to manage the births of unmarried mothers.[7] Women physicians like Harriot Kezia Hunt and Ruth Gleason saw themselves as family counselors and often asserted that only to women doctors would patients confide "heart histories" and that such confidences would transform both their health and the state of their souls.

Then as now, however, conversations between doctors and patients began not with ethical questions but with issues of complaint and diagnosis. Today, the medical interview is organized as a series of steps, taken in an obligatory order: The patient's chief complaint is elicited and placed within the context of the present illness. The physician takes the patient's past history, family history, and some social history—sometimes called a patient profile—and then reviews, in greater or less detail, the physiological systems. The interview concludes with a physical exam, although sometimes questioning overlaps with the direct examination, and sometimes the two segments of the initial encounter are separated. The direct examination is followed by other tests. All these investigations are written up in the patient history. Theoretically, the interview ends with the doctor offering a diagnosis and treatment plan. Because these critical issues are negotiated over time and are often unsuccessfully communicated, the diagnosis may survive more clearly as a notation in the patient history than as a shared understanding between doctor and patient.[8] Medical anthropologist Howard Waitzkin, while declaring that the origin of the structure of the medical interview is "currently a mystery,"[9] suggests that it was formulated in the late nineteenth century and associates it with German scientific medicine.[10]

In the mid-nineteenth century, neither the structure of the medical interview nor the form of the history had been stabilized. Since the doctor-patient interview was an extremely complex interaction, it is not surprising that patients had to be taught to carry out their part in it. And mid-nineteenth-century literature for patients is so full of guidance that talking to the doctor must not have been easy, especially for women. Popular medical texts offered stories of young girls who suffered from ignorance of the onset of menstruation, of middle-aged women who called in a physician for the birth of a child nine months after their periods stopped, never having heard of menopause. One response of physicians, newly organized in the fledgling American Medical Association, was to compel speech, often with threats of even more shameful consequences. Thus, the Code of Medical Ethics adopted by the National Medical Convention in Philadelphia (1847), warns patients to "faithfully and unreservedly communicate to their physicians the supposed cause of their disease" and never to "be afraid of thus making his physician his friend and adviser." Women were particularly enjoined against allowing "feelings of shame or delicacy to prevent their disclosing the seat, symptoms and causes of complaints peculiar to them."[11]

But such candor could have its price: even in the twentieth century, patients' truthful responses to questions can expose them to a "humiliation ritual," in which the physician evaluates the quality of the patient's compliance.[12] Further, it was not at all clear just how forthcoming the nineteenth-century patient was expected to be. Immediately after encouraging the patient to make the physician his friend, the Code of Ethics cautions him against wearying his physician "with a tedious detail of events or matters not appertaining to his disease." The patient should answer the doctor's questions, and not "obtrude the details of his business nor the history of his family concerns."[13] How was a patient to know whether her personal and family concerns were "tedious details" or the secret causes of her disease, which she was bound to reveal? The physician's "interrogatory" would substitute for the patient's "minute account," so that the direction, topic, and pace of the medical interview were all in the physician's hands.

Given the strong tendency of mid-nineteenth-century medicine to diagnose women's illnesses as reproductive and the strong sanctions against speaking in mixed company about sexual matters, women might well have withdrawn from the contradictory injunctions of the medical interview and maintained that reserve which was always correct. Reformers who sponsored women's medical education in the nineteenth century hoped that women physicians would preserve both women's modesty and their health. Samuel

Gregory founded the New England Female Medical College in 1848 to protect women patients from predatory and corrupting male doctors; Gregory's intemperate remarks made few friends for the new college among regular physicians. And the founders of the Woman's Medical College of Pennsylvania often spoke of women's difficulties describing their symptoms to doctors; the first announcement lamented:

> How often does it occur, that the intolerable anguish attendant on disease, has been insufficient to induce the sufferer to make known the nature of her malady; either from too strict a sense of delicacy, or dread of exposure? In the education of intelligent and respectable females for the exercise of professional duty, all such difficulties will have been obviated, and she may, in hope of relief, communicate freely to one of her own sex, those secrets and sorrows, which nothing on earth could induce her, under other circumstances, to divulge. This is not an exaggerated picture in human life; limited indeed must be the observations of any one who is not familiar with some similar instance.[14]

In one of his commencement addresses, Woman's Medical College Dean Edwin Fussell claimed that the college had been founded to preserve modesty:

> Sensitive plants shrink from the common touch! Many sensitive women were seen suffering and dying, rather than shock what they felt to be the sacredness of their womanhood. . . . It is needless here to enquire, whether it is a healthy sensitiveness, or a morbid one, which causes a woman to endure pain, and die of disease, rather than receive aid and relief from a source which would shock her womanly feelings. . . . The existence of the evil being seen, and the necessity for its removal being strong; this College was instituted to provide a remedy; for this object it is in operation now.[15]

Although many reformers thought that women physicians should not treat male patients, common wisdom held that women caregivers were best at talking with all patients, even young men. In Louisa May Alcott's *Hospital Sketches,* based on her experience as a Civil War nurse, she recounts a conversation with a surgeon who casually commissioned her to tell a soldier of his impending death, since "women have a way of doing such things comfortably."[16] Although such a "comfortable" talk would never be recorded in hospital records, both male and female physicians left extended accounts of their talks with patients. Writing in the great age of the realistic novel, physicians who trained students or instructed the general public transposed the conventions of fictional conversation to compose instructive cases for the education of students or the edification of the general public. These stories are not empirically accurate records of doctor-patient conversation, but they do represent what physicians thought they were doing when they were talking well with patients.

21

We can begin with an example from a prominent male physician at mid-century. Charles Meigs, a gynecologist teaching at the University of Pennsylvania School of Medicine, presented patient interviews in his lectures to medical students; some were frankly fictional and idealized; others were presented as records of real cases. Whatever the medical issue, the central question in these conversations was often the physician's authority. Only that authority could enforce the vaginal examination, which Meigs called (appropriately enough, in those prespeculum days) "examination by Touch." In the published collection of his lectures, he recounts an interview with a patient who had been sick six and a half years and whom he diagnosed as suffering from a uterine polyp and proposed to examine and treat. The woman replied:

> "But I cannot let you do it."
> "You ought to have it done; at least, you ought to have it examined, for, though I am very sure of finding the polypus, I have never yet had any sensible sign of it. I only judge it to be there."
> "I cannot."
> "Very well, madam. You have bled six years and a half; you are greatly reduced; your blood is thin as water, and if you go on much longer, there is fear you will have a dropsy, and then lose your life. Would that be wise, or foolish?"
> "I can't help it; I cannot think of being examined."
> "Very well, it is your affair, not mine. I have no other advice for the present than that you should carefully revolve the prospect before you, and, if you should change your mind, you can let me know if you should desire to see me."[17]

The patient's voice in this interview may owe as much to the iterated "ce n'est pas ma faute" of *Les Liaisons dangereuses* as to any words spoken to Meigs; he threatened dire consequences to the patient but refused to argue with her.[18] He did not support his claim to superior knowledge; he gave no evidence of the polyp but stated that he could "judge it to be there." There was no shielding of the sensitive plant; Meigs, in fact, professed indifference as to whether his advice was followed or not. Medical knowledge was presented as a source of certainty that need not explain or defend itself.

Not all Meigs's conversations with patients turn on such bare assertions of authority. In his treatment of a fictional patient named Helen Blanque, also included in his published lectures, Meigs portrays himself as a man of science and culture, playfully and paternally educating the patient.[19] Meigs found Helen

> reposing in a luxurious *fauteuil* of the richest crewel work. She was arrayed in a beautiful *negligee,* and her slippered feet rested on a low ottoman. The apartment was richly furnished with mirrors, and chandeliers, and candelabras, and carved sofas, with chairs of every form and hue.[20]

No more Laclos; Meigs gives us a Balzacian interior, littered with signs of cultivated gentility. Meigs greeted Helen:

> "Good morning, my dear Helen; I hope you are not very sick; and indeed I must think you are not, if I may judge by your fair face and bright eyes. What can you possibly want with a doctor? Don't you know it is a very dangerous thing to meddle with people who go about the world with their pockets full of lancets, blue pills, and iodine?"[21]

Miss Blanque complained of weakness; she had been sick two and a half years, fainted when she shopped, couldn't dance or go to church, and found that life was no longer worth living.

> "Tilly vally, child! there is little the matter with you. You are not half as ill as you think for, and that I shall soon show you."[22]

After this bracing remark, Meigs asked after his patient's age, prior health, and age at the onset of menstruation. He determined that her periods had been regular and inquired about their duration and intensity; we are, for the first time in this conversation, in the territory of the standard medical history. Blanque claimed that her periods had diminished since her illness; she lamented, "It's leaving me. I'm growing old."[23] Meigs replied that she was a veritable flower-bud, asked about her sleep, digestion, bowel movements, and exercise, auscultated her chest, estimated the volume of her inhalations, counted her breaths and her pulse, inspected her color, and inquired about her weight—all diagnostic procedures that bespoke scientific precision. (In contemporary records from the Jefferson Hospital clinics, it is very rare to read such counts of vital signs.)

Meigs promised to cure Helen, so that she would have "two cheeks like the sunny side of an apple; and those pale lips shall pout like twin cherries." He asked if she could "move about"; Blanque protested that she could barely stir, but Meigs had her climb to the second story, took her pulse, and explained her accelerated heartbeat, inquiring, "Do you understand that, or is it all Greek and Hebrew to you?" Blanque did not follow Dr. Meigs: "Indeed, indeed, I hav'n't the least notion of it except that it tires me to death to go up and makes my heart palpitate like the fluttering of a pigeon. It's very strange."[24]

Finally, Meigs offered to instruct Helen Blanque on the cause of her disorder. Blanque transformed herself from a fluttering pigeon to a fearless daughter of the enlightenment: "If you address my common sense, you will command my most implicit faith and compliance. Women, who seem to be a sort of human Parias—who have lost caste—are always flattered and soothed by being treated as if they were really reasoning beings; for when so treated they seem to have regained their caste."[25] Meigs lectured Blanque on the composition and formation of the blood; her own, he said, was too thin and watery. He prescribed exercise—six miles of walking a day—but this therapy was a small part of Meigs's performance. He read from a fifteenth-century copy of Seneca left conveniently lying about, recounted stories of prize fighters in training, told the story of Galatea, and quoted from *Macbeth*. This talk, Blanque declared, already half cured her, and, relieved that she had not been forced to show her tongue, bled, blistered, or dosed, she promised that her father would gladly pay a handsome fee.

In later lectures, Meigs countered critics who found this conversation "indelicate" by reminding them that it was fictional, and he explained that, while Blanque presented symptoms usually associated with a prolapsed uterus, he delayed an internal examination because he "held conscientiously to abstain from any unnecessary inquiries or modes of inquiry."[26] In her case, since a systemic treatment had been succeeded, there was no need to proceed. (Blanque's reality wavers in these accounts; the fictional patient's cure vindicates the fictional treatment.) Meigs had offered his students an almost comically malleable patient with whom he enacted a common class membership, just as his conversation with the patient suffering from a uterine polyp enacted his assumption of class superiority. For Blanque, Meigs was an all-purpose generic professional, taking by turns the role of scientific observer, patient but exacting teacher, and kindly clergyman. The sources of the doctor's authority include his status as an upper-class gentleman, his ability to read and name all the paraphernalia of gentility with which the patient is surrounded, his easy movement from the medical interview to complimentary banter, his knowledge of "the world" beyond the boudoir (as in the boxing example), his ability to interpret the physical signs before him and to elicit such signs experimentally, and finally, his knowledge of physiology. Meigs's professional authority is a gentleman's learning, displayed lightly, offered in polite conversation. The doctor compliments his Helen, but there is no doubt that he is in charge; they joke, she complains, but in the end she submits. Helen Blanque, obligingly running up and down stairs, volunteering the details of her menstruation, is as compliant as Petruchio could have ever wished Katherina. After a few ineffectual protests, she cedes control of the discussion to the physician. Having summoned him, having insisted on her fragility, she listens to him with delighted attention and resolves to order her life according his advice. Meigs's authority also rests on what he refrains from doing: especially, he does not do a vaginal examination or even look at Miss Blanque's tongue; he does not quarrel with her avocations or her life choices but only asks that she take exercise.

Blanque's "cure" rests entirely on her coming to believe that she is not sick, that she is entirely capable of walking six miles a day. Ronald Chenail's contemporary analysis of doctor-patient conversations describes the work of "frame construction": both parties must agree whether the patient is to be understood as sick or well, and that understanding is as consequential for the patient as many of the physical signs of health or illness.[27] Meigs is at some pains, in this fictional interview, to contain Blanque in what Chenail would call the "gallery of health," to interpret her symptoms as the effects of inactivity and youth rather than as signs of a physical ailment. Meigs's repeated descriptions of the restored, radiant Blanque are therefore therapeutic interventions; the physician imagines the patient as healthy so that she can leave off being sick. The physical examination would shockingly violate the frame of health, since only a serious illness would justify such an intervention. Meigs's postponement of the examination in favor of general systemic treatment conserved Blanque's understanding of herself as healthy.

We might expect, given the connections between euphemism and obscenity, that wherever such performances of modesty and delicacy are enacted, a different site permits different (and plainer) speech. And doctors, as men of the world, spoke freely to each other about the body, particularly about women's bodies. That speech may have served as a rite of passage for male medical students; it was certainly one of the reasons why the medical coeducation of men and women seemed impossible to physicians. Sociolinguists call such ways of speaking "registers"; these repertoires of speech performance are marked by their own systems of word choice, syntax, oral genres, and rhetorical forms. And the records of nineteenth-century medical schools offer many examples of this worldly register of medical discourse. One student notebook, kept by Dr. W. Fulton in 1866, records the lectures on gynecology given by Professor Wallace at Jefferson Hospital.[28] The notes, kept in a meticulous hand, earnestly record Wallace's witticisms; a later reader marked the more racy passages with penciled exclamation points. We find, for example, Professor Wallace's claim that "that little cervix will throw more practice into your hands, than will all the rest of the body put together" and his account of one of his ancestors "who now sleeps beneath the shadow of St. Stephen's Church died aet. 104, and had but one child, and that, when she was fifty-three. 'Had it not been for her great ovarian power,' said he, 'I would not stand before you to-night to tell the tale.'"[29] Wallace spoke of pessaries, of gonorrhea, of married women infected with syphilis by their husbands, of cleanliness and cold water syringes; everything normally socially unspeakable became, in the lecture hall, a fit topic of conversation. Nor did such talk end in medical school. The Philadelphia *Medical and Surgical Reporter* for May 31, 1884, includes an article titled "Women Are Dirty Creatures, Anyhow!" reporting on a discussion of gonorrhea at the Philadelphia County Medical Society. The editor comments:

At first we were staggered by the ungallantry of the remark, and wondered at it. A few words more, and we not only realized the full force and meaning of the remark, but felt that it was so eminently true that a few words of advice on the subject would be most opportune. The remark was meant for the vagina, and our friend [the physician giving the report] went on to ask how many women ever syringe out the vagina, unless ordered to do so by a physician, and yet how few women are there who have not some kind of a vaginal or uterine discharge? The old university resurrectionist, Nash, used to say (more forcibly than elegantly) that every man with an elongated prepuce had a cheese-factory at the head of his penis; by which he meant to convey the idea of the accumulation of smegma which occurred in those so formed, unless they were very particular about washing the glans. So our friend referred to the accumulation and decomposition of the various discharges in the vagina, which must necessarily result in making this cavity a very foul place indeed.[30]

Such conversations are evidence of intense horror and fear of women's bodies. They also permit pleasure in transgressive speech; the physician who knows the body is allowed to speak about it, to name its parts and describe its discharges; he may thereby offend against "elegance" or "gallantry" but not against decency. And medical experiment or scientific curiosity could be a transparent cover for sexual curiosity. An 1883 letter by S. E. McCully in the *American Journal of Obstetrics* reports his questioning of women patients about their experience in masturbation. McCully described his "experiments" to settle the perennial question of whether women ejaculate fluid at orgasm: the vagina was washed, a rubber cap placed over the cervix, and "an orgasm is induced." McCully defended his experimental technique: "My experiments have been conducted with great care, taking into consideration all secreting glands in the neighborhood. . . . Several times no ring or sac was used, and my index finger was placed against the most dependent portions of the cervix on these occasions, so as to be able to carefully detect every motion of the organ, while my thumb was in contact with the clitoris."[31]

It was particularly difficult, given these conventions (and subversions and abuses) of free speech, for male physicians to imagine themselves consulting with women physicians. The embarrassment of joint consultation was one of the central reasons for the Philadelphia County Medical Society's resolution against the Woman's Medical College of Pennsylvania. Consultation with a woman physician was contamination; a doctor who consented to such talk should be expelled from the society. When Joseph Lister was asked by Peter Bell, secretary of the Royal Infirmary of Edinburgh, for his views on medical coeducation, consultation was one of his chief reasons for refusing to entertain the possibility: "Being thrown into intimate association with [members of the opposite sex] for consultation & aid in professional emergencies, would, I fear, lead in the long run to great inconvenience & scandal."[32]

26

When Elizabeth Blackwell began practice in New York, she asked a "kind-hearted physician of high standing" to advise her in managing a severe case of pneumonia. She accompanied him into the parlor after he had examined the patient. Blackwell recounts her surprise at the other physician's confusion:

> I listened with surprise and much perplexity, as it was a clear case of pneumonia and of no unusual degree of danger, until at last I discovered that his perplexity related to *me*, not to the patient, and to the propriety of consulting with a lady physician! I was both amused and relieved. I at once assured my old acquaintance that it need not be considered in the light of an ordinary consultation, if he were uneasy about it, but as a friendly talk.[33]

All of Blackwell's skill in reframing was called for here; the physician who first learned the register of consultation as the performance of free (and possibly indelicate) speech cannot transpose that talk into a register acceptable for conversation with a lady. Blackwell suggested an alternate register, that of the friendly talk, in which "women have a way" of putting men at ease and making the conversation go smoothly. Her invitation was accepted, and all went well; they consulted without having had a consultation.

In Meigs's examination of the fictional Helen Blanque, the physician attends to *fauteuils*, embroideries, and rare editions, to the apparatus of feminine daintiness that is metonymic to sexual delicacy; at other times, in other settings, he turned the register of polite conversation inside out, and precisely those organs that had been unnamed became fascinating. At each moment, the physician and his interlocutors know of the existence of an alternate register; we can read in Helen Blanque's thanks to Meigs for not asking her to "poke out her tongue" an acknowledgment that the interview might have gone differently, and in the editors' admission of ungallantry, a recognition that their free speech was a professional privilege. Consulting with a woman physician made explicit what had been tacit; such extraordinary talk would have required the male physician to negotiate disparate registers consciously.

Meigs's discussions, Wallace's lecture notes, and the difficulties of consultation suggest that male physicians employed an armamentarium of devices for producing compliance: the patient could be left to herself or cosseted; spoken about with coarse bluntness, or pruriently, or with baffled sympathy; instructed in physiology or left in ignorance of her true diagnosis. This variety of tactics speaks of a situation in which women did not easily cooperate in medical investigations. Wallace had to counsel his students to "question and crossquestion your patient every time,"[34] and the modeling of those questions was an important element of clinical education.

But these tactics were not always successful. However much Meigs might have imagined a "blank" patient, ready to be inscribed with his own version of popular physiology, midcentury women did not simply comply with their

27

male physicians: they read medicine; they had opinions about their ailments and their treatment; they had something to say, but if all else failed, they could take recourse in the strictures of propriety and fall silent.[35] While medical ideology stipulated the doctor's control of the interview and the primacy of his medical knowledge, the gaps in that ideology and the evidence of hospital records suggest that the doctor's control was uncertain, that the salience of his knowledge had to be continually negotiated, and that the patient could strategically offer her own knowledge of her body. The conversations composed by Meigs tell us as much about the desires and hopes of male physicians as about how their female patients acted.

A different sense of nineteenth-century doctor-patient conversation can be reconstructed from medical histories written in hospital settings. Meigs's account offers images of medical authority relentlessly brandished and never effectively resisted, of treatment based on medical knowledge, mediated by the physician's personal power. The medical histories from hospitals offer a sense of the constraint of cross-gender conversation and of the avidity with which doctors took up the freedom of all-male professional conversation. These accounts of medical conversations speak powerfully, therefore, about what male doctors hoped for and feared in their conversations with women patients. The realities of actual conversations and the hopes and fears of women doctors were both somewhat different.

IMAGINED CONVERSATIONS II: THE HEART HISTORY

Everyone agreed that it was easy to talk to a woman physician. No writer imagined her "questioning and cross-questioning" her patients, as Wallace counseled her male counterparts, and even the strongest opponents of women's medical education conceded that women patients would confide in her. It is not surprising that early women physicians claimed a distinct professional practice founded on the unconstrained confidence between patient and physician. On this ground, women physicians developed and deployed distinct forms of professional authority. Patients were described as telling a "heart history," of which the woman physician was an understanding, but unswervingly moral, auditor. Her response to the heart history established the exigency of her authority, intimate and inexorable.

Attention to the heart history cohered with women physicians' common (but not universal) preference for conservative therapies. Often, graduates of the Woman's Medical College invoked the *vis medicatrix naturae,* and they advocated systemic treatment rather than harsh remedies; medication, rather than surgery. But such conservatism was very widespread among nineteenth-century physicians.[36] Whether this quietism is understood as an

28

effect of clinical empiricism or as a response to the competition of sectarians with their benign baths and homeopathic doses, women physicians who opted for conservative treatment were squarely in the mainstream of their contemporary practice.[37] In the accounts of their own medical practice written by such physicians as Harriot K. Hunt and Rachel Gleason, however, conservative treatment becomes a kind of talking cure, so that the telling of the heart history is not an adjunct to care but virtually its central therapy.[38] And the heart history could also support quite invasive and heroic measures.

What we might call the canonic form of the heart history can be found in the writing of Harriot Kezia Hunt. In histories of women and medicine, Hunt is usually described as the first American woman to make her living as a physician, although there were surely herbalists, Thompsonians, and botanical practitioners before her. Her *Glances and Glimpses* gives a detailed account of her decades of medical practice, from her training by Anna Mott in 1834 in the use of vegetable remedies through her years of medical practice in Boston.[39] Although she applied for admission to the Harvard Medical School several times, she was repeatedly turned down, and her only medical degree was an honorary one granted by the Woman's Medical College of Pennsylvania.[40] Conversation was central to Hunt's therapy, and *Glances and Glimpses* reports many conversations between Hunt and her patients. In the whole book, Hunt never offered any treatment more intrusive than a "champoo" or a tonic, but she conducted a number of remarkable conversations: a mother was induced to allow her sickly daughter to go to dancing school; a nervous woman was sent out to the fields to sit with her cow; a widow was counseled to look to her own financial affairs rather than trusting the executor of her husband's will. Hunt was proud of hearing so many "heart histories of women," which "were revealed to us [only] as women. . . . From male physicians the causes of the diseases of women, as well as the extent of those diseases, are often concealed!"[41] She felt that she should speak freely to her patients: "I never feared to use the utmost boldness of speech; for I certainly felt that volcanic eruptions of condemnation were safe remedial agents, when love had melted the lava."[42] One case, that of a melancholy middle-aged woman, illustrates the complexity of Hunt's practice:

> She began to tell me of the inroads disease had made upon her, of sleepless nights, loss of appetite, etc. etc., but I found my thoughts wandering from the body. I wished to search the spirit,—approached gently and said, "tell me something of your mother"; here was a key which unlocked the heart. "I lost my mother in early childhood and never was a child again—no one understood me, no one cheered me, no one shed around me the halo of love." Away in the distance of thirty-five years did I trace the causes that had sapped health and destroyed happiness—a gushing, noble nature had been restrained and crushed; it yearned for utterance, but no kindred spirit echoed back its thought or shared

its emotions, icy conventionalities choked thoughts struggling for expression. The secret was revealed, she had been educated in that *proper* circle, where *soul* is termed sentiment; suspicion, censure, and ridicule had driven her within herself.[43]

The patient's loneliness had not been relieved by religion or marriage; she had been estranged from her only child, a daughter who was distant from her until the child's final illness:

> During her [the daughter's] last illness her interior life opened—her mother learned too late that there was a wealth of soul in that artificial being which she had never dreamed of. The father went through the usual forms of grief, the funeral was grand, the monument was artistically beautiful. The mother was left in utter desolation—health failed. Reader, could you have seen the light that passed over the deep shadows of her face, as I spoke of spiritual communings not as a theory, but as a fact, not as an ideal, but as real. Her nature was hopeful, buoyant, but it had been crushed; when the voice of faith touched her ear, it penetrated her soul; hope sprung to life, instant resurrection came. The time between her mother's removal and the birth of her child seemed annihilated, her early love returned, the maternal kiss she received was mingled with the one she gave, and mother and child were guests within; then came a deep sense of responsibility, of the importance of living true to her new found life; duty and usefulness were adopted as her watchwords.[44]

More than one of Hunt's interviews turns on a wild psychoanalytic question about the patient's mother, her probing inflection of the conventional query about the patient's family history. Hunt's therapy was based on the continuity between past and present, between what is suffered and what is done, so that the daughter and the mother, for her, inhabited the same body. She offered her patient the chance—perhaps her first chance—to talk about loss and grief.

That is not all that Hunt offered; when she suggested to the patient the possibility of "spiritual communings, . . . not as an ideal, but as real," she proselytized for spiritualism, an immensely popular practice in reform and feminist circles.[45] Hunt was herself a Swedenborgian and promoted the belief that direct communication with the dead was possible. This intervention was perhaps unorthodox but was not improper by nineteenth-century standards; women physicians were expected to edify their patients. The 1852 annual announcement of the Woman's Medical College asked, "Who so proper as woman, in whose heart religion so readily finds a home, to point the sick or dying sinner to repentance and a Savior here and unending consolations hereafter?"[46] Since there was no canon of moral neutrality for a nineteenth-century physician, Hunt was quite correct in offering her beliefs at retail to her patients.

Not all doctors relied so heavily on therapeutic conversation; not all heart histories were so readily or so fully offered; not all therapies were so mild. At the twelfth annual meeting of the Woman's Medical College of Pennsylvania Alumnae Association (1887), Elizabeth Keller presented the history of a patient suffering from nervous illness who cooperated wholeheartedly with her heroic treatment.[47] Keller's patient had entered treatment nine years ago, at twenty-one, for painful menstruation. After several years, "she said that . . . there was another source of suffering that she could not explain, that was separate and distinct from the menstrual pain." The patient felt sudden pain walking, using a piano pedal, or on the steam cars, leaving her exhausted. She feared that she would go insane; she could not bear her music, or any strong emotion. In the fifth year of treatment, Keller reports, "I inquired further in regard to this feeling which she called intense suffering, and asked her the question plainly, whether she had ever indulged in the habit of self-abuse; to which she replied, 'No.' She answered with a great deal of earnestness, and I had no reason to believe that she was telling me an untruth."[48] The patient became convinced that her father was a stranger "cohabiting with [her] mother," and she was eventually hospitalized for mania: "She was under treatment, but was believed to be a hopelessly insane woman. Everybody had a counterpart,—that was her principal trouble—everybody was false, nothing true about her."[49]

Her family could not afford hospital fees and took her home, where she grew worse, thinking that "every woman was a man, and every man a devil."[50] Keller diagnosed the patient as suffering from "reflex insanity," caused by a disorder of the ovaries, and proposed surgical treatment—not an unusual treatment for mania but not the systemic approach associated with women physicians either.[51] Like the many patients studied by Nancy Theriot, patients who demanded gynecological surgery, Keller's patient "wanted it, begged for it,"[52] and administered the ether to herself. Keller removed both ovaries, ligaments, and Fallopian tubes. The patient's first words on awakening were, "If I have these delusions, do not try to persuade me. I find I can reason now myself." The ovaries and tubes were found to be abnormal; in the discussion after her paper, Keller declared that the patient was a virgin but suffering from a "very sensitive, morbid condition, set up by the degeneration of the ovaries and tubes. I believe that girl's sufferings were due to orgasm, and it was that, which led to her insanity."[53] *Orgasm* is sadly ambiguous; for nineteenth-century physicians, it did refer to sexual release but also to any state of turgor or excitement; the patient's "tortuous and congested" Fallopian tubes could have been at issue.[54] Keller's "no reason to believe she was telling me an untruth," however, now reads as a doubled negative hedge: the patient had lost her sanity (temporarily) and her ovaries (permanently) to masturbation that she could not speak about, even though she spoke vividly and directly about her experience of the world and her body.

This case is striking in the directness and precision with which Keller records her dialogue with the patient. In her retrospective account of nine years of treatment, the patient's report of another source of suffering and her avowal that she could reason now herself are quite distinct. Keller valued the voice of this patient in all its unreliable singularity and had learned, perhaps from novel reading, to record that voice in terms we recognize, even as she interpreted the patient's doubled world as a symptom of her inflamed tubes, even as she set aside the patient's disavowal of masturbation, even as she claimed no therapeutic role for either the patient's history or her response. Of all the patients described by either male or female doctors in these case histories, Keller's is the most realized, the most complex in her relation to the physician. She trusts the physician and is avid for treatment, but she may not have told the truth. She gives a vivid account of her illness but will not give up the story of its cause. Alone among these patients, she refuses the doctor's discourse: ". . . do not try to persuade me. I find I can reason now myself."

The telling of the heart history could also offer a woman physician opportunity to intervene in her patient's reproductive life. In the nineteenth century, this intervention would have been seen not as irregular but as responsive to central concerns of women physicians. All women physicians knew of Madame Rastell, the New York abortionist whose reputation as a "female physician" made their own work morally suspect. It had been Madame Rastell's profanation of motherhood, in fact, that finally determined Elizabeth Blackwell to overcome her repugnance for the body and become a physician.[55] Early graduates of the Woman's Medical College, writing on such topics as medical jurisprudence and criminal abortion, specified ways of determining whether abortions had been induced and ways of resisting patients' pleas for help in obtaining one.[56] Rachel Gleason, a water cure physician who, with her husband, ran a popular sanitorium in New York State, told women who came to her for abortions that a woman who married was obliged to accept children as they came, and she disputed their belief in the legitimacy of abortion before "quickening," when the fetus could be felt moving. She offered "no advice" to women who wanted to avoid having children for reasons of health, commending them only "to a husband's consideration, and the counsel of a conscientious family physician," chillingly urging them to be "true mothers," whether "among the weary ones of earth, or those so worn that the dear Lord gives them an early release from mortal care."[57] But Gleason's control of her patients' reproduction was all the more effective because she offered an understanding ear to the transgressor:

While writing this chapter, a young wife called; she had a sick face, and eyes expressive of great mental agony. "I have done wrong," she said, "and am very sorry; I have come to you for counsel. I had excellent health until a few months ago, when my monthly period not coming so soon as expected, I began to be fearful I was pregnant, and as we had two little children, and my husband's means are moderate, I did not want any more just yet; so I sent to the doctor to give me some medicine to bring on my menses, thinking if I was in a family-way it would do no harm, as it was only a few days over my time. The doctor said he thought I was pregnant, and it was a pity to have another baby when this one was so young, and that he would use an instrument to bring me around all right, which would do no harm; that there was nothing wrong in so doing. I yielded, and have never been well since."[58]

The patient offered her story without any urging or even a direct request. Gleason is someone, at least in her own account, to whom the patient can comfortably confess wrongdoing with the assurance that repentance will bring forgiveness. Like Harriot Hunt's disconsolate mother, she is cured without any conventional medical intervention: "During this conversation, hope dawned in her darkened countenance, and she said, 'You have done me good, and I will try to get well, and will welcome the little ones, few or many.'"[59] Like Meigs, Gleason wrote the story of the patient she hoped to have. Like Meigs, Gleason expected to change the lives of her patients— and in rather more substantial ways than by having them take long daily walks. Like Meigs, Gleason did not represent her patient as offering any serious resistance. But unlike Meigs, Gleason saw the patient's story as the initiator and the vehicle of cure.

Gleason's account suggests that, while they practiced a conventional range of therapies, women physicians also understood their medical practice as support for, and regulation of, motherhood. Conversation between the woman patient and the woman physician negotiated the patient's assent to motherhood and secured her participation in the transmission of feminine care from mother to daughter. The woman physician served as a bridge, a supplement for maternal care that might have been compromised, absent, or rejected by the patient. Such a self-understanding was of course contradictory: it simultaneously ascribed to the woman patient enormous power, a psychological equivalent of Professor Wallace's "ovarian power," and contained that power within a social space so constrained that it seems sentimental to call it a sphere.

In the regulation of motherhood, and in such other practices as child-rearing, household economy, dress, amusements, and choice of occupation, the heart history opened the subjectivity of women patients to the interventions of their women physicians. Those interventions were both productive and problematic. Neither Hunt nor Gleason nor Keller forced treatment upon patients; none of their interventions would have been considered unethical by nineteenth-century canons. In all these accounts, their willingness to hear and understand their patients is palpable. While many patients did confide in male physicians—we need only think of Thomas Kirkbride, director of the Insane Department of the Pennsylvania Hospital—we cannot simply discount the reports of both doctors and patients that heart histories were more easily related to women physicians. And the therapeutic force of the heart history is always invested in the physician's response, in her education of the patient to a deeper sense of responsibility or a livelier willingness to take risks. In writing about such conversations, women physicians represented their hopes; the more quotidian narratives offered in hospital case histories present a different image of the medical conversation.

IMAGINED CONVERSATIONS III:
HOSPITAL CASE HISTORIES

Surviving accounts of the medical conversation are not transparent records of what passed between doctors and patients. Hospital medical records follow their own generic constraints, and were designed to guide students, record treatment, or aid memory rather than to capture the give-and-take of colloquial talk. These texts leave an indirect record of the conversation between the patient and a doctor and a record of the apprentice doctors' education as medical writers. I have drawn on such records in the archives of two Philadelphia medical institutions: the Jefferson Hospital, a distinguished male institution with a rich surviving archive, and the clinic and hospital associated with the Woman's Medical College of Pennsylvania, for which a narrow group of records has been preserved. These accounts are also doubtless marked by the student writers' desires to entertain or instruct an audience, to look good in the story, to perform the role of the good student, and to clean up and regularize the speech of all concerned. Nevertheless, they offer the best sense we are likely to get of how patients constructed their bodies and their illnesses and how male and female physicians inflected those constructions.

Contemporary studies of doctor-patient conversations offer some guidance for reading these texts, although they do not necessarily capture the range of interviewing styles or take into account recent reforms in the conventions of the medical interview. Contemporary ethnographers of doctor-patient talk have recorded hundreds of hours of such talk and have transcribed, annotated, and analyzed their data.[60] Research has focused on the diagnostic interview, structured by a series of questions asked by the doctor.

34

The doctor may simultaneously examine the patient and review his or her medical records. Whether doctor or patient is male or female, the usual interview lasts about eight minutes. The patient's story is subject to possible interruption when the doctor follows out a line of thought suggested by the physical exam or asks a question prompted by its findings. In the interview, doctors ask many more questions than patients, and their questions are almost always answered, while patients' are sometimes ignored. Doctors' interruptions and questions often reestablish their control of the direction of the conversation. And the questions asked by doctors differ from those asked by patients. Doctors often chain questions together or offer a forced choice ("Is this real pain or weakness?"). Answers to their questions can be interrupted by new questions.[61]

Two stories struggle for the floor in a medical interview: the patient's story of illness and the doctor's story of diagnosis. Each can interfere with, contradict, or distract from the other. Patients want to tell stories, to articulate the development and changes of their symptoms, while doctors use the interview to pursue a serial and necessarily disconnected investigation of specific themes:

D: How long have you been drinking that heavily?
P: Since I've been married.
D: How long is that?[62]

Replies are interrupted when the doctor responds to what she feels or sees, opening a new line of questions. The medical interview is inherently discontinuous, since the patient experiences the symptom as a history, while the doctor attempts to localize it within a segmented body. Over the course of an illness, the dynamics of doctor-patient conversations change. During initial consultations, the patient is likely to present relatively inchoate events, which are negotiated into a diagnosis through subsequent interventions.[63] During these negotiations, in both subtle and marked ways, categories of power and blame are invoked: patients are "good" or "bad," innocent or responsible for their illnesses, curable or not. These evaluations and other information presented by doctors are taken in, misunderstood, or reorganized. Such struggles and discontinuities are not surprising; it would be strange if a conversation initiated by a person who perceives something wrong in his or her body, carried out in mixed registers of vernacular narrative and specialized scientific knowledge and moderated by a highly trained and hurried professional, did not operate all the ideological and imaginary variables of gender, class, agency, and family romance, did not provide rich resources for both drama and fantasy.[64]

These contemporary studies foreground the strangeness of a ritual conversation that we have learned to consider as normal. Foucault's analysis of the centrality of confession and surveillance in the formation of the early modern subject suggests that these practices, developed in the clinic, were deployed throughout the disciplined society.[65] Although this account must be supplemented with a reconstruction of the agency of physicians and their patients, the records of nineteenth-century hospitals offer striking images of doctors learning to see patients through the lens of medicine, a formation that is repeated as each new medical student learns to take a medical history.

Even in the most fragmentary records, traces of doctor-patient conversations can be found in nineteenth-century documents. And at the middle of the century, it was not unusual to keep sketchy records, especially in hospitals. (Marie Zakzrewska reported that male doctors were astonished that the New York Infirmary for Women and Children kept written records on every patient.[66]) But hospital clinics and dispensaries, particularly if they were associated with the Quakers, often kept a running record of cases, and students kept notes for their own use. A casebook belonging to J. W. H. Reber, a student at Jefferson Medical College in 1866, offers typically laconic notes on physical examinations. The notes begin with the patient's presenting complaint and include short discussions of the present illness, a limited review of systems, and a prescription. Reber does not often note a diagnosis; indeed, in midcentury American medicine, such general diagnostic categories as "dyspepsia" or "weakness" were quite common. A typical Reber note—we could take it as the baseline of nineteenth-century medical narratives—reads:

> Woman. Spasmodic c cough, debility of respiration on left side. Congestion of bronchial membrane. Treatment—Laudanum in very large doses, Dovers powders and ipecac [——][67]

This rudimentary case note suggests that when the teaching physician presented the patient, he also specified complaint, diagnosis, and treatment. Students may have listened to the patient's lungs or may have been offered a description of chest sounds. The prescribed treatment was a model for their future practice. These elements—complaint, diagnosis, signs of disease, and treatment—are the minimal constituents of nineteenth-century case notes. They can be inflected with very minimal variations: Is the patient described as a woman or a lady? Is the patient's age or nationality given? How is the patient's reproductive status noted? What is the relation between the complaint and the diagnosis? Does the treatment assume an ongoing relation with the patient, or is it understood as a single intervention? However, to trace out the signs of doctor-patient conversations, we must turn to the more developed histories found in clinic notebooks.

The clinic notebooks, kept by medical students, were records of the medical and surgical clinics at which patients were given demonstration treatment. The notebooks may have been reviewed by the attending physician or his assistant, a post normally taken by a promising recent graduate. None of the entries was signed, but the patient histories are free from blots or corrections, suggesting that they have been recopied from rough drafts. Histories are followed by periodic notes of treatment, usually medication, sometimes in different hands. Often, although not always, the record ends with an account of the patient's death or condition on release. One notebook from an 1853 Jefferson surgical clinic offers detailed accounts of various trauma patients; circumstantial accounts of their accidents are sometimes augmented with fairly full medical histories and reviews of systems. We read, for example, of one WW, identified as a "colored man":

> A house painter aged 43 years states that he fell from a ladder at 5½ while painting the second story window shutters of a house, the ladder then falling across the right leg.
>   On examination I found a transverse fracture of the tibia just below the tubercle and a longitudinal fracture dividing the tuberosities and running up into the knee joint. The patient states that he has taken four drinks of brandy since 1 oclock and that he is in the habit of drinking porter for dinner every day; seldom any stronger drink. He states that he has been in the habit of urinating very frequently night and day for more than eight years otherwise he enjoys very good health, never being much disturbed by this desire to urinate.[68]

After three weeks of painful treatment for his fractures, the patient observed that "the quantity of his urine [was] beginning to increase a little," and he was found to be diabetic. He received the standard treatment—cod liver oil and a diet of meat and milk—but began to fail; a month later, he was described as "evidently sinking." He died; what was interesting to this surgical student, however, was his fractured leg. The bone was examined in an autopsy and found to be healed; his friends "demanded the body almost before the wound was sewed up from where the bone had been taken." The writer finds the case "most interesting as showing that fracture into the knee attending joint does not always involve amputation. The bone is a most valuable one and is in the hands of Dr. Norris but *is the property of the Hospital Museum.*"[69]

This history recounts a battle between doctor and patient for the literal ownership of the patient's body and the analogous conflict between doctor and patient over what counts as interesting. The patient's completely untreatable diabetes did not blunt the surgeon's triumph at having healed a difficult fracture; his catastrophe was irrelevant to the physician's technical triumph. But beneath the official story, we can trace another series of conversations; it was WW himself who first advanced the theme of diabetes by mentioning frequent urination and who raised the possibility of a diabetic crisis by noticing increased urination. While the doctor experimented with framing WW's as a story of alcoholism, the patient's account, sadly, became salient and ultimately prevailed.[70]

Many of the Jefferson clinical notebooks record similar negotiations between doctor and patient: each partner advanced a frame for the narrative of illness; and it was by no means a foregone conclusion that the doctor's would prevail. A notebook recording treatment in an unspecified clinic of the Jefferson Medical College for 1866–69 offers the following account:

> HR, Epilepsy
> Monday, Nov. 4th, 1867. Aet 16.
> History. Had convulsions since she was four years of age, with the exception of two years from the 14th year to a few months ago. March a year ago was the first appearance of catamenia—during the year before the catamenial change the attacks ceased. For the last nine weeks menstruation has been irregular.
> At first, the attacks occurred several times in a week; during the last three weeks they have been daily. No aura of epilepsia but she knows when attacks are coming on by a sensation of agitation. In the attack she becomes stiff, would fall but generally gets to sofa &c. Bites her tongue to bleeding; good deal of spasm. Attack lasts generally fifteen minutes. Screams at beginning: seldom goes to sleep after spells.
> Appetite poor. T.[ongue] not coated. B.[owels] regular.
> Has good deal of head-aches. Sight good. Memory poor. Gait unimpaired. Four years ago, following violent attack of epilepsy, had paralysis of left side, which was marked for six weeks. Left hand still partially paralyzed.
> No affection of heart.
> Diagnosis. Epilepsy from organic brain change.
> [Four prescriptions are written here.]
> Monday, Nov. 11. No convulsion since Nov. 4th.
> Monday, Nov. 25, 67. Had four convulsions since Nov. 11th, one Nov. 16th; two Nov. 18; one Nov. 21. These occurred near setting in of menstruation, which has been absent for three months.[71]

This account suggests how, in the course of the medical interview, patient and physician negotiated control of the topic. In the first paragraph of this history, the narrative of the patient's complaint is scrambled and discontinuous, moving from the first appearance of the complaint to the present, back a year and then two years, and then to the immediate past. These scattered remarks may well reflect two different stories, told by patient and physician. The patient presents herself as having frequent epileptic attacks and tells her story from its beginning: she has had continual convulsions with only a brief period of relief at puberty. The doctor investigates the epileptic attacks as related to the patient's menstruation—an entirely conventional line of inquiry, but one which punctuates and syncopates the patient's narrative by reorganizing it around the onset of puberty and the regularity of the patient's monthly periods.

Both narrative lines are introduced in the first sentence of the history: the patient "had convulsions since she was four years of age, with the exception of two years from the 14th year to a few months ago." The present illness is framed: we know when it began, how long it has continued, and how it is situated in relation to the "now" of the interview. The physician's inquiry then unfolds episodically while the patient answers his questions. The narrative of this paragraph is both fragmentary and doubled, with the patient's account of her seizures ("since four years," "with the exception of two years," "a few months ago") laid over the physician's reconstruction of her menstrual history ("March a year ago," "during the year before," "for the last nine weeks").

In the second paragraph of the history, the patient responds to a request for information about the seizures, and the narrative vectors become strong and direct. The story is located in time and space: the attacks happened in rooms with sofas, and they were seldom followed by sleep. The patient's consciousness provides narrative focus: she knew when an attack was coming and screamed at the beginning. This patient had substantial narrative resources and got on record an account of her epileptic fits that ignores the diagnostic terms that the physician put in play: she did not have an epileptic aura, but she just knew when a fit was coming on. Her account is augmented with information that she herself could not have known directly, which could have been supplied in the interview by an accompanying relative or which she could have heard from her family: she bit her tongue, the fits lasted fifteen minutes.

This remarkable history is followed by a review of systems and what appears to be a simultaneous physical examination; the doctor inquires about the patient's digestion and inspects her tongue, eliciting the further history of her paralysis. Such a comprehensive review of systems would be, for a contemporary analyst, axiomatically associated with a lack of clinical experience.[72] The initial diagnosis of epilepsy is confirmed, the patient is given a prescription, and she returns for several subsequent Monday clinics for desultory investigations of the relation between her epileptic seizures and her menstrual periods. Those investigations never become conclusive, are never resolved; the story of reproductive disturbance that the physician was attempting to tell withers away, while the patient's robust tale of nervous disorder organizes her treatment.

This sixteen-year-old patient was quite adept at directing the course of the interview and went on record with an account of her experience as she understood it. The line of investigation that mid-nineteenth-century medical practice would have suggested never got off the ground; the doctor's story of convulsions related to a menstrual disorder was encapsulated, as it were, in the segmented time of the initial paragraph and was never integrated into the story of this illness.

At other times, the voice of the patient is firmly elided. Returning to the laconic clinical notebook of J. W. H. Reber, we read of the following case of "Mania-a-Poter":

> *Patient—Male. Diagnosis.* Man habitual drinker suddenly stopping to drink, on account of superstition. Taken with disease two days ago. Violent motions of body, with screaming; destroying everything about him. Talking nearly all the time, with various images before him.
> *Treatment.* First approach with caution, talk gently to him, and gain confidence, if that will not answer strapping to the bed or floor must be resorted to.
> Then a stimulating treatment combined with narcotics.
> Whiskey then a narcotic (morphia) to bring on a gentle sleep.
> Digitalis or veralium veride when the pulse is too strong and numerous.
> Beef tea and a nourishing diet.[73]

This account speaks of the patient "talking nearly all the time," but we have none of his words, no idea which "superstition" prompted him (foolishly, in the eyes of the physician) to stop drinking. The central voice in this account is that of the professor, who delivers the case as a series of imperatives to the medical students. The lecturer's presentation is relentlessly didactic in its control of the narrative voice; the student's attention is directed to a story of treatment in which the delirious patient, whether by cautious talk or by forcible restraint, is subdued to a gentle (and alcoholic!) slumber. The doctor's talk is a device, a way to quiet the patient. Unlike Keller's maniac, this patient passes silently before us; we have only a record of the noise he made, "destroying everything about him."

What is common to all of these Jefferson cases is the doubled frame that emerges in any but the most elliptical case record. Sometimes control of the treatment remained in the hands of the doctor, as in the case of delirium tremens, where the patient's frame is only indicated ("on account of superstition"). Sometimes, the patients' framing of their condition prevailed in fact, but a different frame organized the medical narrative, as with the diabetic house painter. Sometimes both frames remained inconclusively active, as with the sixteen-year-old epileptic. While none of the doctors writing these cases was interested in the patient's heart history, in none of them is the patient's voice simply silent. These histories confirm that, when physicians like Meigs recounted conversations with patients who simply surrendered to the physician's guidance, these physicians were offering not only their hopes but also their fantasies. The patients who actually presented themselves in clinics and hospitals were much less tractable interlocutors.

It is difficult, but possible, to juxtapose these texts with surviving records of the conversations between women doctors or medical students and their patients. The student records we have from the Woman's Hospital of Pennsylvania, the clinical facility associated with the Woman's Medical College, are not comparable to Reber's notebook. Rather, they are patient histories taken on admission to the Woman's Hospital, roughly comparable—with some important differences—to those preserved in official notebooks at Jefferson. These are hospital rather than clinic records; only women patients were admitted, and no trauma cases came to the hospital. And, a "clinic book" ascribed to Dr. Kersey Thomas survives from the early years of the Woman's Medical College. In 1852, before the foundation of the Woman's Hospital, the Woman's Medical College operated a clinic; since women students were barred from all the hospitals and clinical lectures in the city, the clinic was their sole opportunity for bedside training. In the clinic book, Thomas, the attending physician, and two student clerks recorded patient visits and treatments for 1854–55.[74] Case notes in the clinic book could be both terse and opinionated; they were not dutiful students' memoranda but the professor's extensions of clinical teaching. Dr. Kersey Thomas's account of a patient seen January 20, 1855, for example, reads: "MM [address] Aet 70. Escaped being victimized by Wall's mag. syrup. Old adhesions in the ant and lower portions of pleura of both lungs. Present disease bronchial irritation extending as low as upper third of right lung. Treatment Hives syrup as a tonic."[75] Another prescription follows. This patient is presented pedagogically as someone the class should rescue from quackery. Like Reber's laconic account of a patient with spasmodic cough, the note focuses on what is generalizable in the case.

We might distinguish Reber's note from Thomas's by looking closely at each text's deictic system. For text linguists, *deictic system* refers to features of language that are oriented to a particular speaker and her audience; the deictic system includes pronouns (*I* versus *you*); demonstrative adjectives (*here* versus *there*), demonstrative pronouns (*this* versus *that*), and verb choices (*come* versus *go*). By extension, we can speak of a text's deictic system as including everything that orients reader and writer both to one another and to a series of objects constructed in the discourse; the deictic indicates points of readerly attention and establishes their boundaries. If nineteenth-century medical education can be seen as moving from discursive, text-based teaching to practical, clinical teaching, that development emerged in the language of the classroom as the articulation of a more directly demonstrative deictic system. The discursive teacher speaks *about* something ("Typhus has three symptoms"), while the clinical teacher *shows* something ("Note the three symptoms of typhus in this patient"). Later, in the practice of Mary Putnam Jacobi, we will meet an exuberant development of textual deictics; in reading these earlier examples, we might ask first of all what objects are

41

being pointed out and what relationship they construct between reader and object. In the example from Jefferson Hospital, the patient with spasmodic cough is written up by Reber as a series of signs and symptoms; his attention focuses on what is generalizable in the patient and what is replicable in the patient's treatment. The patient at the Woman's Medical College clinic is articulated, however, in a narrative of professionalism; she demonstrates what it is to be treated by a quack, what constitutes bad practice. Reber's account orients the student to the patient; the clinic book orients her to professional practice: the Woman's Medical College student should imitate Thomas rather than the quacks who dosed the patient with Wall's syrup. Such imitation and the identification that might support it would have been read as signs of women's capacity to take up and pass on the knowledge offered by their teachers, a capacity that, in mid-nineteenth-century Philadelphia, was in doubt. Thomas's note suggests that his readers would become like him, impossible as that might have been in the nineteenth-century gender economy, that they would not become like some lesser physician, and that their coughing patients would benefit from that transformation.

Another unsigned note, probably also by Thomas, records the treatment of a Mrs. D., aged twenty-two:

> Disease cancer of rectum of many years standing. Mistaken by other physicians for hemorrhoids who treated it by ligatures, secharatics etc, increasing its growth and prostrating the sufferer.
>
> Becoming a clinique patient Jan 15th. Treatment sedative and tonic. No hope of cure. Her strength is gradually giving way before the march of her fatal disease. Swelling of the limbs. Buboes in inguinal region with transient neuralgic pains in various parts, mark its course. Pain and irritability of the part allayed by local applications of nit. silv. Constitutional treatment. Quinonia alternating with Iron tr. Opium to obtain rest with nutritious diet.
>
> By this plan of treatment her sufferings have been allayed and life made more endurable.[76]

The note records continued treatment with palliatives until the patient died on March 12; the body was autopsied, and the tumor "preserved in the college." (The Woman's Hospital, like Jefferson, was constructing the "pathological cabinet" that was, for scientifically advanced hospitals, a step toward close study of how disease affected particular organs and tissues.) Like the victim of Wall's syrup, this patient was presented as having been mismanaged by other physicians. The note began with a diagnosis rather than a presenting complaint, moved to a wry history of the patient's mistreatment, and then projected the difficult future that Thomas would attempt to soften. The note itself articulated a very complex time frame: the treatment was presented both projectively, as something that would only slow "the march of her fatal disease," and also retrospectively, "her sufferings have been allayed."

42

Thomas's narrative might have allowed students to read the patient retrospectively while they were treating her; this patient was one of the few who arrived at the clinic with a serious illness, and her treatment may have been difficult for the students. Or the note may have been edited and transcribed after the patient's death. Thomas, deploying a scientific deictic, directed students' attention to physical signs, relating the progress of the patient's neuralgic pain to the course of her cancer, and prompted them to integrate their knowledge of those signs to a professional *habitus* that would have avoided her early misdiagnosis. The case narrative, therefore, maps out both a body ("in inguinal region," "in various parts") and a therapeutic practice ("local applications," "to obtain rest," "this plan of treatment").

A final history, by an unidentified writer, is quite singular:

> July 11th //55 Mrs. M. M. age 32.
> Sick with poverty and general illness [this sentence struck out.]. Probable prolapsis—though no manual examination. Complains of pain in left side between fourth and sixth ribs and of general lassitude with the usual symptoms of prolapsis on standing.[77]

The transgressive general diagnosis, "poverty and general illness," survives clearly under erasure; it is possible that the student clerk wrote this sentence and that the attending physician struck it out. The conventional diagnosis of prolapsed uterus is supported by the patient's complaint and is assimilated into the "usual symptoms"; it is as if the writer herself had very little faith in the efficacy of the diagnostic system she was operating; her encounter with poverty and disease was not at all convincingly mediated through the diagnostic routine of searching for uterine displacement.

The Woman's Medical College clinic book records conversations, not between doctors and patients, but between Thomas and his students. It shows how he directed their attention to the patient as someone who had been ill-served by the profession that these students were about to enter. In all three of these notes, we read criticisms of current medical practice—an entirely regular refusal of quack medicines, a complaint against the previous treatment of a patient, and a transgressive diagnosis. The comparable clinic books from the Jefferson Hospital show no similar criticism of current medical practices.[78] Instruction at the Woman's Medical College, then, may have been seen, at least by Thomas, as oppositional to conventional medical practice. The clinic was understood as a refuge to patients suffering from self-dosing or conventional medicine. This sense of the institution as insurgent, however unsupported by distinct strategies of treatment, would have informed students' self-understanding as new doctors, different from those in practice, but better. We shall encounter this dissenting voice again, in the theses written by students at the Woman's Medical College. Much more distinctly than any expression of care or connection, a willingness to criticize conventional medicine, to hold themselves at a distance from the profession they were joining (or training others to join), separates the students and teachers at the Woman's Medical College from those at Jefferson. Although similar critical reflections marked the rhetoric of irregular schools like the Penn Medical University, they are extremely rare in the institutional discourse of regular medicine.

The clinic books from Jefferson Hospital and those written at the Woman's Medical College clinic, however, are similar in important ways. All of them offer an account of the patient's chief complaint, history, current illness, and treatment, although sometimes in unconventional order.[79] The cases in all the clinic books are organized as teaching exempla: The accounts draw students' attention from physical signs to an understanding of the causes and the progress of disease. They record the treatment of particular patients for particular, limited audiences, and they are also directed toward the readers' future treatment of similar patients. In the clinic books of both hospitals, the student's attention is focused on signs of disease rather than on the general "system" of the patient. While none of the clinic books were published, all were used, even disseminated; the medical student Reber kept his clinic notes throughout his career, and all members of the class at the Woman's Medical College would have read the notes provided by Thomas and the clinic clerks. The writer, whether a student or a physician, offered the written history in its unblotted penmanship, regular phrasing, and the proper performance of professional *habitus* as evidence of fitness for the profession or as a model of professional performance to which students might aspire. As the conventions of French clinical medicine became more widely accepted, the individual patient history was put to different use: when doctors ceased to explain disease as a breakdown in the patient's general constitution and began to diagnose specific illnesses as disorders in physiological processes, the patient's medical history ceased to be an investigation of his diathesis, or predisposition to disease, and became a tool in differential diagnosis or a means of coordinating the work of health care providers.[80] Even more dramatic changes in the hospital record followed the dissemination of German systematic rationalism: if illness was seen as the quantifiable divergence of some discrete system from its normal parameters, then the hospital record could plausibly be reduced to a telegraphic series of measurements of pulse, respiration, temperature, and laboratory results.[81] Hospital case records then became operational rather than demonstrative; they were vehicles for organizing the care of individual patients, of limited pedagogical value. The story of illness they told would (they hoped) be enacted as the patient was treated and responded to treatment—the happy story relentlessly inscribed in such contemporary charting conventions as "problem-oriented records."[82]

If we move from the brief records of the clinic books to the early accounts of patients at the Woman's Hospital of Pennsylvania, we can trace the early stages of this transition as it was inflected by a women's institution. The patient histories taken at admission to the Woman's Hospital during its first years of operation, in the late 1860s, were often gnomic and never as candid as the earlier clinic accounts. But these vivid case records offer a lively sense of the new institution's entry into practice.

No. 540
Admitted June 16th, 68
MN—mother of a family had been suffering for about ten days from abundant sanguineous discharges, dependent upon the abortion of a three months ovum and the retention of the placenta. The placental mass was found protruding from the os uteri: but so soft and friable that it broke down under the slightest touch. It was removed in successive portions by the fingers and the placental forcep. Discharges ceased. Wine of Ergot and Serringinous tonics were administered and the patient was discharged June 18 in satisfactory condition.

No. 542.
Admitted June 17, 68
AS had just been delivered of a child in a station house on her way to the hospital. Suffered no inconvenience from the journey. Made a rapid recovery and was discharged in satisfactory condition June 30.[83]

From the fall of 1868 until 1875, students at the Woman's Hospital were taught to take more formal comprehensive histories and to perform detailed physical examinations. The prescribed form used in these histories seems to have encouraged a particularly open conversation between the student physician and the patient, in which the patient located herself in her family and personal history and in which her understanding of her condition was given remarkable weight. Although the topics of the history were conventional, their arrangement was not. The interview began with inquiries about the patient's family, investigating the health of her parents and siblings. Next, her age at first menstruation and her subsequent menstrual history were determined; the patient evaluated her general health and gave her history of pregnancy and births. Only then was her present complaint determined and the story of her current illness told. Upon admission, the patient was examined: pains were specified and located; tissues and orifices inspected; glands palpated. Pulse, respiration, and bowel movements were investigated, and a urinalysis was done.[84]

Consider the following history of a young woman of eighteen who came to the hospital complaining of paralysis in September 1875; the assistant E. H. Pollard took her history:

> Married. Bookfolder by occupation. Mother of one child. Both father and mother died of consumption. Brother and sister living. She commenced to menstruate at 14. Was regular up to pregnancy. Patient reports good health up to birth of child. Baby born May 1st, 1875, one hour's interval between rupture of membranes and expulsion of child, had pains for six days—baby weighed 10 pounds. She had severe frontal headache for four days after confinement, followed by many convulsions with unconsciousness of nine days, so that patient is unable to give a very accurate account. On recovering consciousness, there was more or less paralysis of all the extremities and tongue, but none of the face.[85]

Two days after admission, the patient was examined, and among other notes, the physician reported that she "can dress herself, but cannot comb her hair on account of weakness at wrist." The patient was diagnosed as suffering from a prolapsed uterus, retroversion, and endometritis, treated by medication and faradization, and released five weeks later, "improved."

Although it was an internal examination that determined both the final diagnosis and the treatment of this patient, the patient's diagnosis and treatment rest on her own account of her condition. Her paralysis is reported as she might have described it, in terms of what is easy and what is hard for her. The doctor listened to the patient's account of her illness and incorporated it into her history; uncorrected and unembellished, at precisely the time when, in many hospitals, such transcription of the patient's language was becoming rare.[86] The history's account of the onset of the patient's illness is limited to what she herself knew directly. We have a full and circumstantial account of her labor but no idea what happened during the nine days when she was unconscious.

Another history, taken in 1876 by A. L. Brindle, demonstrates a collaboration (or perhaps a contest) between physician and patient to describe the patient's course of illness. The patient was thirty-nine years old and would be diagnosed with uterine fibroids:

> Family History. Father died phthisis pulmonalis. Mother living but affected eventually. Has had two brothers and four sisters; all died when young.
>
> Began to menstruate when 16 yrs old: has always been regular. Was married when 18; had one abortion when 4 mo.s pregnant. Patient was always healthy till 5 yrs ago when she began to feel tired and weak constantly: also had pain in left lumbar and iliac regions: suffered great pain during menstruation for more than one year; pain then ceased. About three years ago she noticed that her abdomen was growing larger. One year ago Patient had pneumonia. About four months ago she again had pain during menstruation. About 3 mo.s ago, patient noticed a blood discharge from the bowels: also had watery discharges from bowels. These periods of discharges alternate with periods of constipation. Dur-

ing periods of discharge she has soreness over the epigastrium and everything she eats distresses her, after making her deathly sick and causing her to vomit.[87]

The comparable history of the young epileptic at Jefferson suspends two competing narratives of illness—a sequential narrative associated with the patient and a retrospective narrative constructed by the doctor. This Woman's Hospital history simply adopts the patient's narrative frame, and we read a continuous story told in her terms.

The lexicon of the history is also collaborative. The patient's story is sometimes translated into medical language, as in *pain in left lumbar and iliac regions*. At other points, the language hovers between technical discourse and ordinary talk: the ordinary reader of medical advice would know such expressions as *periods of discharges alternate with periods of constipation,* a phrase that could have been uttered by either physician or patient. And there are also moments when the colloquial register takes over: we do not know whether the patient herself said that her food made her *deathly sick* or whether her description elicited that vernacular evaluation from the medical student; in either case, colloquial vigor has overcome any attempt at technical precision. This history is a narrative deploying both ordinary talk and a specialized medical vocabulary to construct the story of an illness. Such mixed registers are, in contemporary practice, common in the histories written by inexperienced medical students, and it is possible that Brindle's transcription of the patient's story and language was as much a sign of her inexperience as an expression of the Woman's Hospital's orientation toward its patients.[88]

The Brindle case is not an isolated example, and the stories offered by patients could shape the more scientific sections of their histories. Some patients' theories as to the causes of their illnesses are reinscribed in the history. Such a history was written in 1876 about a patient who was a visitor from Cincinnati, born in Prussia; Emma Gaslow was the hospital assistant, but the history is not in her handwriting.

> The patient's parents are living and healthy, she has three sisters and two brothers living and well.
> The patient commenced to menstruate in her fifteenth year and has always been regular, with the exceptions of her pregnancies. She was healthy until the last two years. She has given birth to three children; the first of whom is living in Germany and is healthy, the second child died at six months of age from some enteric disease, the third child was premature and still born. The patient menstruated last in January, 1876 and she believes herself to be pregnant now. During June and July of this year had some kind of a fever, but she was not sick enough to be confined to her bed. She continued to work, but had attacks of dizziness, and at one time, some three weeks since she became unconscious and fell in the street. The physician attributed said attack to weakness, dependant on

her condition. During her convalescence she says she passed three days without voiding urine, from inability to urinate, and from the time of that distention of the bladder she dates the cystitis.

Here, the examining doctor translates the patient's history into technical terms, so that her dead child suffered from *some enteric disease*. But the patient herself specifies her current state (*believes herself to be pregnant now*), gives the cause of her illness (*from the time of that distention of the bladder*), and offers the report of her former doctor's diagnosis (*weakness, dependant upon her condition*). All these critical elements of the history are ascribed to her, whether the precise words are hers or not. The patient has presented herself as a complete package, with a history, a record of consultation, a diagnosis, and a theory as to the cause of her illness. That package survives, more or less intact, in the official history. The examining doctor did verify pregnancy by measuring the fundus of the uterus and examining the breasts for milk. She treated the patient for a month with medication but never quarreled with her diagnosis or the story she told.[89]

Compared with the clinic notebooks from Jefferson Hospital, these cases offer a much more direct sense of the patients' speech, of their own stories of illness, and of their negotiations of their cases with physicians. These differences may be more—and less—than simple reflections of gendered conversation styles. After all, many of the Jefferson patients had suffered traumas; the notebook presents a florid collection of nineteenth-century industrial, shipboard, and traffic accidents, none of which encouraged relaxed or expansive conversation. Further, the specific inflection of this medical genre practiced at the Woman's Hospital was extremely hospitable to patient narratives; the assistant's first questions located the patient in her family and placed the current illness in the context of a life lived among others. Rather than opening with the current illness, so that the patient's history is organized around the presenting complaint, the histories elicited at the Woman's Hospital take their own course, knitting together relevant and irrelevant events. Finally, the separation of the physical examination from the history offered the patient greater control of the illness narrative; the physical signs of illness are first inscribed as they are perceived by the patient and only later verified or augmented by the physician.

These modest and relatively formal differences in the ways that patients were encouraged to speak represent a difference in medical practice, if not a difference in medical care, that characterized the day-to-day work of the women physicians associated with the Woman's Medical College of Pennsylvania; there is some evidence that similar norms characterized the work of women physicians at the Boston school, with which the Woman's Medical College was associated.[90] It is important to emphasize that we are dealing here with a difference, not necessarily an improvement; both good and bad therapeutic regimens can either accept or ignore patients' understandings of their illness, although many readers of this book will share with me a current cultural preference for patient collaboration and education. In terms of nineteenth-century medical techniques, these 1868–75 admission histories at the Woman's Hospital are as remarkable for their consistent urinalyses, counted pulses, and temperatures given in degrees as for the relation they suggest between doctors and patients. But rhetorically, this difference in relationships is extremely significant, suggesting that as medicine was elaborating its professional and scientific practices and working out the relations between them, more than one model of how doctors and patients might talk was in play. The conversations between young doctors and their patients at the Woman's Hospital of Pennsylvania suggest possibilities of a more collaborative and open relationship between the doctor and patient, broader possibilities for the construction of medical knowledge, and a democratization of expert competence. The fact that these possibilities distinguished a practice that also used the most advanced technology available suggests that neither the triumph of clinical empiricism nor the later hegemony of experimental physiology need have come at the expense of traditional medicine's attention to patient stories.

AFRICAN AMERICAN WOMEN PHYSICIANS AND THE MEDICAL CONVERSATION

If gender was a vexed issue in conversations between doctor and patient, race could be even more intractable. We have seen how WW, the diabetic patient at Jefferson, contested his doctor's story of triumphant surgery and how his family continued his resistance when they claimed ownership of his body. Such misdirections were common in interactions between African American patients and white doctors. Toward the end of the century, the African American physician Rebecca Cole wrote for the clubwomen's publication *The Woman's Era* an account of W. E. B. DuBois's report on his research for *The Philadelphia Negro*. DuBois had argued that African Americans suffered high mortality rates from consumption because they were ignorant of hygiene. Cole countered that high rates of consumption among African Americans were artifacts of white doctors' unwillingness to take the histories of African American patients. She observed that "hosts of the poor are attended by young, inexperienced white physicians. They have inherited the traditions of their elders, and let a black patient cough, they immediately have visions of tubercles, let him die, and he writes "Tuberculosis" and heaves a great sigh of relief that one more source of contagion is removed."[91]

While white physicians could be unwilling to listen to stories of African American patients, these patients continued to prefer white doctors to the newly trained African American professionals. A survey of the Baltimore African American community in 1882 showed that only 1 percent of insurance holders used African American doctors.[92] And given the role in which white regular medicine cast African American doctors, such reluctance was understandable. Pioneer African American physicians were seen as emissaries, bringing the gospel of hygiene rather than the most advanced medical care to the African American poor. Just as women caregivers were considered suited to the work of having "comfortable" conversations on difficult matters, African American physicians were assigned the difficult work of hygienic proselytizing. Rebecca Cole herself began her careeer as a "sanitary visitor" attached to the Blackwells' New York hospital. As Elizabeth Blackwell wrote in her autobiography, Rebecca Cole's work was to "give simple, practical instruction to poor mothers on the management of infants and the preservation of the health of their families."[93] While Cole might well have sought out just such an engagement with the New York African American community, in Elizabeth Blackwell's appreciative account no hint remains of the young woman who had excelled at the rigorous curriculum of the Institute for Colored Youth, with its required courses in Latin, Greek, and mathematics.[94] And at Cole's graduation from the Woman's Medical College, Mary Scarlett, the commencement speaker, implied that, while valuable, work such as Cole's would not be the best possible use of a woman's medical education. Scarlett conceded that

> could proper hygienic influences be brought to bear upon the denizens of filthy localities; could they be induced to cleanse their houses, alleys, streets, and their own bodies and apparel; to open their windows and admit freely the pure air, cook their food properly, and obey well-known laws of health, a much better condition of both mind and body would be secured. . . . If any lady graduate feels that it is peculiarly her mission to labor among this class of people, or that she can in this way make herself more useful than in any other, let her enter into the labor, realizing that "each individual in this world has a work to perform which no other person can do so well."

But she declared:

> Ladies, this is not the chief end and aim of educating women medically. A great need is felt in society—in all classes of society—for competent medical advisers of the same sex. It is among the most sensitive, pure and refined, whether rich or poor, that your professional skill will be brought most into requisition.[95]

We have only fragmentary and indirect accounts of what the work of a sanitary visitor might have been like; the work of Rebecca Lee Crumpler is a valuable source for reconstructing those interactions. Rebecca Lee Crumpler was the first African American woman physician; she graduated from the New England Female Medical College in Boston (1864) over the objections of some faculty, who, "owing to the deficiencies in the academic education of Mrs. Lee and the slow progress she has made in her professional studies . . . have hesitated very seriously in recommending her."[96] After graduation, Lee practiced in Richmond, Virginia; she vanished from the historical record and has only recently been identified as Rebecca Lee Crumpler, who practiced in Boston and then in Hyde Park, Massachusetts.[97] In 1883, Crumpler published *A Book of Medical Discourses in Two Parts*, the only book by a nineteenth-century African American woman physician I have been able to identify.[98] (See figure 1.) Crumpler's practice was oriented toward the care of children, and her *Book of Medical Discourses* focused on infant care. Crumpler presented the book as a revision of her "long-kept journals," although its thematic organization suggests that any journal entries had been thoroughly reworked. The *Book of Medical Discourses* is a work of sanitary education by other means; it also serves as a tool for basic literacy:

> I desire to present different subjects by the use of as few technical terms as possible; and to make my statements brief, simple, and comprehensive. Indeed I desire that my book shall be as a primary reader in the hands of every woman; and yet none the less suited to any who may be conversant with all the branches of medical science. If women are permitted to read and reflect for themselves, it is hardly possible that they will say it is uninteresting to them, or that it should only be read by men.[99]

Crumpler's *Medical Discourses* records her half of the remarkable medical conversations that she had with patients; she is extremely frank in her recognition of the material difficulties they faced. We read: "It is just as important that a doctor should be in attendance before the birth of a poor woman's child as that he should be present before the birth of the child of wealth," of the "custom of old-fashioned people, as they style themselves, of giving newborn babes castor-oil and molasses, or soot tea (for that irrepressible belly-ache), and urine and molasses, to clean them out," of children entrusted with the care of a younger brother or sister, of hungry children given a meat rind to chew, of children who failed to thrive because their mothers were under-nourished during pregnancy, and of the difficulty of treating cholera with a change of diet, since "the expenses of the articles mostly ordered by physicians render a trial almost out of the question," of a seamstress working a treadle machine who "allows herself but little time to eat or sleep. And, what is more than all, [she] frequently gets angry with the machine, unstrings it, and gets it in as bad condition as she has her own nerves."[100] Crumpler wrote for readers who could not simply resolve to "obey the well-known laws of

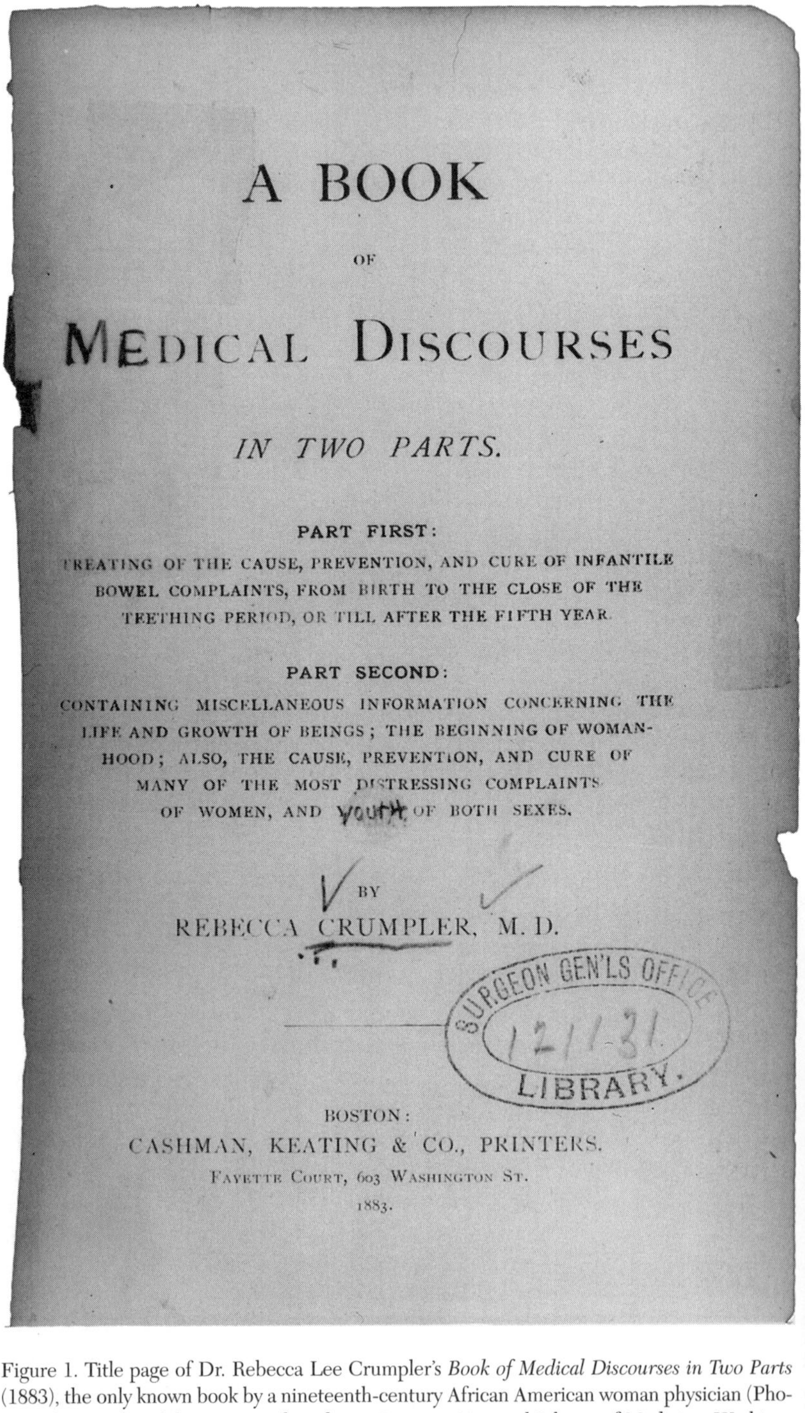

A BOOK

OF

MEDICAL DISCOURSES

IN TWO PARTS.

PART FIRST:

TREATING OF THE CAUSE, PREVENTION, AND CURE OF INFANTILE
BOWEL COMPLAINTS, FROM BIRTH TO THE CLOSE OF THE
TEETHING PERIOD, OR TILL AFTER THE FIFTH YEAR.

PART SECOND:

CONTAINING MISCELLANEOUS INFORMATION CONCERNING THE
LIFE AND GROWTH OF BEINGS; THE BEGINNING OF WOMAN-
HOOD; ALSO, THE CAUSE, PREVENTION, AND CURE OF
MANY OF THE MOST DISTRESSING COMPLAINTS
OF WOMEN, AND YOUTH OF BOTH SEXES.

BY

REBECCA CRUMPLER, M. D.

BOSTON:
CASHMAN, KEATING & CO., PRINTERS.
FAYETTE COURT, 603 WASHINGTON ST.
1883.

Figure 1. Title page of Dr. Rebecca Lee Crumpler's *Book of Medical Discourses in Two Parts* (1883), the only known book by a nineteenth-century African American woman physician (Photograph courtesy of the History of Medicine Division, National Library of Medicine, Washington, D.C.)

health," in Mary Scarlett's words, but who contended with a radical shortage of all the means of health, including information.

In the face of this shortage, Crumpler offered, first, the succor of her book, pointing out that "books on the laws of health . . . could never injure the mind and morals; but would, if read aloud in the family circle half as often as trashy novels are thumbed over, prove a blessing more lasting than gold." Crumpler spoke in a familiar voice, which also rectified the times when she had been silenced, giving the advice she longed to give "at times, and places, that it was not deemed my business to speak."[101] When she did speak, Crumpler did not mince words. She described treating a sick infant:

> About a dozen years ago a neighbor of one of my patients, thinking it for the best, gave catnip tea to her three-days'-old son. I was hastily summoned, and on arriving in the room where everything a few hours before was so tranquil, I suspected that catnip tea had been around. Of course no one would own up until, after I had staid by the little victim fifteen hours without sleep, finally succeeding in checking the frequent discharges and thus saving the child's life,—shame caused the disclosure of the cause of the mischief. The tea had not been given for food, as the mother had a full supply; but as the babe was moving about, it was thought that a little catnip tea would make it sleep.[102]

This passage echoes with Crumpler's colloquial assertion that "catnip tea had been around" and places her as an untiring investigator, whose discovery of the cause of the illness parallels her heroic care of the child.

But in the *Medical Discourses*, objects are as eloquent as either the doctor or the patient. In her attention to the material surroundings of her patients, Crumpler evokes household goods with remarkable vividness and specificity. She wrote of the newborn's first bath, with "a great cake of perfumed soap purchased long, long before, for the occasion."[103] (Crumpler herself recommended using melted lard or sweet oil rather than alkaline soaps.) And, with that soap, we encounter the parents' hopes for the baby, their preparations for the birth, the social ceremony of the first bath. In her "better mode of washing the new born," Crumpler urged that the baby be kept covered with a white wool blanket, "not necessarily new, but pure, never having been used about fever patients, or about the dead."[104] The baby enters a world of scarcity and limit, where objects carry the history of death and disease. The caregiver will protect the baby from those possibilities, even when the world around it cannot be made new but only, and provisionally, pure.

Crumpler's book is virtually silent about race; she never mentions her own race directly and refers to it only by implication in a late chapter, where we read, "The laboring men of my race, generally speaking, take much better care of the horses intrusted to their care than they do of their own health. Were men just as particular about what they themselves eat and drink, and how they dress and sleep, the deaths of young men of thirty and forty years would not be so common. Those who are not careful of their health die early in this climate, and their offspring *die earlier.*"[105] In a letter included in the National Library of Medicine's copy of *Medical Discourses,* Crumpler specified her purpose as the general "prevention of pauperism" rather than any project of racial improvement. (See figure 2.) Race was, and was not, central to Crumpler's medical practice, just as gender was, and was not, central to the practice of white women physicians. Her book offers us a densely mediated account of nineteenth-century doctor-patient conversations: talks constrained by the perceived contradiction between race and medical skill, shaped by mutually acknowledged conditions of scarcity and misinformation, talks in which the implements of care speak of their own history.

MEDICAL CONVERSATION AND THE CONSTRUCTION OF GENDER

Medical conversations took place in the presence of the patient's suffering body; they were among the physician's central means of establishing both authority over and care of that body. They were therefore affected by all the social forces that mediated authority: class, race, education, and gender. Also in attendance, real or virtual, were the patient's family, the doctor's sense of good medical practice, norms of "decency," and a flock of curious medical students. In that setting, the medical conversation offered doctor and patient both singular resources and limitations. If the patient were female and the doctor were male, the patient also often faced an intractable double bind: she must speak freely to the doctor about her reproductive organs, parts of her body that she should not otherwise name. But that impossible speech situation also offered the patient resources of indirection, silence, and evasion, strengthening her formidable powers of determining the conversation. The doctor, for his part, was expected to maintain authority over the patient, standing as surrogate for the more proper authority of husband or father.

If the female patient were treated by a female physician, she would have had a wider scope for telling her story; it is certain that she faced a less constricted speech situation. In some circumstances, the woman patient might also have been able to incorporate her story into the narrative that directed her medical treatment or been able to tell a story in which previous doctors had been mistaken or inattentive. But the greater freedom of speech offered by such settings also increased the avenues of subjection and control: the understanding woman physician who heard her patient's heart history could also regulate her family life and her reproductive behavior. And the physician, male or female, African American or white, could take up the role

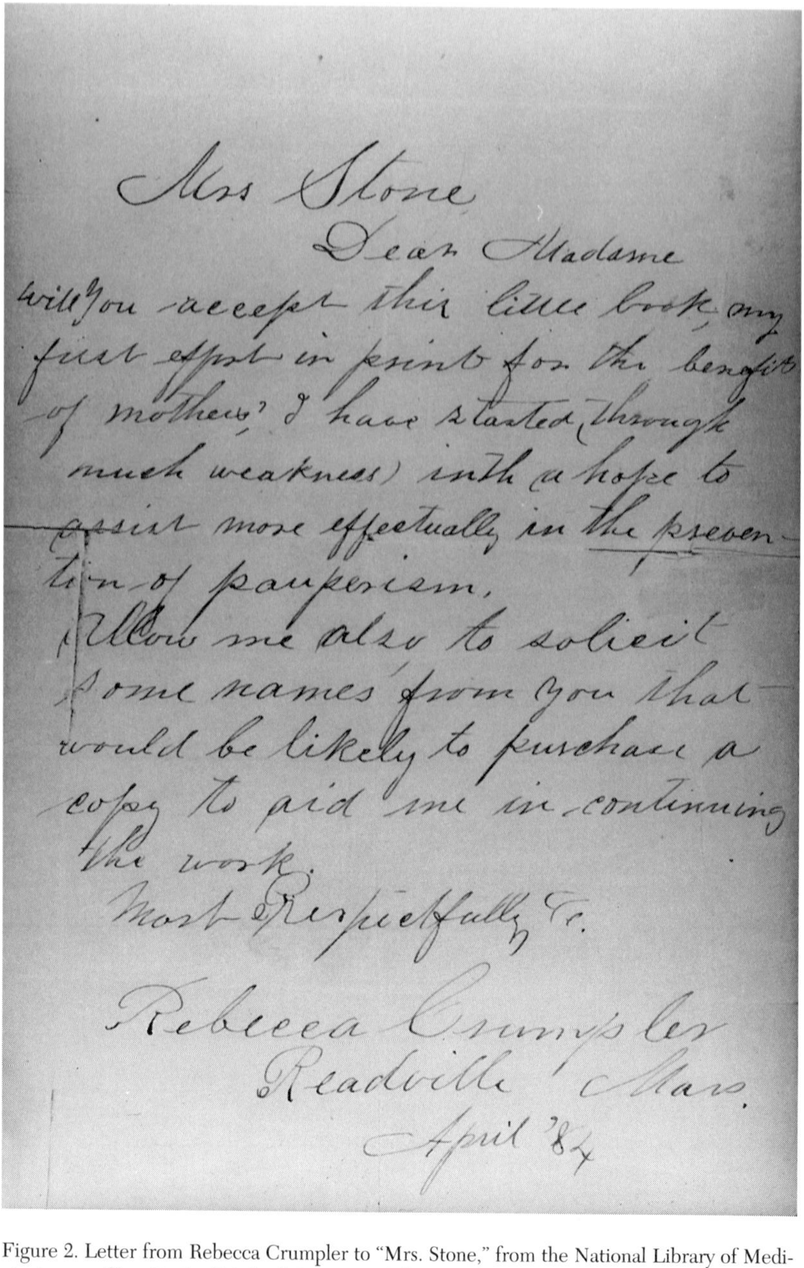

Mrs Stone,

   Dear Madame

will you accept this little book, my
first effort in print for the benefit
of mothers? I have started (through
much weakness) with a hope to
assist more effectually in the prevention of pauperism.

Allow me also to solicit
some names from you that
would be likely to purchase a
copy to aid me in continuing
the work.

  Most Respectfully &c.

   Rebecca Crumpler
    Readville Mass.
     April '84

Figure 2. Letter from Rebecca Crumpler to "Mrs. Stone," from the National Library of Medicine's copy of her *Book of Medical Discourses* (Photograph courtesy of the History of Medicine Division, National Library of Medicine, Washington, D.C.)

of interrogator or refuse the patient's explanation. Patient and doctor were implicated in relations of exchange and inhabited a favored scene of fantasy. Physicians fantasized utterly compliant patients; patients fantasized utterly attentive physicians.[106]

As a gender performance, the woman physician's role was complex. Her presence in the profession was justified by the difference that made her problematic: patients would feel comfortable talking to her about things they would not discuss with male doctors. But, as a student being trained by male physicians, the woman doctor had to shape a way of being a doctor that was like her teachers'. For some students, in some places, the social dissonance of gender could be displaced in a strategy of cross-dressing; the woman physician was remarkable, not because she was a woman, but because she avoided the errors of conventional medicine—even though her practice was otherwise quite conventional. For the established woman physician, an openness to the patient's heart history placed her as a regulator of the patient's morality and religion, a role that does not seem to have been problematic for nineteenth-century women physicians. Nineteenth-century women physicians were defined as different from male doctors; patients were invited to experience their therapy as distinct. And clearly, some women physicians talked to their patients differently, wrote their patients' histories differently, and performed the discourses of medicine in a style that allowed them more access to—and more control over—patients' subjective experience.

3

Invisible Writing I
Ann Preston Invents an Institution

Nothing from the first thirty-seven years of Ann Preston's life suggests that she was interested in medicine, let alone that she would become dean of a medical school. In a letter to her teacher and lifelong friend, Hannah Monaghan Darlington, the twenty-year-old Preston reported some casual botanizing,[1] but most of her letters concerned political issues and recent literature rather than amateur scientific pursuits. She was active in the very lively intellectual and political life of Chester County, which was, like the western New York "burnt over district," no rural backwater but a center of advanced thought. The county had not only organized the Farmer's Library but also a lyceum visited by well-known speakers, a literary society, and an antislavery society, for which Preston served as secretary.[2] Ann Preston herself wrote poems, including a commemoration of the burning of the Pennsylvania Hall by a proslavery mob in 1837 and a published book of children's poetry, *Cousin Ann's Stories for Children*.[3] She was politically active; she probably wrote for the West Chester *Bee*, a temperance paper, circulated a petition against capital punishment, and addressed the West Chester Women's Rights Convention, arguing against any arbitrary definition of women's sphere.[4] Benjamin Fussell, a physician and supporter of women's medical education, was a near neighbor, and his nephew, Edwin Fussell, also a physician and a neighbor, married Ann's friend Rebecca Morris. Preston nursed sick family and friends; she was deeply affected by her younger sister Lavinia's death. In a letter to her friend Lavinia Passmore, she wrote about another young woman "who appears to be dying with a terrible and loathsome disease": "Allas for 'the ills which flesh is heir to.' How strong would that spirit be that has to endure the probations of this world. I gazed upon that poor woman, and realized that 'all flesh is grass and the loveliness thereof as the flowers of the field.' I felt that beings capable of such intense suffering had the strongest claims on each other for mutual sympathy and kindness."[5] It was not unusual for nineteenth-century American women to draw moral lessons from their all too frequent encounters with fatal illness. But Preston's response enacts her sense of mutual vulnerability and speaks of an ethic of responsiveness in the face of death, a responsiveness which marks the best of Preston's medical writing. Hers was not an attachment to medicine, and still less an attachment to science; her sense of calling was rooted in the fragility of the body. One of the projects of Preston's medical career would be to animate the institutional genres of regular medicine with this sense.

At the age of thirty-seven, Ann Preston began her medical education. She was the oldest girl in a family of ten, seven of whom were still alive; her youngest brother was nearly twenty. Preston had been freed from family obligations and was occupied with teaching, privately studying physiology and hygiene in order to lecture on those subjects. After hearing of plans for the Woman's Medical College, she decided that it was both right for women in general to learn medicine and possible for her in particular to do so.[6] She took the Philadelphia physician Nathaniel Moseley, whom she would later refer to as "a capable modest, and agreeable young man," as her preceptor, studying informally in his clinic. When the Woman's Medical College of Pennsylvania opened, she enrolled, describing herself as "restful in spirit and well satisfied that I came." She dismissed rumors that the college would close and remarked, "There is a considerable and increasing apparatus and the Professors seem enthusiastic and to have their hearts in their business."[7]

The college did reopen, and Preston listened to the second round of lectures, wrote her thesis, "A Disquicition on General Diagnosis," passed her examination, and received her medical degree with the first graduating class in 1852. After graduation, she returned to the Woman's Medical College of Pennsylvania and heard its round of seven lectures for a third time while herself giving lectures on physiology to general audiences. Sarah Mapps Douglass, an inveterate lecture-goer, described one of these lectures in an undated letter: "I work very hard just now, and recreate by attending Ann Preston's lectures. I cannot describe the pure intellect and enjoyment they give me. How marvelously has God fashioned these poor bodies. How imperative the duty that they be used to his glory!" In a subsequent letter, she wrote, "I like Ann Preston as a teacher of Physiology. I have heard very eminent professors but she excels them all in bringing great truths clearly."[8] Others were less impressed. Anna L. Wharton, in an 1856 letter to her husband, Joseph, regretted having missed Preston's free introductory lecture but was dissatisfied with the subsequent talk:

> The audience was choice, very select, mostly Friends, orthodox and Hicksites, and the room was crouded. There were several pictures of the human body in different positions hung up, a skeleton and a figure in the middle, or nearly so, of the platform, covered over with a chintz bag. . . . I liked the lady's maner and ease, and was very much interested in what she communicated, but I knew most of the things she told us about. Indeed there were very few that I had not gath-

ered from my own reading and experience. The main subject to day, after giving the structure of the human body, was "Digestion." She explained the "modus operandi" very minutely and satisfactorily but as to the practical end of the business, like many another, she had not much to say, and so we came away with just as much enlightenment on that point as we went. As to food, she told us we could not depend on general rules, but each one must judge for herself, and knew better what suited her and what did not than any one could tell, which thee knows accords with my convictions. The next lecture is to be on the "lungs" and I hope to gain some knowledge that can be put into practice.[9]

The decently covered chintz manikin will return to our story; for now, we should note the continuity between the lectures Preston heard at the medical college and those she gave to a lay audience interested in questions of health. Wharton was readier to discount Ann Preston's opinions than to change her own. For both writers, decorum was an issue: both Wharton and Richardson are relieved that the lectures were inoffensive.

Preston's third year at the Woman's Medical College would have brought her in contact with a whole new cadre of teachers. The 1852–53 academic year was a watershed for the college; physicians suspected (quite rightly) of irregular tendencies left and were replaced by others whose opinions were beyond reproach. Preston's old preceptor, Nathaniel Moseley, sympathetic to the Eclectic Longshores, was replaced by Seth Pancoast, member of the Pancoast medical dynasty. Seth, however, strayed from the fold, writing such works as *Blue and Red Light or Light and Its Rays as Medicine . . . How to Apply the Red and Blue Rays in Curing the Sick and Feeble* (1877); *An Original Treatise on the Curability of Consumption by Medical Inhalation and Adjunct Remedies* (1855); *Onanism-Spermatorrhea* (1858); *Porneio-Kalogynomia-Pathology* (1858); and the *Ladies' Medical Guide and Marriage Friend* (1859).[10] Pancoast only lasted the year, when he was replaced by Preston's old neighbor Edwin Fussell. One of the school's founders, Joseph Longshore, resigned in March of 1853; Livezey and Harvey followed within months, and all were replaced by more regular physicians. Finally, Preston herself was appointed to the chair of Physiology and Medical Institutes and became the first woman to hold a chair in medicine in the United States.

From that chair, Ann Preston taught until the end of her life in 1873. While the college was closed during the Civil War, she raised money to found the Woman's Hospital, where students could receive practical training. In 1867, she was elected dean of the new college. She is rightly revered in its official memory as a woman who had devoted her substantial intelligence and energy to its foundation, ensuring by her own efforts that the medical education of women would be one of the "revolutions which never go backward."[11] (See figure 3.) Preston is also an exemplar of one strategy for nineteenth-century women's medical writing: cross-dressing or masquerad-

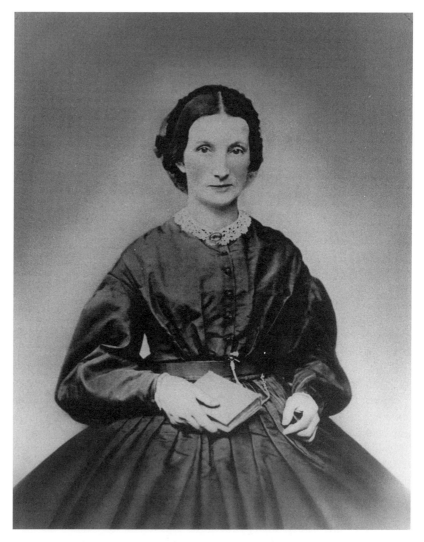

Figure 3. Ann Preston, M.D., ca. 1850 (Archives and Special Collections on Women in Medicine, MCP Hahnemann University)

ing. She was scrupulous in the regularity of her medical opinions and argued that women were as likely as men to become good physicians. Differences between men and women, in Preston's view, simply led women to specialize in such underrated fields as hygiene or to orient their practice to women patients, so that gender differences benefited the profession as a whole. Like the cross-dressed actor, the woman physician occluded her gender in order to perform it. Such performances, of course, have their price, as Judith Butler recognized:

> Identification is always an ambivalent process. Identifying with a gender under contemporary regimes of power involves identifying with a set of norms that are and are not realizable, and whose power and status precede the identifications by which they are insistently approximated. This "being a man" and this "being a woman" are internally unstable affairs. They are always beset by ambivalence precisely because there is a cost in every identification, the loss of some other set of identifications, the forcible approximation of a norm one never chooses, a norm that chooses us, but which we occupy, reverse, resignify to the extent that the norm fails to determine us completely.[12]

In Preston's case, the project of being "just like" male regular physicians reached its limit in such crises as the jeering incident when women medical students who entered the Pennsylvania Hospital amphitheater were publicly harassed or the Philadelphia County Medical Society's decision to exclude women physicians not only from membership but also from consultation. It is not accidental, perhaps, that those incidents prompted Preston to a more combative rhetorical strategy.[13] But the bulk of her writing was ordinary, the steady, quotidian production of institutional texts for the Woman's Medical College.

ORDINARY INSTITUTIONAL WRITING: WOMEN DOCTORS AND THE GENDER MASQUERADE

Preston's was a voice deeply situated in her institution. She was appointed to committees to write memorial resolutions, to revise the bylaws, and to write a history of the college.[14] She often sat on the committee drafting the "essay" for the college's annual announcement.[15] She took her turn as introductory and valedictory speaker, opening and closing the school year.[16] Her lecture "Nursing the Sick and the Training of Nurses" and her letter to the Philadelphia *Medical and Surgical Reporter* on the medical education of women were both printed and used to publicize the college and its associated hospital.[17] After the Woman's Hospital was established, it was often Preston who wrote its annual report. Except for the public statements written during crises, none of this writing attempts heroic acts of persuasion. None of it makes, or pretends to make, any contribution to medical knowledge. Much of it was anonymous; Preston did not sign the announcement essays, and we do not know how much of her work on annual announcements survived editing sessions by the faculty. The history of the college was not to see the light of day until the seventeenth annual announcement, when

Preston had become dean. And one of Ann Preston's most important texts, her personal journal, has simply vanished.[18]

Preston's institutional location was singular; her adherence to institutional routine obscures that singularity. Very few nineteenth-century women controlled regular medical establishments, and only the Blackwell sisters had direct responsibility for both a hospital and a medical school. At an anniversary celebration for the Woman's Medical College, one of the speakers declared, "Ann Preston was the College; the College was Ann Preston."[19] Such a transubstantiation was not easily or commonly available to nineteenth-century women, who were active in social and political organizations but seldom in charge of institutions of science or education.[20]

Ann Preston resolved the central rhetorical problems that faced both the college and its graduates. She offered a way for the Woman's Medical College to present itself as a pioneering institution and also to insist on its utter regularity; she devised a strategy for women physicians to assert a professional credibility while maintaining their conventional gender identification. Preston acknowledged and represented women's medical education as an epochal innovation but steadfastly refused to treat their medical vocation and training as anything but the natural result of social progress. As an institutional rhetoric, this stance modulated the Woman's Medical College of Pennsylvania's transformation from a somewhat irregular institution marginal to medical education into an entirely regular medical school controlled by women. As a personal rhetorical performance, Preston's stance offered a model of dignity, reserve, and courage that is still compelling.

Preston's first introductory lecture (1855), given a year after she had been appointed to the faculty, offers convenient examples of her favored rhetorical tropes. During her first year on the faculty, the college had written bylaws, purged its remaining irregular faculty, and established procedures for admitting students and examining them on their theses, consolidating itself as a regular institution. Dean William Johnson, who had guided many of these changes, suddenly died in December 1854; his place was taken by Harvey, who would be succeeded by Fussell in September 1856. It was therefore a somewhat chaotic institution to which Ann Preston welcomed a sixth class—certainly an institution which had seen conflict and would see more. But to the newly arrived students, Preston invoked the passage of time as a sure, secular, and inexorable ally:

> The sage poet, not very long since, gravely enunciated the fixed, long sanctioned fact, that
>
> "Just experience shows in every soil,
> That those who think should govern those who toil";
>
> but while the world was complacently humming over the couplet, hard-handed, clear-headed men went to the ballot box, and through continents ran the electric

words—"All men are created equal," and "governments derive their just powers from the consent of the governed."[21]

Preston's understanding of change, even of revolutionary change, is strategic: change does not come about by argument but through a realignment of the system. Such an understanding placed a heavy burden on those "hard-handed, clear-headed" individuals of either gender who undertake innovation, but for Preston, that burden did not include an obligation to argue. As an advocate for temperance, women's rights, or abolition, Preston was willing to work at persuasion. As professor of physiology at the Woman's Medical College, she chose to educate women physicians rather than to argue for their right to medical training. Repeatedly and in many contexts, Preston maintained that the equity of admitting women to the medical profession is "beyond controversy":

> You and I feel that "our true sphere is that circle which we are able to fill"; that it was fixed by God in the capabilities and adaptations of our nature; and we can well afford to look with quiet pity upon those self-elected arbiters, who, gratuitously, have taken upon themselves the labor of marking out for us its boundaries.[22]

> Ladies, we should gain nothing by meeting such as these in argument. Prejudices are not amenable to reason. Your business is, not to war with words, but "to make good" your position "upon the bodies" of your patients by deeds of healing.[23]

> Despite of opposition, we think it may be truly said, that public sentiment in this country already decides that woman, in studying the science, and practicing the art of Medicine, is not stepping outside of her fitting place.[24]

One would scarcely think, reading these remarks, that crowds of medical students had gathered to jeer at students from the women's college who attended clinical lectures or that the Philadelphia County Medical Society was still decades away from admitting women. One would scarcely think that Elizabeth Blackwell was sitting idle, waiting for patients, or that Zakrzewska was arguing with Samuel Gregory about the need for a microscope in the New England school. Preston's story of progress was efficacious for its primary audience, the students and graduates of the Woman's Medical College. She regularly offered them an image of their studies as a historical movement rather than as a marginalized fad and of their own role as serious intellectual workers, willing to make good upon the bodies of their patients the worth of their education. Preston did not offer arguments about their own gender identity; neither did she demand such arguments from them. Her caution was as sensible and reserved as her advice that graduates should continue to sleep, exercise, and enjoy a social life: she wanted these women to live and succeed, and so she constructed a narrative in which their success was already ensured.

Students of the Woman's Medical College of Philadelphia wrote theses that deployed similar narratives to form a place for themselves in a profession which was anything but welcoming. Preston's rhetoric had refunctioned for them the narrative of progress that was a staple of reform discourse, so that it became a sanctioned epideictic for the new women's college. Preston avoided the triumphalism of the college's founders, who claimed a resounding permanence for the school in its second announcement; she asserted instead modest but inexorable progress. This narrative offered students two positions in the story of impending victory: As spectators, they could objectify themselves as agents of universal progress. But, in their daily practice as physicians, students need only attend to the work before them and, in particular, remember such "despised things" as prevention, hygiene, and temperance. The higher civilization would advance through their quotidian efforts.

Preston's strategic refusal to enter controversy and her reliance on a narrative of universal progress place her within the tradition of female speakers in the abolitionist movement, particularly her close friend Lucretia Coffin Mott, an active supporter of the Woman's Medical College of Pennsylvania. Both women shared a commitment to Hicksite Quakerism, with its decentralized organization and its abolitionist ethics. Lucretia Mott's extremely active rhetorical practice in the antislavery and women's rights movements, in fact, was an extension of her Quaker preaching ministry; Hicksites in particular saw preaching as an intuitive faculty open to women.[25] Like Preston, Mott spoke of women's rights as an inevitable trend rather than a topic for argument. In her reply to Richard Henry Dana, who had asserted the importance of gender differences, Mott declared, "I have not come here with a view to answering any particular parts of the lecture alluded to, in order to point out the fallacy of its reasoning." Instead, adducing scriptural examples, she concluded:

> Let woman go on, not asking as a favor, but claiming as right, the removal of all the hindrances to her elevation in the scale of being—let her receive encouragement for the proper cultivation of all her powers, so that she may enter profitably into the active business of life; employing her own hands, in ministering to her necessities, strengthening her physical being by proper exercise, and observance of the laws of health.[26]

In Preston's 1855 introductory lecture, the argument from progress led, as it often did for Preston, to an argument from consistency: if women patients speak of their bodies to male physicians without impropriety, then it is proper for them to speak about their bodies to women physicians. Preston's strategy for framing this argument was characteristically cross-dressed: she kidnaped one of her most formidable opponents and spoke through his voice. Preston quoted a "Professor in one of the most popular medical schools of this city and country," who had said that the difficulty of giving good medical care did not come from any want of medical competence, "but from the delicacy of the relations existing between the sexes."[27] This quotation would have been familiar to Preston's audience; the writer was Charles Meigs, the creator of the compliant Helen Blanque. In his *Woman; Her Diseases and Remedies,* Meigs wrote that women's delicacy was a great obstacle to effective treatment. While many female complaints could be easily treated in their early stages, they later became incurable:

> All these evils of medical practice spring not, in the main, from any want of competency in medicines or in medical men, but from the delicacy of the relations existing between the sexes of which I spoke; and in a good degree also from want of information among the population in general, as to the import, meaning, and tendency of disorders, manifested by a certain train of symptoms.[28]

Preston passed over Meigs's statement that he had reason to take pride in the modesty of American women, because "in this country generally, certainly in many parts of it, there are women who prefer to suffer the extremity of danger and pain rather than waive those scruples of delicacy which prevent their maladies from being fully explored."[29] Nor did she remind her audience that Meigs was an active opponent of medical education for women. Rather, Preston dressed her argument in Meigs's text and made him serve as a supporter of the Woman's College—as, indeed, his son would in real life. The argument from consistency had a venerable history in the women's rights movement. Susan B. Anthony argued that, if laws written in the generic masculine could be used to tax women, they also permitted women to vote.[30] Preston was adroit at embedding the argument from consistency, at inflecting it to render ridiculous any argument of biological or spiritual inferiority, at placing it in the mouths of her opponents.

However, Preston's claim for the propriety of women physicians was relatively moderate. She did not argue, as Harriot Hunt or Samuel Gregory had, that it was indecent for women to be treated by men or that male physicians were ordinarily coarse. Preston, in fact, was seldom critical of male physicians, speaking only of "the delicacy of the relations" between the sexes, even on those rare instances when her considerable satirical gifts were unleashed. Rather, she freely admitted the shortcomings of both women physicians and their educational institutions: "We do not deny the fact, ladies, that while this opposition exists, women cannot possess the advantages *in some directions,* which are accessible to their brothers. . . . Nor are we disposed to deny, that some women may, and do engage in this department, whose abilities and acquirements do not pre-eminently qualify them to adorn it."[31] But women would not always be denied the clinical advantages open to men, and the ranks of male physicians offered a "full share" of the underprepared. Critics of women's medical education, not male doctors, were dismissed as "pretentious" or "coarse and ignorant," eliding the fact that male physicians were the most vocal opponents of the Woman's Medical College.

The study of medicine itself, for Preston, became a narrative of progress. In the 1855 introductory lecture, she addressed the entering class directly, in the second person, in future tense:

> You will pursue the study of *Chemistry*. . . .
> You will study the *anatomy of the Human body* with its wonderful revelations of design and adaptation! . . .
> You will study the nature of healing and preserving agencies in the *Materia Medica* and in *Hygienic rules*. . . .
> You will find these subjects points of chrystalization, around which, all the knowledge that has been gained in other departments of learning and observation will naturally arrange itself; and the higher the general intelligence and mental tone of the student, the more beautiful and interesting will become these special studies.[32]

Beauty and interest were, for Preston, the signal attractions of medical study. Here, the academic course forms a narrative of progress: just as society progresses to higher and higher levels of refinement, so the student comes to finer and finer "points of chrystalization." The course of study is a persuasive trope: just as society demonstrates its progressive capacities by accepting women physicians, the student demonstrates her fine mental tone and high intelligence by her absorption in her studies.

Preston's cross-dressed rhetoric consistently refunctioned the tools of the domestic sphere as the proper apparatus of professional medicine. Preston spoke of the special talents that the students of the Woman's Medical College should bring to their practice of medicine. Not surprisingly, these are of a virtually domestic character: "We hope for that nice appreciation of the influence of habits and daily surroundings upon the constitution, which is so much wanting in medical practice."[33] Preston recodes such traits as "nice appreciation" and attention to the everyday as specifically professional qualifications. Habits and surroundings influence the constitution and are sources of health and illness; in attending to them, the woman physician is simply being a good doctor. Preston translated women's customary attention to domestic surroundings into the nineteenth-century medical habitus of attention to the peculiarities of setting, climate, and soil.[34] And she interpreted women's medical work as an extension of teaching—a profession in which women had already been accepted—since women doctors could act as "interpreters" of nature's "secret oracles."[35]

Preston, inveterate cross-dresser, has sketched out a role for medicine which would have been associated with feminine domesticity: the doctor is the manager of daily life, the teacher of good habits. That role is assigned to the medical profession in general and is also seen as a special contribution from women and as a replication of the power of (a feminine) nature. Commonplaces of midcentury medicine—the laws of health, the importance of "despised things," the healing force of nature, the teaching obligation of the physician—are excavated from the normally masculine rhetoric of the profession and mined for feminine themes. Preston constructed from these commonplaces an alternate image of medical practice, in which women were most radically feminine in their entirely regular performance of a male profession. Medical domesticity was presented as a professional obligation:

> Sound advice is the staple in which the physician should deal, and impressed as you are with the importance of those "despised things" which here also have been chosen to confound "the mighty," and reverencing profoundly the indications of Nature, you will study to make your practice an enlightened cooperation with her healing and preserving forces.[36]

Preston presented herself as a figure of the future success of the college's students. She spoke directly to the class:

> Ladies, in welcoming you here to-day, let me extend to you the warm hand of sisterly sympathy. I know the heart of a woman, and especially that of one entering upon a new and untried course, like that before you.
>
> I know your fears and misgivings. There is much to be mastered; you know not whether success or failure is before you! But you have entered upon a course right in itself, and sanctioned by your own hearts, and there is nothing to dread.[37]

We should not underestimate the significance of this moment: never before had women medical students been welcomed by a faculty member who could give them sisterly sympathy. Preston presented herself as an icon of womanly regularity—in contemporary terms, as a female man. She used her own subjectivity in aid of an institutional project. Preston ordinarily did not speak or write personally, in what we now call "her own voice." As in this introductory lecture, she offered herself as a sign, a masqueraded sign, that self-formation as a woman doctor was possible. This was a moment fraught with dangers for unwomanly self-aggrandizement: Preston claimed the status of a responsible intellectual woman, entitled to a position of power and trust. She performed her own role by foregrounding her uncertainty, modesty, shared hesitation, by remembering her doubt and insecurity. The fact that she is speaking offers the promise of success; the words she speaks portray her as hesitant and modest.

The rhetoric of Preston's institutional discourse, of which the 1855 introductory lecture is a fairly typical example, focused on the project of forming women as subjects capable of medical work. Within that project, science is morally edifying, and professional labor becomes domestic care. Everything transgressive or unwomanly about medicine was translated into a feminine register, so that medical habitus, culturally determined as male, becomes a performance style of conventional femininity. In unfolding the complexities of this rhetoric, we might remember Preston's early understanding of the claims of suffering. The terrible and loathsome disease she encountered, mentioned at the beginning of this chapter, might well have been syphilis; both the patient's disease and her culturally imposed shame mark her gender emphatically. Preston experienced this tragic encounter with the gender economy, however, as a prompt to compassion, not as a special duty of women, but as an expression of common humanity. Bodies, in this context, appeared not as male or female but as "beings capable of . . . suffering." That inflection of human species being implies a reciprocal claim for "mutual sympathy and kindness" operating alongside the gender economy but following quite a different logic.[38]

Preston wanted to educate women physicians animated by such a calling. The gender masquerade that she modeled for them was strategy for insisting on their gender regularity while taking up practices normally barred to them. Since there is no material social position outside gender, only such a doubled formation, reflecting and confusing gender performance, could accomplish Preston's project of responding to human bodies as simply suffering, responding with a sympathy and kindness that were simply mutual. A subject formed by such an education would have been most pressingly feminine while undergoing an exigently masculine training. These tropes and strategies would be repeated in many of Preston's other published addresses. In valedictories, Preston assured graduates of the support of the enlightened; in introductory lectures, she offered them her personal sympathy and help.[39]

Preston's public talks defined the institutional rhetoric of the Woman's Medical College, both for the initial audience of entering and graduating classes and for a broader public. Lectures at the beginning and end of the term were well attended and routinely published. The faculty minutes for November 15, 1859, for example, note that Preston's introductory lecture was heard by "an attentive audience of both sexes."[40] Commencements of the Woman's Medical College could be daunting events: the mayor of Philadelphia sent fifty police to the first commencement to ward off threatened disruptions; in many years, particularly during the war, no public commencement was held. Since speeches of any kind by women to mixed audiences were by no means commonplace at midcentury, Preston's bare willingness to address an audience was a demonstration of the institution's commitment to its project.[41] She adroitly constructed a professional register homologous to that of regular male medicine and modeled for her students a strategy of discourse and conduct that was both professional and conventionally womanly. Marjorie Garber has asked whether, since "successful treason is not 'treason' but 'governance' or 'diplomacy,' " it might also be true that "successful cross-dressing, when undertaken as a constant rather than episodic activity" might no longer be cross-dressing but a different kind of gender performance.[42] Preston's institutional rhetoric provided students and faculty at the Woman's Medical College with a basic set of tropes and a durable ethos for the individual rhetorical performances that would be demanded of them.

These rhetorical inventions shape the "essays" published in the annual announcements of the college. Preston's first essay, in 1853, makes no mention of the special suitability of women to the healing offices of the bedside and gives no particular rationale for the college.[43] Instead of proclamations, we read of a lengthening of the term of study, the provision of dispensary and pharmacy, and the acquisition of new apparatus. Here, the college offers to make good upon its body its equality with the regular male establishments. No argument or controversy is engaged; the propriety of the college is assumed, placed beyond controversy.

The sixth annual announcement (1855–56) was to set the pattern used during the next three years, a crucial and delicate period in the life of the college. This announcement was sent to a committee that included Preston; she read the text to the faculty at one meeting, and it was "read, amended and adopted" when the meeting continued on the next day.[44] None of the early publications of the college received such scrutiny from the whole faculty, although several of them are quite remarkable documents. The cross-dressed 1855–56 announcement is marked by the characteristic figures and arguments of Preston's rhetoric. Like her public addresses, it makes modest claims in sober language: the medical education of women is a mark of social progress, and a particularly feminine medical practice is actually identical to that of males. The essay surveys changes in the faculty and the student body, but it also focuses on the economic advantages of medicine as a career for women: Graduates in practice had been so successful that "it will be long before the supply can equal the demand." In fact, women physicians were doing better than women teachers, since women patients were anxious to employ them, and many male physicians welcomed them. Those "influential and eminent" men greeted women doctors "as co-labourers in a field where there is room and need for both sexes, and in which their interests cannot be antagonistic."[45] While Preston had elsewhere explained the hostility of the medical profession as the reaction of a threatened monopoly, this text places an assertion of common interest, of a mutually beneficial division of labor, in the mouths of male physicians—exactly the kidnaping strategy Preston had used in the 1855 introductory lecture.

The prosperity of the Woman's Medical College graduates was given as a warrant for a proleptic upgrading of the college curriculum, presented here as evidence of its regularity. The extension of the sessions to five months was credited to "both . . . [the faculty's] own sense of duty and . . . the general sentiment of physicians, as expressed in the resolutions of the National Medical Association." Women would be trained to a "standard of requirement as high, and . . . term of study as extended, as those of the best medical schools"; in fact, the faculty protested licensing the "ignorant and unqualified of either sex."[46] The five-month term was said to be modeled on recent developments at the University of Pennsylvania; the University of Pennsylvania School of Medicine had extended its term in 1847, before the foundation of the Woman's Medical College of Pennsylvania. The most recent, striking reorganization of the medical curriculum had been that of the Penn Medical University of Philadelphia, undertaken by Joseph Longshore, an Eclectic. In 1855, the Penn Medical University established a term that lasted from October through June and guided a student through a series of twenty-four graded lectures, extending over sixteen to eighteen months.[47] The assertions of rectitude of the sixth annual announcement may have been directed toward this rival; no open controversy, of course, was engaged.

The announcement described, at greater length than the previous essays, the facilities of the dispensary and clinic, the museum, including its anatomical, pathological, and materia medica departments, and the chemical laboratory. The exclusion of women from hospital instruction was passed over in silence. But the anatomical laboratory, often described at length in previous announcements, was barely mentioned.[48] Students were assured "unsurpassed" accommodations for boarders, to be secured by the dean before the student's arrival. This was an institution so sure of its path that it could be silent about it. The fact that the Woman's Medical College was opening new territory is apparent on every page of the announcement, even in the offer to secure accommodations in advance so that students need not risk the impropriety of staying in a public hotel. The college, however, advertised itself not in gendered terms but as a progressive, scientific, medical institution. In establishing a pathological cabinet, the Woman's Medical College of Pennsylvania was marking its aspiration to join the scientific avant-garde; the New York Hospital, after all, was only in 1855 appointing a paid curator to their pathological cabinet for "the elucidation of the nature of disease and the instruction of the medical profession," and the Pennsylvania Hospital was still debating establishing a cabinet.[49] There is no mention in this announcement, as there had been during the early years of the college, of ladies attending the college for a "finishing education," or coming to lectures to study chemistry or physiology as a "liberal art," or using their medical educations to treat their families, although the college included such students for many years. Instead, students and alumnae are referred to in purely professional terms, avoiding gender as much as possible: we read of *the students,* of *those who have graduated in this institution,* or *the class.* Indeed, if it were not for the title page of the announcement, one might think that the college had only a general, benevolent interest in the medical education of women.

A similar strategy of cross-dressing marked many of the writings of African American physicians during the last half of the nineteenth century. The short-lived *Medical and Surgical Observer,* founded to improve communication among graduates of African American medical schools, advertised itself as providing medical information "from a colored point of view" but did not mention the race of any of its writers or refer to race in any medical discussions.[50] And in Rebecca Crumpler's *Medical Discourses,* the first discourse arrives at its final pages before Crumpler mentions "our women," "our men," and the desire to "raise up children who shall be an honor to that noble race with which we are identified, in point of strength and longevity."[51] Once the race or gender of the divergent physician was identified, the rest of the text presented a relentlessly normalized surface. That regularity functioned as a powerful argument for professional credibility.

Rosi Braidotti argues convincingly that Western discourses locate power in embodied subjects that are necessarily gendered, and she advocates "a new form of materialism that places emphasis on the embodied and therefore sexually differentiated structure of the speaking subject. . . . In feminist theory one *speaks as* a woman, although the subject 'woman' . . . is not an essence defined once for all but rather the site of multiple, complex, and potentially contradictory sets of experience."[52] Preston's practice suggests the paradox that, in the emerging profession of nineteenth-century medicine, one of the most effective strategies for the feminine speaking subject was to deploy a masculine discourse while paraleptically insisting on her feminine body. She offered these tropes to students, presenting them in the college annual announcements as impersonal injunctions, phrased in the hygienic discourse of a settled institution. And what an institution the Woman's Medical College of Pennsylvania is in these pages—not six embattled and underpaid faculty members, but a school of unimpeachable regularity, competing with the University of Pennsylvania School of Medicine and avidly following recommendations of the National Medical Association, a group that would not admit them as members.

The whole institution was engaged in a gender masquerade, an adroit version of the strategy Preston had modeled for students at the college. The students would be regular physicians; like the most advanced regular physicians, they would develop scientific interests. They had no special qualms about dissecting, requiring only assurances that the "material for dissection" would be "abundant." They would have professional careers, earning good

71

money from the open market of women patients. No inflated claims needed to be made for them; things were stable, would "continue to improve."[53] It was a reliable performance, one that the college repeated often. The 1859–60 annual announcement, which Preston also helped draft, hews very close to the mark of 1855. It opens with modest assurances that "the prospects of the Institution are more cheering now than at any previous period of its history," marks the formation of the Board of Lady Managers and the increased demand for "well educated female physicians," and claims that the college wants to graduate not many students but a few well-trained physicians—a prudent aspiration, since only one student would receive her diploma in the 1860 class. The lengthening of the term of study, still credited to the example of the University of Pennsylvania, is pronounced successful, and the college again affirms its desire to meet standards "in all respects as high as those of the best medical schools in this country." We hear again about the dispensary, the clinic, the museum, the laboratory, the anatomical laboratory, and the "unsurpassed boarding."[54] The Woman's Medical College of Pennsylvania announced itself as a progressive and scientific institution that happened to train women, enjoyed broad public support, and followed conventional models. That rhetoric normalized and contained an experiment in medical education; only in a few other American cities were women learning medicine in their own institutions, and in neither Boston, New York, nor Baltimore was the local medical establishment so unrelentingly hostile as in Philadelphia.

From the time Preston took up the college's deanship in 1867 until her death in 1872, she oversaw the production of announcements in which this rhetoric was tested. The eighteenth annual announcement, her first as dean, includes a historical note—perhaps the note she had been commissioned to write when she entered the faculty. Never again reprinted, the history is a soberly progressive account of women's medical education, including a rare explicit mention of the breach with the Penn Medical University, an admission of the limitations of the Woman's Medical College, and a plan to remedy those limits through new clinical opportunities. The succeeding announcements focus almost entirely on concrete educational and institutional plans: clinical opportunities, bequests and their dispositions, the new progressive course, a schedule for laboratory and clinical courses offered in the new additional spring term. The crises that the institution faced during these years—rejection by the Philadelphia County Medical Society, the jeering incident—appear only obliquely, as "difficulties" attending clinical lectures at Pennsylvania Hospital[55] and in an appendix to the eighteenth annual announcement reprinting the faculty's response to the jeering incident. Announcement "essays" grew progressively shorter through this period; any vestiges of triumphalism were ruthlessly shorn from these pages; Preston's rhetoric had become a normalizing discourse for the embattled institution.

HIDING IN PLAIN SIGHT: CROSS-DRESSING AND GENDER PERFORMANCE

The cross-dressing strategy that Preston devised for her college was one that she had come by honestly, very early in her life. During her days as an abolitionist, Preston had been connected to activists in the Underground Railroad. Her Chester County house was not on its normal route, but one day (we do not know the year) she was asked to hide an escaped slave. Eliza Judson told the story, which is worth quoting at length, at Preston's memorial:

> One morning a man came running with the information that the slave-catchers were in the neighborhood. His house, the point at which the woman was last concealed, was being searched, and they would be there next. To Miss Preston's question as to what she should do, he replied that she must devise her own expedients, as he could not remain to advise or assist, but must hasten on and arouse the neighborhood, to assist in the rescue.
>
> Miss Preston was alone, but with great coolness and forethought, she locked the woman into the closet, went to the pasture, caught a horse, harnessed him to the carriage, then hastily dressing the woman in her mother's plain shawl and Quaker bonnet, carefully adding the two veils often worn by plain Friends when riding, she started with her in the direction from which the slave-catchers were expected with the ostensible purpose of attending meeting, it being Sunday morning.
>
> Soon the slave-hunters came in view, riding rapidly towards them, came close to the carriage and peered curiously in; but seeing only a young girl and an apparently elderly woman, in the dress of a plain friend, leisurely going to meeting, they rode rapidly on, to continue their search elsewhere. The great danger was past; Miss Preston carried the woman to the house which had been recently searched, where she was comparatively secure. She eventually reached Canada in safety.[56]

Preston "devised her own expedient" by using the distinctive and somewhat radical dress of a "plain friend," a Hicksite Quaker, a group marked by its insistence on local independence and its antislavery stand; neither she nor the escaped slave was likely to blend into a crowd. But in Chester County, plain dress would not have been unusual; placing herself and the woman she was charged to protect in an eddy of the rhetorical mainstream, Preston found a way to normalize her exceptional project, just as she sought security in a house that had recently been searched. Preston's strategy for evading the slave-catchers was not to argue with them, but to hide from them by provoking their curiosity. Presenting themselves as exotic northern Quakers, Ann and the fugitive escaped; to their pursuers they seemed strange, but not dangerous or even interesting.

Preston's strategy had its costs. Judson, in her memorial, quotes an entry from Preston's journal from October 8, 1861:

> I have been sad for my country, because it is so slow to learn the wisdom which would bring prosperity; sad for my disabled mother and desolate home; sad in the prospects of the Institution to which I have given so much of my time and my strength, for there now seems no possibility of success; and I fear that, after all these years of toil, we may be doomed to succumb to the weight of opposition.[57]

Preston went on to search for "inward encouragement," but it is striking to read here, in a private document, an admission of the very possibility of failure that her institutional rhetoric excluded. Maintaining two such different perspectives in the same body, however protected by masquerade, could not have been easy. Preston was hospitalized for "mania" from September to December 1862 in the Insane Department of the Pennsylvania Hospital.[58] Her friendship with the head of the hospital, Thomas Kirkbride, was held up to scandal years later, in a pamphlet written during the jeering controversy. And it is only from this pamphlet and from scattered interviews that we know about Preston's illness, since none of her preserved correspondence mentions it.[59] Preston gives her most direct account of illness and dependency in her lecture "Nursing the Sick and the Training of Nurses," given on May 21, 1863, soon after the end of her hospitalization. The specificity of her language in this talk suggests a prolonged encounter with suffering but characteristically translates that experience into professional advice.

> Ladies, sick people are like children. They feel what they want without reasoning much about it. Let us now, while in comparative health, fortify ourselves by self-discipline and self-renunciation, all that we may; let the children be trained to endurance and self-restraint, let home discipline be thorough, and let no weak tenderness give present gratification at the expense of future suffering; but in the sweet name of mercy, spare the racked with illness—the smitten of nature—all your homilies and wise reproofs. The sick bed has its own teachers—teachers as stern as justice—and needs not our additions; and they who will not try to humor the little harmless whims and notions of the sick, who indulge in sharp words and tones and looks, and will protest and argue before they are willing to stop the rattling of the windows, the grating conversation, or any other disturbing thing . . . may indeed be fitted for some rough work in this work-day world, but they are surely out of place in that chamber which weakness and suffering should ever make sacred. "Don't cross me," said a sick friend, whose temper in health was the sweetest, "I can't bear it"; and they soothed her in her need, and soon she could bear crosses.[60]

74

Preston might have had more than one feeling about such passivity. She reported her two ideas of perfect physical pleasure: eating quantities of strawberries, and "sailing in a little boat, away down, down a smooth stream." During her vacation, Preston recorded in her journal that she had had her fill of both pleasures and found them a vexation to the spirit.[61]

THE MASQUER UNMASKED: ANN PRESTON
AND THE RHETORIC OF CRISIS

During two great crises of the Woman's Medical College of Pennsylvania, Ann Preston publicly took up the controversy over women's medical education. The jeering incident and the 1867 Philadelphia County Medical Society resolution on women physicians were both turning points in the life of the college. At these moments, the protective cross-dressing of Preston's rhetoric gave way to what Marjorie Garber calls a "category crisis," a "failure of definitional distinction, a borderline that becomes permeable" in a problematic way.[62] And at these junctures, Preston's rhetoric was anything but bland. Her response to the 1869 jeering incident will be relevant to the last chapter of this book; I turn now to her letter against the 1867 Philadelphia County Medical Society resolution on women physicians. The 1867 resolution was a serious, if temporary, defeat in the college's long struggle to regularize itself, a struggle resolved only when the first woman was elected to the society in 1888. In 1858, the society had voted to bar "the faculties and graduates of female medical colleges" from membership and even to forbid its members to consult with them.[63]

Under Preston's guidance, during seventeen years of unceasing regularity, the women's college had quietly courted the Philadelphia medical establishment. Such mild innovations as movement therapy, offered at the hospital for a single year, were quickly quashed.[64] Leading physicians such as Alfred Stillé, J. Forsyth Meigs, and Henry Hartshorne had been enlisted as consultants to the Woman's Hospital; S. Weir Mitchell was one of the external examiners certifying graduates from its nursing school.[65] In 1866, Hiram Corson, who had secured the admission of women doctors to the nearby Montgomery County Medical Society, asked the state meeting of the Pennsylvania County Medical Society to withdraw its endorsement of the 1858 Philadelphia resolution; he was only narrowly defeated. In March 1867, Preston and Emeline Horton Cleveland joined the president and secretary of the Woman's Medical College corporators in appealing for a recision of the 1858 resolution. There was support for recision, however ambivalent, within the Philadelphia County Medical Society. Seconding the motion, one Dr. Butler admitted that, regrettable as it might be that women wanted to become physicians, it was clear that they were entering the field, and so they must be made as competent as possible.[66] Just when it seemed that the Philadelphia County Medical Society would recognize the women's college, a circular from Mark Kerr, professor of materia medica at the Woman's Medical College, was shown to the meeting. It was an advertisement for Compound Asiatic Balm, just the sort of cure-all that the county medical society, and Preston herself, condemned as quackery and fraud. The society stopped in its tracks, confirmed the repressive resolution of 1858, and augmented it with the usual arguments against women doctors: women, debilitated by their monthly cycles, were unequal to the physical demands of the profession; the practice of a profession would interfere with the woman doctor's home obligations, including that of "giving healthy milk to her infants"; most of all, women doctors should not consult with male doctors: "Will women gain by ceasing to blush while discussing, every topic as it comes up, with philosophic coolness, and man be improved in the delicate reserve, with which he is accustomed to address women, in the sick room?" Women physicians could neither treat men nor limit their practice to women, since no family could tolerate two physicians without "misunderstandings and heartburnings."[67]

Preston's careful, patient planning had come to naught, torpedoed by a scandal that took her genuinely by surprise, an unexpected and embarrassing exposure, a violent disruption of the masquerade of regularity. Preston first secured Kerr's resignation and then published "Women as Physicians" in the Philadelphia *Medical and Surgical Reporter* (May 4, 1867). It was her most positive and passionate assertion of her right to a medical career.

The letter begins by renouncing Preston's favored strategy; now, at last, she would not avoid a fight: "Although shrinking from all controversy, and seeking the quiet path of duty, the time has come when fidelity to a great cause, seems to demand that I should speak for myself, and for the women with whom I am associated in this movement, and give a reason for the course we are pursuing."[68] She then summarized the four main points of the Philadelphia County Medical Society resolution and answered them in order. To the objection that women are unable to support the work of the profession, she answered that women had been practicing medicine for a dozen years without damaging their health. She countered worries about the "home influence" of women physicians by observing that half the women in Philadelphia must work, and work hard, for their living; a woman physician could at least support herself well and run less risk of exhaustion. To fears of collisions and "heartburnings," she adduced again the argument from consistency: it was already very common for different members of a family to use different doctors. The final argument, the argument against indelicacy, received a fuller and more careful refutation. Preston's response was an assertion of reciprocity: women patients were routinely treated by male doctors, and it was not uncommon for "some tender experienced mother or elder friend" to mediate with the doctor for a young woman. If these conversations were proper, then conversations with women physicians were proper; in fact, women physicians would shield the "sensibilities of shrinking women."[69]

Neither the Philadelphia County Medical Society resolution nor Preston's reply mentioned the Kerr scandal specifically; Preston fought her battle on the broad grounds of women's right to practice medicine rather than the narrow one of regularity. And that broad issue is framed directly, in terms of calling and obligation, terms that recall Preston's early encounter with the mutual human claims of sympathy and help.

> When once it is admitted that women have souls, and that they are account-able to God for the use of the powers which He has given them, then the exer-cise of their own judgment and conscience in reference to these uses, becomes a thing which they cannot, rightfully, yield to any human tribunal.
>
> As responsible beings, who must abide by the consequences of our course for time and eternity, we have decided for ourselves that the study and practice of medicine are proper, womanly, and adapted to our mental, moral, and physical constitution.[70]

This is a remarkable assertion of the emancipatory powers of individual-ism, coupled with the Quaker doctrine of inner light. Preston claims only to represent women doctors; she does not offer to speak for women in general. And she does not exactly argue for the propriety of their course, but argues only for their right to decide questions of propriety. This focused argument takes on the whole apparatus of the "separate sphere": if each woman could, on reflection, decide what was appropriate to her without consulting any "human tribunal," then it would be impossible to enforce the hegemonic notion that women's influence, authority, and power began and ended in the home.[71] And both the calling and the accountability Preston claimed for women are militantly located outside gender. Women are identified as "souls," as "responsible beings." It is as if, on this level of commitment, the cross-dressed blurring of categories that Preston effected was seen as an ulti-mate subjective truth: vocation, obligation, the choice of life, all operate out-side gender. The subject who chooses is a mortal being, not a man or a woman. Preston justified this subversion by invoking the inviolable authority of religion: since women are accountable to God alone and must answer for their choice of profession "for time and for eternity," they need not answer to the county medical society. Women facing such terrific sanctions would not find the censure of regular male physicians so serious; medical educa-tion, rather than a right granted to them, was their obligation, an exercise of divinely given powers for which they will be held accountable.

Preston refuted the charge that women physicians were not as well trained as men and discussed the final point in the medical society's resolution: that no other country than the United States permitted women to practice medicine. Preston pointed out that if women did not enjoy the advantages of a clinical education, their exclusion had been enforced by the very members of the county medical society who had refused them entrance to clinics and hospitals. She deployed the rhetoric of progress, pointing to women who had traveled to Europe for medical education and to the founding of hospitals for practical education. And she argued from consistency, pointing out that there are badly trained men physicians as well as badly trained women physicians. Preston refunctioned the argument that the United States is singular—always a double-edged sword—by basing the right of women to practice medicine on the "propriety of republican institutions."[72]

Preston's final paragraphs invoke the "advancing civilization of the age" and name the medical education of women as a "revolution which [will] never go backward." She asserts that "for us it is the post of restful duty—the place assigned to us, as we believe, in the order of Providence, and we can do no other than maintain it." It seems appropriate to read that *us* as editorial; Preston maintains that divine will placed her as first woman dean of a medical school. She does not fight for herself, she says, but on behalf of emerging women doctors, and she fights "not because we are ignorant, or pretentious, or incompetent, or unmindful of the code of medical or Christian ethics, but because we are women." The separate sphere argument has been refunctioned: being a woman is not a reason to renounce medical practice or to passively submit to the county medical society's resolution but a reason to "protest" "against injustice" and to enter public controversy.[73]

Preston's reply to the Philadelphia County Medical Society takes up the ideological materials available to her—ideas of individual obligation, of progress, of American exceptionalism, of a separate sphere for women—and transforms them into an argument that recognizes communal responsibility, suggests an ethic of reciprocity, and dismantles any fixed understanding of feminine essence. This reply is also in some ways the most personal and direct of Preston's surviving works. Preston uses here many of the tropes and arguments—consistency, reciprocity, progress, republican virtue—she had developed in the institutional rhetoric of the Woman's Medical College. In official documents, Preston offers these tropes paraleptically: she is not going to argue but is simply going to assert these themes as signs of the undeniable justice of her cause. In a more public setting, speaking for herself, Preston deploys the same topics aggressively. But at the end of the letter, instead of arguing that the Woman's Medical College should be recognized as a regular medical college, Preston proclaims that she will struggle for women doctors "because we are women." At this category crisis, the masquerade abruptly ended; Preston's response was characteristically doubled, since gender was irrelevant to the obligations of a "responsible being" and also the avowed ground of her resistance.

This text produced in a crisis refunctions Preston's institutional rhetoric. The Woman's Medical College of Pennsylvania had steadily divested itself of any deviation from uncompromising regularity. Its official documents, under Preston's guidance, insisted that the college was fostering a medical practice identical to that of the male profession, but somehow simultaneously uniquely feminine. When there was nothing to do but to fight, as in this instance or later in the jeering controversy, Preston made a case with the materials at hand and transformed those materials in the process. Her organizational contributions to women's work in the medical profession were substantial, but not least among them was the construction of a rhetoric that allowed women to avoid or enter controversy, to claim and enact their gender or to bracket it, to locate themselves within the medical profession or to project its progressive transformation. This fluid, combative, achingly anonymous and adroitly cross-dressed rhetoric gave women a voice with which to be doctors, a voice that later women physicians would elaborate, complicate, and contradict.

4

Learning to Write Medicine

Nineteenth-century medical students saw the thesis and its associated examination as a demanding rite of passage.[1] Even though the thesis required nothing more than a workmanly review of current medical knowledge, it was still a major task for a student. While Joseph Longshore waited to be examined on his thesis by the University of Pennsylvania School of Medicine in 1834, he wrote to his brother Thomas that he suffered from "unpleasant forebodyings, the existing combat between contending mental emotions, that create sensations, and feelings—to give an expression of which, the pen of the most sentimental genius would be incompetant."[2]

Joseph Longshore's trepidation was not unreasonable: the thesis, like contemporary gatekeeping performances, would be judged by its grammar and spelling as much as by its display of disciplinary knowledge. The Regulations of the Medical Department of the University of Pennsylvania did not prescribe that theses should make a contribution to medical knowledge but only that they should be on a medical subject; neither did the regulations specify a level of research.[3] But they were quite specific about the mechanics of presentation:

> VIII. The Essay must be in the candidate's own hand-writing, and must be written uniformly on letter paper of the same size, the alternate pages being left blank.
> IX. General bad spelling in a Thesis, or general inattention to the rules of grammar, will preclude a candidate from examination for a degree.[4]

Nineteenth-century discussions of the role of the thesis in the formation of new physicians and in the boundary work of the profession suggest it imposed special exigencies on a student. The medical lectures that were the core of nineteenth-century medical education were not, properly speaking, classes, since students did not recite, answer questions, write papers, or take examinations. The medical thesis was the first and only time a medical student's writing was evaluated. It was therefore the student's sole chance to display control of the body of knowledge that had been transmitted in the lectures and the faculty's sole chance to monitor the student's competence and regularity.

Nineteenth-century physicians, worried about the relatively low standing of their profession, wanted medical students who were well educated—and, of course, properly genteel. But since anyone, even an unlicensed physician, could practice medicine, and since no previous education was required for admission to medical school, it was impossible to restrict the profession to a learned elite, although the most powerful physicians continued to be well-educated members of the middle and upper classes.[5] The thesis required students to approximate, at least, the discursive norms of a learned profession. Physicians' worries about the status of their profession often emerged as worries about the prose style of the thesis. Then as now, a student's compliance with the rules of "proper English" served as evidence of the correct class background or, failing that, of a proper disposition toward social norms. Daniel Drake, writing in 1832, worried that physicians would leave illiterate instructions:

> Even at this late period the profession abounds in students and practitioners who are radically defective in spelling, grammar, etymology, descriptive geography, [and] arithmetic. . . . Nothing is more common than to commit gross violations of [grammar and spelling], in the directions which we write for our patients; and, what is still more humbling to the pride of the profession, not a few of us never learn to spell the names, either of the medicines which we administer or the diseases which we cure.[6]

Repeatedly, in the nineteenth-century literature on medical education, professional control and professional status are connected to literacy: if regular physicians were to be distinguished from irregular practitioners and quacks, only those candidates whose literacy was beyond reproach could be admitted. Nonstandard orthography could discredit medical reform, irregular ideas, or an interest in the medical education of women. When the *Boston Herald* wanted to damn Samuel Gregory, founder of the Boston School for Midwives, Nurses, and Female Physicians—by all accounts a singular man—they quarreled with his pronunciation, finding him "a poor plagiarist [who] speaks in a slovenly, monotonous, and halting manner, and cannot pronounce even the commonest English words correctly."[7] It is in this context that we should read the medical faculty's insistence on a thesis in the candidate's "own handwriting" and on conventional spelling and grammar.[8]

For many physicians, and for most medical schools, literacy implied at least a taste of latinity. While the requirement that a candidate for medical school should know Latin was not commonly enforced, and few students exercised the option of writing their theses in Latin, a failure to write Latin told against a physician, especially if she was a woman. In the 1870 debates of the Medical Society of the State of Pennsylvania on the recognition of graduates of the Woman's Medical College, one Dr. Hamilton supported his assertion that the faculty of the Woman's Medical College were generally incompetent by showing that they were poor Latinists:

> . . . notwithstanding the declaration in reference to the high qualifications of this female medical college, . . . I have not long ago met with two or three prescriptions, written partly in Latin, partly in English, and partly in Latin that I presume she understood, but no Latin scholar could understand. This was written by a female practitioner of great celebrity in this city. Now it is only a very short time since I saw another prescription by one of the female professors; it was in the same condition.[9]

While not all physicians unhesitatingly identified good Latin with medical competence, all agreed that good English, as demonstrated in a hygienically correct thesis, was essential.

Finally, the thesis was not only a simple demonstration of medical knowledge but also an exercise of the student's powers of expression. The medical essay was not clearly distinguished from a belletristic one. At Geneva College, theses were judged by "comparative clearness, force, and correctness of style"; the best was awarded a gold medal. When Andrew Boardman, an 1841 Geneva graduate, felt that his thesis had been unfairly passed over for this award, he supported his case by quoting a medical professor's praise of its stylistic merit. The professor had compared the winning thesis with Boardman's, claiming that while the winning thesis had "nothing original, no striking views or sustained argumentation: the style is verbose, unequal, and sophomoric, full of scraps of Latin and allusions to heathen mythology," Boardman's was "grave, thoughtful, and argumentative, indicative of an observant and sagacious mind: the style is clear, forcible, and mature, and though the positions are bold, they are maintained with courtesy."[10] Boardman published his thesis; most medical school regulations permitted such publication with the permission of the examining professor. And a fair number of published theses can be found, slim volumes in stiff covers, neglected in medical archives. Unpublished theses by mid-nineteenth-century medical students, both men and women, remain filed in folders or bound in groups in the archives of medical schools. They do not seem ever to have been consulted as a source of information; it is likely that, like a contemporary master's degree candidate, the nineteenth-century medical student wrote a thesis without having read one and expected his own work to remain unread.

As an academic genre, the thesis is oriented to both the past and the future. It summarizes the student's education, serving as a culminating performance, and it anticipates a future in the profession. In the 1850s, when women began the formal study of medicine, students wrote theses after a relentlessly didactic medical training; once they had been examined on the thesis, they were immediately qualified to practice medicine. Few of the students writing medical theses would have treated patients in any systematic way; very few of them would have enjoyed any clinical training beyond large hospital lectures in which physicians presented and treated cases. Only the most elite graduates of the most elite institutions could look toward further training as a hospital house officer; others sought clinic or dispensary appointments, out-of-door appointments to relief institutions, or association with a professional mentor. The role of physician, for which the thesis was an audition, was one most students had never attempted.

The most common subjects for theses were diseases, symptoms, treatments, or organs; they are expository and quite general in their content. But theses could take up a range of medical discourses, from experimental reports to avuncular advice. J. Dickson Bruns's 1857 University of Pennsylvania thesis, *Life: Its Relations, Animal and Mental,* is an essay in natural philosophy, moving from Kant to vitalism, arguing for a hierarchy of the races and languages according to their powers of abstraction.[11] Empirical research also appeared in theses; Elisha Kane's *Experiments on Kiesteine, with Remarks on Its Application to the Diagnosis of Pregnancy* (1842)[12] recounts Kane's experiments showing that pregnancy could be diagnosed by a film that formed on the urine of pregnant women. Both Bruns's and Kane's theses were considered worth publishing; Kane's was cited by Oliver Wendell Holmes as "an actual accession to the treasures of science."[13]

Women's medical schools modeled their graduation requirements strictly on those of male schools; women medical students wrote theses to demonstrate medical knowledge, literacy, and belletristic adroitness. The annual announcement of the Woman's Medical College of Pennsylvania first mentions a thesis in 1852, after one class had already graduated and the irregular professors had been purged. The regulations stipulate that the candidate, at the time of application for the degree, must present a thesis written in her own hand, along with her graduation fee. The thesis was to be, in the familiar phrase, "upon some medical subject," and the regulations warn that "general bad spelling, or inattention to the rules of grammar, in a thesis, will preclude a candidate from examination for a degree," criteria copied, almost verbatim, from those of the University of Pennsylvania.[14] The five women in the first graduating class of the Woman's Medical College (1851) wrote theses on topics similar to those produced at the University of Pennsylvania School of Medicine or the New York College of Physicians; they took up a disease, injury, or medical practice to display the student's control of the material presented in lectures or textbooks. Theses were evaluated as much for their regard for conventions of writing as for their level of medical information. In 1859, the faculty minutes record such comments as: "spelling not very good and matter and shape not very clear, but passable," "very well written and very good but not original in its thought," or, from Ann Preston, "a few errors in spelling and grammar but . . . a very good treatise on the subject."[15] Subsequent generations of women medical students added to the files of successful theses; taken together, these texts may well constitute the largest body of scientific writing produced by women in the nineteenth century. Women physicians did not publish their theses, although many graduates of the Woman's Medical College went on to publish in the alumnae journals of the school or in the regular medical literature.[16] A careful comparative reading of the theses written by male and female medical students has much to teach us about the ways women physicians wrote the medical discourse that formed their scientific understanding of the body and about how they themselves embodied the habitus of their profession. Later in the century, African American women entered the medical college; their theses form a cognate body of early, understudied, scientific texts. I have read the 17 theses produced by white Woman's Medical College graduates in 1852–53, transcribing 10 of them for close study and analysis; a selection of the 161 theses written by the University of Pennsylvania School of Medicine class of 1851, closely studying 5 of them; and 4 of the 5 theses written by African American graduates of the Woman's Medical College from 1867 to 1888. Taken as a group, these theses demonstrate a full range of nineteenth-century medical performances, including varieties of gender performance. For purposes of rhetorical analysis, I divide the theses in two registers: a discourse of health and a discourse of medicine; the two registers are distinguished by lexicon, preferred syntax, overall organization, and presentation of the reader and the writer. Theses written in the discourse of medicine, the more common of the two registers, typically concern a disease, an organ, or a course of treatment and position the student as an apprentice writing to more knowledgeable professors. But, in any class, some students wrote theses addressed to the public or to patients, offering advice on health. They elaborated an alternate register—the register of health. The register of medicine is retrospective: the thesis demonstrates that the student has done the work set by his medical school. The register of health is prospective: the thesis looks forward to the student's future role as counselor to families.

At the University of Pennsylvania School of Medicine in 1851, 161 students graduated; most of their theses concerned a disease, organ, or mode of therapy. But twenty-four theses concerned issues of general health or therapies so diffuse as to be modes of hygiene rather than specific medical treatments ("Water," "Sunshine").[17]

THE REGISTER OF HEALTH

Thomas Corson's "Essay on Health versus Fashion" was based on nineteenth-century common sense, advising that the reader preserve health by renouncing fashion in matters of diet, exercise, dress, and amusements; it can serve as a typical example of the register of health as it appeared in the University of Pennsylvania theses.[18] Thomas Corson (1828–79) was a member of an important medical family; his father practiced medicine in New Hope, Pennsylvania, and his relative Hiram Corson would be among the most effective supporters of medical education for women. After receiving his degree, Thomas Corson practiced briefly in Jonesville and Morrisville before settling in Trenton in 1854. He was active in the Medical Society of New Jersey, serving as its president in 1869; in his presidential address, *Physician and Patient*, we hear the hortatory tones he had used nineteen years earlier, in "Health versus Fashion."[19] In both texts, Corson took up the role of family counselor; in his thesis, he moralized, offered concrete advice, ruefully confessed his own addiction to tobacco. This performance, to contemporary eyes, seems strange; we are not accustomed to the nineteenth-century conventions that prompted a twenty-three-year-old to claim such mature authority.[20] For Corson, that decorum seems to have come easily. Some of Corson's rhetoric was indebted to the lively nineteenth-century literature of advice, gentility, and good conduct, but he took up an exceptional range of issues, moving through the whole round of daily life, giving directions that were both stern and concrete for dress, diet, ventilation, and exercise.

What is absent from Thomas Corson's thesis is medicine in anything like the forms we know it today or even those of Kane's thesis. In "Health versus Fashion," the body we encounter is not the finely structured, densely layered series of tissues of French physiology.[21] Still less does Corson present the segmented body of systems and organs that scientific medicine would render visible later in the nineteenth century.[22] Corson's lexicon for the body is relentlessly colloquial; he writes of the *stomach*, the *stomach and intestines,* the *muscles and muscular systems*, the *chest*, the *lungs*, the *heart*, the *spine*, the *blood*, and (quoting from an unnamed source) the *pelvic regions* and the *lower extremities*. Corson's vocabulary establishes a body which is recognizable, a vernacular body. While contemporary writing in the register of medicine described the body as a series of nested structures, so that organs are divided into regions and tissues are divided into layers, Corson's body resembled a schoolroom map: each region is its own state; there are no subdivisions, no fine structures. This is not the body of scientific medicine but the body as we know it, the body as we might teach it to a young child.

For contemporary text linguists M. A. K. Halliday and J. R. Martin, nominalization is a central feature of mature scientific prose: an action (*food di-*

gests) becomes an object (*digestion*), which can be elaborated and modified (*disturbances of digestion, digestive processes*).[23] In Corson's thesis, physiological functions become nouns (*digestion, respiration*), but these nouns are seldom modified, nor are propositions about them embedded within further statements. Corson's *digestion* never leads to *disturbances of digestive functions* or *remedies for disturbances of digestive function*. In mature scientific writing, such nominal chains allow a text to study and refer to both temporal processes and concrete objects. Halliday asserts that "the device of nominalizing, far from being an arbitrary or ritualistic feature, is an essential resource for constructing scientific discourse."[24]

Corson's thesis, on the other hand, is rich in terms for the body as a whole. He speaks of *various life-functions*, of the *whole frame* or the *whole physical frame*, of the *whole system, organic actions*, the *human organism*, and, tellingly, of the *economy* and of *ourselves corporeally*, terms drawn from law. In these legal metaphors, health is a unitary state ordered by laws, seen as undifferentiated codes of prudent behavior. We read of *laws of health, hygienic and physiological laws, sources of hygiene*, and *laws of hygiene*. Corson's terms for disease are equally general, including many variations on *morbific* (*morbific agents, effects*, and *influences*), iterations of the covering term *disease*, and common ailments such as *dyspepsia, phthisis, pneumonia, bronchitis, anaemia, gout*, and *crasis of the blood*. The body as represented in Corson's thesis is a collection of palpable and evident parts, subject to diseases that are (or were, to the nineteenth century) immediately given to the senses.

Corson's thesis, therefore, exemplifies the broad quietist tradition of early nineteenth-century medicine. Although there are many ways to tell the story of how medicine changed in the United States during the nineteenth century, one of the most productive is seen in the account given by Charles Rosenberg in his history of the American hospital, *The Care of Strangers*.[25] For traditional medicine in the early nineteenth century, the body was an economic system, and disease was an imbalance of input and expenditure. The body took in air, food, and rest; if these sources of strength were compromised, it responded with fevers, inflammations, and swellings. One disease could turn into another.[26] Equilibrium could be reestablished with heroic courses of bleeding and purging; by midcentury, doctors had grown skeptical of these measures and favored the milder systemic treatments Corson advocated: temperance, a moderate diet, exercise, and rest.

Later medical theories, whether based on French clinical medicine or on German pathology, would resolve the body into much more discrete series of organs and tissues and construct diseases as we know them today—as stable entities, each with a unique cause, each to be treated with a preferred specific therapy. Disease would be represented as a disturbance of an organ

86

or tissue rather than as an economic imbalance. Scientific medicine would become remarkably successful, and indeed hegemonic, in the last decades of the nineteenth century, and in all of its inflections, it specified that therapy should consist of the treatment of identifiable illnesses rather than the adjuvant support of the patient's singular "constitution," which was the norm at midcentury.[27]

Thomas Corson's thesis, with its undifferentiated lexicon for tissues and organs, its attenuated list of diseases, and its well-developed set of terms for the economy of the body, could serve as a handlist of terms for traditional or organicist medicine. But although the register of health was especially hospitable to quietist systemic therapies such as diet, rest, and exercise, theses in this register could also popularize advances from Parisian clinical medicine or offer general information on diseases and their processes, understood in less traditional terms.

Halliday has shown that the early texts in the development of a scientific discipline are concerned with scientific processes, objects, and relations but that later texts attend to the act of "doing science." Early in the history of a science, texts posit causal relations among events (A happens, so we know that X happens). A later text draws implications from one event-state to another (happening A is the proof of happening X). As a science develops, personalized forms (Q said; we did) become more rare. The drift toward nominalization, paradoxically, leads to syntactic simplification; nominalized forms do not support complex modifiers. A very common syntactic pattern for mature scientific prose links a heavily nominalized subject to an equally nominalized complement by way of a minimal relational verb: "Griffith's energy-balance approach to strength and fracture also suggested the importance of surface chemistry in the mechanical behavior of brittle materials."[28]

This is the sort of sentence that Corson never writes, that is in fact rare in all the theses in the discourse of health. For Corson, subjects were normally persons or parts of their bodies; predicates were processes or attributes of bodies. The text simply presented unmediated objects to the reader, a strategy which complicated the task of a writer who had yet to establish his own professional authority. Corson argued, for example, that parents tend to neglect their children's physical education and to favor education over health,

> thus laying the foundation for diseases which will afflict the individuals who have been subjected to such treatment while children, during the whole of their after-life. For my part, I would rather have a child who at six or seven years of age should have his muscular system well-developed, and his features darkened by the rays of the life-giving sun, even though he were hardly able to read his primer, than have one who at his age had made surprising intellectual advancement, while his skin was as white as chalk; his muscular system hardly strong enough to carry him, and his whole frame showing that his mind had been devel-

oped to the detriment of his body. Leave the mind alone until the body grows strong, then it will be able to support the effects of strong mental exertion.[29]

The speaker of this passage offers advice which is not information; no plausible reader would find these facts and ideas new or surprising. His advice does not refute any ideas then current about educating children. No potential reader of this thesis, including the public to which it was addressed but which would never see it, would argue that it is appropriate to sacrifice children's health to their education. Instead of information, the paragraph offers surveillance presented as care: the physician watches over the child, shielding him from overly ambitious parents. Corson specified and developed ideas through personification, the development of an ideal character who serves an example—the chalk-faced, overstudious child. Much more complex figures were possible in the middle of the nineteenth century, even in the register of health; much more complex arguments were constructed, even in medical school theses.

These straightforward modes of elaboration proved to be very durable for Corson. Later, addressing the Medical Society of New Jersey as its president, he again used personification to remind physicians to keep their appointments with patients: "As the hands on the dial point to the hour when the visit is expected, the sufferer listens eagerly for the familiar step, which brings with it comfort and consolation; and if the voice which he so much desires to hear is not heard until long after it was promised, he grows fretful and impatient, and his dissatisfaction increases as the leaden hours roll by."[30] This little drama of illness offers no information not implicit in the first sentence of the paragraph: "If the visit is delayed, the patient becomes irritated and vexed." The text advances, not by specifying an argument, qualifying it, or answering objections, but by establishing the presence of its central terms, embodying them as generalized persons: the fretful patient, the pale child. Corson's speech act in the thesis is utterly at odds with his actual situation as a student. The speaker of the thesis is constructed as someone who knows the body and knows social mores; the reader is constructed as the docile object of instruction, ignorant of the laws of the body. But of course, Corson's thesis had as its primary (and perhaps its sole) readers the faculty of the school of medicine, who were not subject to his instruction.[31] The thesis is Corson's audition for the role of physician, prompting his reader in the role of the docile patient.

The role of physician was, of course, gendered at the middle of the nineteenth century, but not in any simple way. "Health versus Fashion" participates in a genre we can trace to Hesiod's *Works and Days:* benign patriarchal advice on the feminine task of ordering the household. But the more minutely Corson's text takes up questions of domestic and social life, the more extravagantly it threatens to wander into the domestic sphere.

> If low-necked and short-sleeved dresses happen to be à la mode, you will see young ladies who are threatened with phthisis and to whom it is all-important that every precaution should be taken to prevent its occurrence, exposing themselves, while thus unprotected, to the influence of cold and damp, thus contracting pneumonia, bronchitis and other diseases, which will act as exciting causes to develope the latent tendency to phthisis which is lurking in their system, ready to appear at the slightest bidding.[32]

Corson goes on to advise "protecting the breast by high-necked dresses and flannel."

Corson's advice is inscribed within the complex nineteenth-century gender politics of tuberculosis, a disease which was frequently fatal and not at all understood.[33] As physician, Corson takes up the position, generally coded as masculine, of subject-supposed-to-know—a position utterly speculative for a nineteenth-century physician faced with consumption. One way of controlling that uncertainty was to translate consumption into the domestic sphere, where approximation and random events were to be expected. But Corson's text is also arranged around the ambiguities of a specifically masculine gaze; the young ladies that he warned not to expose themselves are offered to us in the text, clad in low-necked, short-sleeved dresses; their breasts unprotected, exposed at once to disease and to the gaze of the reader.

Corson implicated himself in domesticity. He inveighed against specific ways of dressing; he recommended specific fabrics and styles. Here, as in the very well-developed discourse of dress reform, a masculine interest in the "feminine mystery" of fashion is normalized; the doctor speaks of feminine things, but only for the good of women. The closer the speaker comes to specific domestic practices, the more homely the material that the discourse handles, the more positive and assertive the performance of masculine authority must be.

There was in the mid-nineteenth century a well-developed, if not especially prestigious, medical discourse on domestic questions. The *Eclectic Medical Journal of Philadelphia* included both domestic and medical recipes in its "Miscellany" section.[34] And physicians writing about the cleanliness of hospitals, the plausibility of the germ theory, or even the details of surgical technique might draw upon a feminine domestic register. Samuel Gross, an extremely important Philadelphia surgeon and a leading critic of women's medical education, wrote in his essay "The Factors of Disease and Death after Injuries, Parturition, and Surgical Operations" that "a blunt, dirty needle, coarse, unwaxed thread, and rude manipulation, are ill calculated to favor reunion [of the edges of a wound]. A bandage applied unevenly or too tightly cannot fail to act prejudicially."[35] Perhaps Gross and Corson insisted on a particularly stringent patriarchal authority because so often they wrote like housewives.

The register of health, then, can be characterized by its relatively restricted vocabulary, oriented as much to states and conditions of the body as to organs, structures, and diseases. The body appears in this discourse as both a collection of familiar parts and a system organized under economic laws. The argument of the text proceeds by adding instances and examples, making present the states of health or disease that have been thematized. Rhetorically, the text claims a serious and searching authority, generally coded as masculine, but this authority operates on the undignified terrain of domestic life, generally coded as feminine. As an ensemble of features, the register of health articulated a professional habitus that was quite powerful and would eventually be adapted to the exigencies of the new scientific medicine. Many features of the discourse of health—representation of a palpable body as an economic system, loose organization of information, contradictory gender performance—are common to the theses written by both male graduates of the University of Pennsylvania School of Medicine and female graduates of the Woman's Medical College.[36]

As we might expect, the register of health, with its attention to issues of domesticity and its occlusion of professional and scientific practice, was both attractive to and problematic for the graduates of the Woman's Medical College of Pennsylvania. They had already transgressed conventional notions of woman's sphere and were excluded from many professional ties and conventions. And indeed, in the first graduating class (1851), three of the seven theses were written in the register of health: Anna M. Longshore's "A Disquisition on Electricity," Ann Preston's "A Disquicition on General Diagnosis," and Angenette Hunt's "A Disquisition on the True Physician."[37] Angenette Hunt was born Angenette Payne in Ithaca, 1819; she was therefore thirty-two when she graduated from the Woman's Medical College. She had been married since 1837 to Dr. Nelson Hunt, her preceptor. After her graduation, the family moved to the Verona Mineral Springs House, which they ran as a water cure resort until the end of the century. Hunt died in 1901.[38] Like Corson's thesis "Health versus Fashion," Hunt's "True Physician" is organized by a very thin vocabulary, oriented toward a material world of health and bodies rather than a discursive world of medical investigation and dispute. But Hunt's performance of gender is more complex than Corson's.

In Hunt's thesis, specialized medical terms are presented, as it were, in brackets, as examples of things that ancient physicians did not know: "They knew nothing of cell germs, or ultimate fibrils,—were ignorant of the circulation of the blood and supposed the arteries to carry nothing but air."[39] Like

Corson, Hunt wrote of an undifferentiated body, of a general economy subject to *mournful catastrophe* and generalized *disease* rather than specific illnesses. The body is not a system of organs and tissues, but *man with all his mysterious relations and connections.* Like Corson, Hunt referred often to general principles of health, such as *rules of health*, the *science of healing,* or more often and more emphatically the *art of medicine.* Borrowing a convention from opening and closing lectures at medical schools, Hunt invoked the history of medicine in her opening paragraphs and referred to Hippocrates twice as her authority for recommending that physicians study the theories of "*all* the schools."[40] But for Hunt, history does not end in the triumph of regular medicine; it establishes a precedent for Eclecticism, the popular branch of irregular medicine that combined allopathic, homeopathic, and herbal remedies.[41] Hunt's thesis, like Corson's, took up the task of correcting deluded opinion, even when the delusion existed nowhere but in the student's thesis. (A writer in the register of health will energetically argue that fatal disease ought to be avoided.)

For the most part, Hunt's thesis concerns groups of physicians and their customary actions rather than nominalized systems or states of the body. Like Corson, Hunt speaks of connections among subjects and events rather than agreements or disagreements among texts and studies. For Hunt, the "true Physician" is one who "humbly confessing his ignorance . . . looks hopefully to a higher state of existence, for a fuller and clearer revelation."[42] Medicine was not, for Hunt, a specialized system of knowledge but a way of intervening in crises that are as much psychological as physical:

> [The physician] often witnesses the darkest tragedies of life & feels his inability to avert the last mournful catastrophe. Confessions, almost too horrible for belief, are poured into his ear—when the poor victim of circumstance & passion—weakened by disease feels the weight of his foul secret too terrible for endurance & recognizing a higher & purer nature pours out his soul in confession as to the supreme being.[43]

Much of Hunt's verbal energy is organized in adjectives, often doubled or written as lists: *the science of healing will rise bright in pristine purity and simplicity,* the physician is *milde and tolerant.* These sentences, like the rest of Hunt's thesis, display the complementary pattern of thin lexis and complex syntax typical of the discourse of health.

Like Corson, Hunt developed and advanced her argument by establishing presence and giving personified examples. Her initial invocation of the long history of medicine, however, situates the true physician in both the traditional past and the imminent future, while the false "counterfeit" physician is a brief corruption of the present. Transitional phrases, therefore, invoke the future as a domain of truth and enlightenment: *the world is growing wiser; when the profession is purified in the hot fire of public opinion; the signs of the age which point so decidedly to the education and elevation of women.* Hunt was likely to move from antiquity to the future, and then back around to the problematic present. Like Preston, Hunt saw progress as a source of vindication, applying this staple figure of reform rhetoric to support a transformed medicine.

But the use of irony is Hunt's most striking innovation in the register of health and her most interesting gender performance.

> The common complaint of many Medical practitioners—that the world is ungrateful, & *they* the *worst-used* men living; causes one to feel that there *is* a pressing necessity for medical reform. But opinions differ—& *my ideas* of this subject may not accord with the views of *those* who consider themselves so *dreadfully ill used.*
>
> Doubtless, such,—sincerely wish a new enactment which should compel people to pay them all the respect and attention which their *modesty* could endure, & in return for pills and plasters, fill their pockets with weighty tokens of gratitude. But alas! The world is growing wiser, and the fulfillment of their wishes seems every day less probable: People instead of reverencing their pretensions & taking their infallibility for granted, seem always on the look out for blunders. If by *a slight mistake* one of the number administers as much Laudanum to a baby, as would be a full dose for a strong man, straight-way a cry is raised against his knowledge or judgement and his bright prospect of favor & fortune is clouded.[44]

Hunt invoked public opinion as the ultimate arbiter of a profession's utility, associating the cause of women physicians with enlightened democracy. Against this background, "the common complaint of many Medical practitioners," is placed as given information, something already known and understood, as if a twentieth-century writer were referring to an overpaid baseball player or to corrupt political campaigns. In fact, while physicians' organizations did complain about the relatively low status of their profession and lamented that both the clergy and the law were held in more esteem, they seldom personalized these complaints, at least in the extensive medical press. Physicians argued that they ought to be more respected, but they did not complain of being the *worst-used men living.* Hunt's hyperbolic version of the physician's complaint transposes it from the sphere of public problems—the status of the profession—to that of private grievances. The august body of physicians becomes an overworked, querulous housewife—or even, by extension, the female invalid—*dreadfully ill used.*

Such irony is very rare in the theses written by male medical students, even when their topics—fashionable dress, the evils of the theater—invited ironic or satirical treatment. And I have never read a thesis in which a male student directs irony at the profession he aspired to enter, as Hunt does here.

92

For Hunt, irony was a way of establishing the authority required for a writer of the discourse of health, an authority not easily negotiable for a woman writer. Just as both male and female physicians struggled to balance their authority with the voices of patients in the medical interview, young doctors like Thomas Corson, with whatever trepidation, advised on child rearing and diet. But Angenette Hunt displaced the language of private, domestic life to physicians and took up a public, secular voice.

Like Corson's domestic advice, Hunt's satire on medicine continues a very old genre; from Montaigne through Molière, from the dangerous doctors of Sterne to the terrifying medicine of Dickens, antimedical satires turn on the physician who does harm to his patient while protesting against his own treatment. But antimedical satire certainly violates the decorum of the medical school thesis. Hunt does not mourn with the distraught mother but laughs at the inept doctor. Hers was a performance of the discourse of health quite distinct from any at the University of Pennsylvania.

Many women physicians writing in the register of health used irony to defend their right to speak, ridicule their critics, and contest the emerging professionalism of medicine. Harriot Hunt, the Boston physician, described the medical consultation, a highly ritualized event, as a "farce played by doctors." Hunt parodied a doctor's explanation of the etiquette of consultation to an anxious family:

> "—no, says the conservative M.D., you desire a consultation; I will bring my friend, Dr.———; we will have a private interview in your parlor; then he will see the patient; we will retalk the matter over; then I will give you his opinion!" Is this not an outrage on common sense and propriety.[45]

In Ann Preston's 1858 valedictory address, she speculated that

> no lordly Turk, smoking on his ottoman, could better depict the depravation which public manners would suffer, if Turkish women, should openly walk, side by side with fathers, husbands, and brothers, to the solemn Mosque, than some among us have portrayed the perversion our society must undergo if woman shares with man the office of Physician.[46]

Women physicians used satire to argue for their own positioned knowledge as a source of medical information. At the end of the century, Rachel Gleason, an Eclectic water cure physician, dismissed the received medical opinion that there was no good reason for nausea in the first trimester of pregnancy: "Certain it is, had these members of the profession vomited for months, casting up everything but Jonah, until every part was emaciated save the abdominal region, such preposterous theories would never have been propounded."[47]

If the medical thesis recalled the conventions of the belletristic essay, Angenette Hunt's irony shows how far those conventions could be stretched. And in their public performances of the discourse of health in books of medical advice or lectures to women on medical topics, women physicians made irony a central trope. The woman doctor was, to the attending audience or to her readers, already different from the doctor who normally lectured or wrote. The very fact of her speaking in public at all, albeit to an audience of women, was transgressive. But she was also a doctor, an authorized speaker. Preston usually performed the discourse of health without overt inflection, in a strategy I have called cross-dressing. Both Angenette Hunt and Hannah Longshore perform travesties of medical discourse: they seem to comply with the norms of regular medicine but actually subvert its standing as received wisdom. The classical tropes of irony and parody organize Hunt's performance: the distance between her compliant words and their satiric intent is patent, available to the reader. Longshore's travesty, as we shall see, was unmarked.

For women physicians writing in the register of health, authority was a vexed issue. Students writing the thesis commonly referred to themselves as novices; their acute awareness of the examining reader was often expressed in their texts. But for Hunt, everything in the writing situation was salient, including the generic masculine pronoun:

> I have used the masculine pronoun in describing the Physician but the signs of the times threaten yet *another* and more extensive innovation on the ancient and honorable science than even the irruption of Homeopathy & public opinion is beginning to prove that there is a female side to *this subject,* as well as most others. It is certain that the health of the world, depends on the women of the world & at least, *some* of the qualities needed in the medical profession—as gentleness, patience quick-perceptions natural instinct which is often surer than science, deep sympathy with suffering—all these belong to the sex in an eminent degree.[48]

Using the double edge of the argument for gender difference, Angenette Hunt transformed a potentially embarrassing question—how could a woman writer describe the true physician without excluding herself?—into an argument for granting her a medical degree. Hunt demonstrated the need for women physicians whose competence would be certified by their ability to argue the need for women physicians. The text, in a starkly material and institutional fashion, authorizes its writer.

This powerful move is unusual for a thesis specified as inaugural. The writer asks to join the profession she satirizes; she asks the targets of her criticism to admit her to their ranks because of the truth of her criticism. In Angenette Hunt's case, this strategy probably carried few material risks. Not only was her preceptor also her husband, but the faculty at the Woman's

Medical College was open to criticism of the established profession. Hunt's narrative of medical progress, in which the exclusion of women physicians was a temporary episode, collocated very strongly with the official rhetoric of the institution. While Hunt's advice on health, like Corson's, was commonplace and (at least for readers interested in homeopathy) uncontroversial, she performed and demanded from her readers a complex gender alignment. She virtually dared her readers to admit her to the profession, but at the same time, she allied with them against a common enemy and presented her challenge within an institutionally sanctioned triumphant narrative.

Woman's Medical College of Pennsylvania theses in the register of health were likely to construct their readers as astute consumers of medical care and to advise them in the choice of a physician; male graduates of the University of Pennsylvania constructed their readers as the direct recipients of hygienic advice. The women's theses are distinguished by a coolly distant and critical relation to the regular profession, by their ironic assertion of their own authority, by their affinity for satire. These are not the global, diffused, "connected" tonalities we associate with "women's ways of knowing." But given the social situations and rhetorical resources of these early women physicians, such strategies were both plausible and productive. Hunt transposed herself chiasmically with the physicians that she ridiculed; they saw women as querulous patients, but she turned that professional derision aggressively against them, portraying them as petulant whiners. Satire on medicine, including for Hunt an interesting willingness to joke about sick babies, supported a critique of regular physicians as badly trained and insufficiently scientific.

Not all the graduates of the Woman's Medical College who wrote in the register of health were so audacious, although each of their theses is interesting. Ann Preston's "Disquicition on General Diagnosis" concerned the personal qualities of the physician required for accurate diagnosis: the physician should know the "laws of health" which "regulate the growth of the minutest hair with as much precision as the laws of gravity balance the starry worlds." Preston's thesis presented the familiar undifferentiated body and thin vocabulary of the discourse of health. Perhaps the strongest commitment of the thesis is to the act of beginning, of opening, loosely collocated with diagnosis, the opening move in treatment. We read at the beginnings of the first three paragraphs: *The first duty of a physician; this preliminary step is the foundation;* and *here, on the threshold of his labors, the wise practitioner.* Of course, it was the writer who had taken up her first duties, essayed a preliminary step, paused on the threshold of her labors; this act of inception is displaced into the content of the text.

In her "Disquisition on Electricity," Anna Longshore-Potts described electricity as a "subtile fluid" that gathers in currents deep in the earth, issuing forth to form crystals and sprout seeds. Too much or too little electricity would surely cause illness, and we should "defend ourselves by more correct habits, and further by diet, and still further by the arrangement of our robes, as to favor a healthful electrical condition." Longshore-Potts argued that electricity resembles "volition power"; one can move the point of a compass by holding it and concentrating on it: "The experiment of the will on the needle also proves a most intricate and beautiful relation to exist between the volition power, the living action of the system, and electricity." Longshore-Potts's manuscript breaks off unfinished, but its final paragraph certainly has strong closural energy:

> Electrical currents pass from the equator to the poles charged with a renewed supply of the forming material gathered from solar light, and heat, which they retain with them in their passage through the etherial space, from their great source the sun, and when these currents of electricity pass from the poles up to the higher regions of the atmosphere, here the effect of what they received from solar influence is most beautifully displayed in that grand phenomenon aurora biorialis, on which the ignorant gaze with awe as forbodings of evil to the human family while the enlightened student [49]

There the text ends. The Longshores, as a family, were deeply interested in electricity, which also figured in Hannah's thesis, although in less florid fashion than in Anna's. Longshore-Potts was especially subject to enthusiasms, even for a Longshore; she would later argue for anticorset leagues that would bury the discarded corsets of newly converted women.[50] At any time, in any context, she would have been exceptional and perhaps just as weirdly prophetic. But extravagant as her thesis was, it was also a quite regular performance of the discourse of health. We find the same attenuated vocabulary for the organs and tissues of the body, the same attention to the body as a whole (*the living frame*), the same thin nominalization (*nutritive functions, curative power, volitional power*), and elaborate conversational syntax. The thesis develops its argument by making assertions about electricity, not by engaging what others have thought or written about electricity; it associates the writer with progress and the familiar hope for a new age. Like Angenette Hunt, Anna Longshore-Potts must manage her own intractable presence in the text: she did not write about *dress* or *fashion* but chose a dignified and entirely undomestic term, *the arrangement of our robes*. She undertook a complex performance of distance from conventional medicine, invoking the evidence of experiment and authority, positioning herself as the physician of the future.

Like traditional quietist medicine or noninterventionist sectarian therapies, the register of health was marked by a thin and nonspecific vocabulary for bodily tissues and organs but a full development of terms for the body as a whole system. Arguments proceed slowly, moving associatively from one topic to the next rather than gathering force through modifications and elaborations of positions; tautologies and synonymous expressions are common. These texts speak of the body and of its practices, of illness and its treatment, rather than of physiological opinion or medical practice as a discipline. They speak in the complex, deeply embedded and elliptic syntax of colloquial talk, and the speech role that they exact of their writers is never simple. It is a mature and hortatory role, patriarchal but also domestic; it can be complicated by being placed in a historical narrative or even by satire.

Some elements of the register of health are absolutely common to both genders; I have not found any difference in vocabulary, nominalization, or syntactic complexity between theses from the Woman's Medical College and those from the University of Pennsylvania. Both speak of bodily events rather than of scientific controversies. Both develop arguments through tautology and redundancy, illustrating rather than qualifying their statements. But there are also clear differences associated with gender between these two groups of texts.

The theses written by women vary considerably in their performance of the medical persona. Corson approximated the voice of a family counselor, a guide to the details of domestic life. This voice was one of many available to male writers of medicine, including those of the scientist, the man of the world, and the brutal realist. It was particularly adapted to the delivery of generalized advice to a docile audience, but it was in many ways inappropriate to a male speaker, to a young male speaker, and especially to a young male speaker whose actual readers were medical experts. Corson, therefore, had to negotiate a complex gendered performance, an exigency he met with embarrassed zeal. But Preston, Longshore-Potts, and Hunt established themselves as speakers for the future, whether that emerging social reality was embedded in the text, as in Preston's insistence on beginnings and inaugurations, or offered as a justification for the act of writing at all. Hunt and Longshore-Potts acknowledged the hostility of the profession they were attempting to enter by dividing their potential audience: conventional physicians, hostile to the medical education of women, would be proven wrong, while enlightened physicians, like the actual readers of the theses, were helping to inaugurate a new age (or to return to a primitive purity of medicine). The Woman's Medical College writers positioned themselves outside conventional medicine but argued implicitly that medicine would be reorganized to include them. Both Hunt and Longshore-Potts delivered somewhat transgressive performances: Hunt satirized the medical profession, and Longshore-Potts may well have exceeded even the broad latitude allowed irregularity in the early days of the Woman's Medical College. But both writers, allied by family ties to the male physicians who served as their preceptors and deft in drawing their audiences into the frame of the theses, passed the thesis without opposing votes.[51]

In tracing these differences and similarities between the texts produced by men and by women medical students, I wonder how much, and in what way, I am seeing specifically *gendered* performances. I am thinking here in Lacan's terms, of genders as positions available to any subject whatever at various times, these positions being taken in relation to the whole apparatus of social role, language, and law.[52] Some elements of gender performance in the theses are patent: the male doctor dispenses advice on good conduct; the female doctor corrects medical distortions of women's bodily experience. These enactments of gender are straightforwardly positional; they depend on a match between the known sex of the writer and the sex-linked social role enacted in the text. Such instances of writing as a man or as a woman illustrate a standpoint theory of gendered medical writing; the writer offers a vision of the world organized by and through experiences that are linked to life as a man (the patriarchal chief of the household) or as a woman (subject to nausea early in pregnancy).[53]

There are many other ways, of course, in which scientific writing can be gendered. The discourse on health is contradictory in its gender positioning, since it enacts a patriarchal authority that is obsessed with a feminine domestic sphere. Feminist scholars of science since Evelyn Fox Keller have also traced the gender politics of a female nature opened to the gaze of a male scientist; in later scientific medicine, that gender positioning would become literal.[54] Scientific medicine, at the end of the nineteenth century, would offer a very wide range of practices, including medical illustrations and norms of dissection, that literalized the male gaze penetrating the female body, seen as a series of layers which could be folded back, opened to view, and analyzed scientifically. Earlier medical traditions, however, had included practices of visualization and concealment, including the display of wax models which represented a female body as segmented into sequentially removable organs; flap anatomies sold to middle-class households that offered paired images of the male and female reproductive organs; or the general reluctance, in early modern anatomy texts, to represent the female body at all (except for the reproductive organs).[55] Women writers within the discourse of health could draw upon this diversified representational economy to establish for themselves a position as authorized speakers.

Writers of organicist medicine had been trained to see the body as a mapped system of regions and organs rather than as a series of layered tissues. But for these writers, the body was also a generalized space, a whole economy, subject to a different style of intervention. Very often, that generalized space was represented as a legal system, codified in "laws of health," thereby invoking the complex gendering of legal and political space in mid-

98

century United States.[56] Law was at once a masculine domain and a territory contested by women, presented as neutral and impartial and therefore subject to claims by any speaker. It might have seemed strange for women in the middle of the nineteenth century to speak of "drawing back the veil from nature,"[57] although later physicians would normalize that rhetoric. But women who had agitated against slavery, defied the fugitive slave laws by working in the Underground Railroad, and campaigned for woman suffrage would have found it natural to invoke the operation of impersonal laws. Here is "strong objectivity" with a vengeance;[58] just as scientific objectivity can be a protection against arbitrary gender politics, a kind of legal objectivity was imputed to nature and claimed by women.[59]

Finally, the women who wrote theses in the register of health constructed not only new forms of the medical persona but new organizations of the medical audience. It was not enough for them to sketch out a way of writing medicine that they could manage as women; they also had to offer their readers, at this early date uniformly male, a position from which to read their work. That position intersected, in ways we can never fully reconstruct, with the quite remarkable domestic space that these writers and their families must have formed. Over what breakfast tables, in what hilarious evening conversations, were these alliances tested and honed? These theses construct a community of marginality, a historicization of medical discourse, that compensated the faculty and graduates of the Woman's Medical College of Pennsylvania by offering them a narrative of medical and social progress. Their classmates who chose to write theses in the register of medicine faced different exigencies.

THE REGISTER OF MEDICINE

The claim to medical authority was negotiated differently in the register of medicine. A student writing in the register of medicine could align herself with medical research and practice that were scientific rather than traditional, or address a more professional audience. Very often, the same text includes both traditional and scientific propositions and practices; such transitional forms were common in midcentury medicine.[60] Margaret Richardson's thesis, "A Disquisition on Phthisis Pulmonalis" (1852), demonstrates the central features of this register, very commonly used in theses from both the University of Pennsylvania and the Woman's Medical College of Pennsylvania.[61]

Richardson's is the most interesting of the early Woman's Medical College of Pennsylvania theses written in the register of medicine; "Phthisis Pulmonalis" can serve as an example of the vocabulary, syntax, arrangement, and gender performance of the register of medicine. Richardson, born in 1818, was thirty-four when she wrote her thesis. Like Angenette Hunt, then, Richardson was much older than the average University of Pennsylvania medical student; she was widowed, well-traveled, the mother of a small boy who would later take a medical degree from the University of Pennsylvania. And she was to enjoy a successful medical career that spanned the century; her obituary described her as the "first and oldest woman physician in Montgomery County" and mentioned a Norristown practice that continued until 1906.[62]

Richardson's four-thousand-word thesis is the longest of those produced by early graduates of the Woman's Medical College of Pennsylvania. It follows a conventional format for describing an illness, moving through the topics of definition, symptoms, causes, prognosis, dissection, and treatment. This arrangement, common in the University of Pennsylvania theses, was not used in any of the women's theses written in 1851 but did organize many of the 1852 theses. Richardson's topic, phthisis, roughly corresponded to tuberculosis, although Richardson did not understand that disease in the way that German medicine would later define it. For Richardson, tubercles were the distinguishing mark of the disease, but they are not prominent in her text. (The bacillus that causes tuberculosis, of course, would not be discovered for decades, and in 1851 nobody suspected that a germ caused the disease.) Richardson's thesis constructs a body distinct from the general economic and legal system of the discourse of health, although many of the treatments she advocated were quite traditionally supportive.

While the register of health was marked by a generalized vocabulary for tissues and organs, Richardson offers a more fully elaborated set of terms. When she writes about the lungs and their associated tissues, we find not only *lung*, but *pulma, pleura, mucous membrane of the bronchia, pulmonary vessels*, and *parenchymatous structure of the lungs*. *Pleura* is differentiated into *pleura lining the cavity of the chest* and *that portion of it encircling the lungs*. The gross structure of the chest is indicated—we read of a *narrow chest*—but Richardson also minutely describes tubercles, *very minute particles, scarcely distinguishable by the naked eye*, or *larger bodies, varying in size form and color, abscesses of various sizes and secreting a brownish or blackish pus*, and *cartilaginous bodies indicating the cicatrization of the ulcerous cavities*. Richardson writes about *lungs* rather than using a phrase like *Laennec's observations of the lungs*, but her lungs are more highly differentiated than Corson's, more finely structured, and susceptible to a more specific derangement.

As Richardson's dissection of tubercles demonstrates, disease processes are also markedly more specific and detailed in the register of medicine than in the register of health, as if Richardson had been influenced by Parisian physiology's search for specific causes of distinct diseases that responded to standard treatments.[63] Richardson's interest in these issues would not have

100

been fostered by her preceptor, Joseph Longshore, who, like his family, preferred water treatments, a Grahamite diet favoring whole grains and vegetables, homeopathy, total abstention, and electrical and spiritual experiments over Parisian innovations. Richardson's detailed and technical interest in disease processes was by no means universal among American physicians, cautious and selective in their appropriations of French clinical medicine.[64]

Margaret Richardson's thesis represented phthisis in ways that a half century later, after the adoption of the germ theory, would have been considered self-contradictory.[65] She did not search for a singular or specific cause of the disease. For her, phthisis was hereditary, although heredity, of course, was not connected with genetics. A hereditary "disposition" by no means guaranteed that any one patient would contract tuberculosis; even an acquired characteristic could be inherited. Since the contagious nature of tuberculosis was not understood, heredity functioned as a parsimonious explanation for its progress through whole families.[66] *Hereditary* denoted not an unavoidable disease process but a tendency, something that one would have to watch, and even something for which one is responsible: "The Scripture declaration that "the sin (disease) of the parent shall be visited upon the children to the third and fourth generation is more applicable to the present instance than to any other of which I can form conception"[67] (punctuation as in manuscript).

But phthisis had many causes besides heredity, including "physical conformation," specifically a "scrofulous diathesis," demonstrated by complexion, body shape, and hair color.[68] Richardson is close here to the medicine of humors, an extremely elastic frame for analyzing the body, and to the enormously influential diagnostic science of physiognomy.[69] Such diagnostic frameworks would have been part of the curriculum at the Woman's Medical College of Pennsylvania. Carpenter's recommended textbook on physiology emphasizes the importance of "constitution": "There is no doubt that, in individuals of the plethoric or 'sanguineous' temperament, the proportion of the whole solid constituents, and especially of the corpuscles, is considerably greater than in persons of the 'lymphatic' temperament."[70]

Richardson also takes into account environmental and occupational causes of phthisis. Milling, limeburning, and stonecutting could irritate the mucous membrane of the bronchia and cause a kind of quasi-phthisis, really bronchitis, curable "by the various nostrums of the age," but threatening, if untreated, to develop into full-fledged phthisis. Other occupations, "those of a studious or sedentary kind," but also "watchmaking, tailouring, weaving &c.," compress the lungs, leading to congestion; the circulation of the blood is suspended "or greatly obstructed," and the lungs are subject to true phthisis. Diseases are interchangeable: bronchitis becomes phthisis, unless "cured" by early treatment before it takes final form.[71]

101

Richardson's text deploys both traditional understandings of disease processes as bodily imbalances and scientifically advanced understandings of specific diseases identified through pathological examination of tissues and lesions.[72] In Richardson's discussion of dissection, she mentions the tubercles: "Postmortem examinations present us with a great variety of appearances of the morbid mass, according to the peculiar character of the disease, or the advancement it had made at the time of death. But in a truly genuine pulmonary affection, tubercles, more or less numerous present themselves."[73] But tubercles, however central to the scientific understanding of phthisis, were useless in diagnosing a live patient. Richardson did not know of Laennec's method of diagnosing the progress of tubercles through breath sounds.[74] Her knowledge of the existence of tubercles offered her nothing to look for or attend to. Indeed, given the absence of any method of imaging the lungs in the mid-nineteenth century, this mark of the disease would have been diagnostically useless to Richardson, "until death enables us to obtain ocular evidence of the facts."[75]

Richardson found a consensus of medical opinion that the "affections exciting the disease," such as bronchial irritation, could be cured before tubercles had developed, but she records a variety of opinions about its later course. Some authorities thought that its progress could not even be slowed; others, that it could remain dormant; still others, that tubercles could be self-limiting. This difference of opinion had consequences for the physician trying to shape the story of the disease; as in the medical interview, narrative was central to clinical medicine. In the case of phthisis, there was no accepted schema, no story that reconciled consumption's many symptoms and courses with its infallible (if diagnostically useless) sign—the tubercles. Richardson, like other writers in the register of medicine, faced the problem of forming a narrative from that fundamentally intractable material. Her frustration is palpable:

> This [variety of opinions] may arise from the discrepant views entertained by different authors upon the real nature of the disease the great uncertainty attendant upon its causes and the utter impossibility of knowing positively what particular structure is involved, or what progress the affection has made, until death enables us to obtain ocular evidence of the facts.[76]

As if in response to the shifting symptoms of phthisis, the disease is sometimes a set of symptoms, sometimes a disposition, and sometimes a lesion; disease is not a stable representation that the doctor can use to think through a case and its therapy, but a symbolic, thrown-together organization of the intractable difficulty of the disease.

In her initial discussion of the symptoms of phthisis, Richardson moves from the domains of physiology and contested medical opinion to present a

102

typical case in its final stages. Her narrative becomes vivid, particular, and sympathetic:

> Diarrhea and colliquative sweats alternate with each other, and great debility and emaciation ensue—oedema of the lower extremities takes place, the features become contracted, the conjunctiva pearly, the hair thin, the nails convex longitudinally and transversely the roots having sometimes a chalky appearance[,] deglutition difficult, the breathing frequent, the voice whispering, the cheeks prominent, the eyes sunken and the countenance assumes an altered expression. During this time the spirits of the patient remain good, and are frequently better than when in health, the faculties of his mind are also sound, in regard to every thing but his own situation, with the daily increase of debility and all the symptoms of approaching dissolution, he feels confident of a speady recovery. Nor can the opinion of his Physician nor the anxious solicitude of those who feel concerned that he should be aware of his real situation affect a change in his futile hopes, until the glassy eye and the projected jaw indicate that the clayey tenement must very shortly become a cold inanimate body.[77]

Each surface of the body speaks, eloquently, of approaching death, in language audible only to the observer; the patient himself is constitutionally unaware of his peril, his delusion being another symptom of the illness. This passage is dense with specific information as it is presented first to the anxious physician and then, only when the unmistakable signs of death appear, to the deluded patient.

Such case studies are not especially common in the medical theses written in the middle of the nineteenth century. Sometimes, as with this cheerful phthisic, students wrote generalized narrations in vivid detail, perhaps drawing upon personal experience. (And in the case of tuberculosis, vivid personal experiences would have been all too common.) Rarely, the writer offers an illustrative anecdote that connects the scientific investigations of the register of medicine to the police functions of the register of health. Kane, for example, offered as proof of the reliability of his pregnancy test a woman whom he had transferred to his hospital's "working ward" on the basis of a negative test, although she

> claimed the privileges of pregnancy in round terms and presented all the other symptoms of that state in confirmation of her pretensions. She still retains the suspended catamenia, enlarged abdomen, etc., though five months have elapsed since the birth of the infant was promised me as a proof of my mistake. Other cases of attempted imposture, some of them ludicrous enough, which were detected by the same means, I have collected in my table C.[78]

For the most part, however, medical theses at midcentury, unlike articles in medical journals, avoided narrative development and did not present case studies. Like other purely academic genres, the thesis diverged from the discursive forms of its profession.

Richardson's text, like the theses in the register of health, faced the problem of positioning both reader and writer within an inhospitable profession. Unlike writers in the register of health, Richardson summarized medical opinion on specific topics; her references, like most of those in theses, are not documented. When opinions clashed, Richardson ingeniously transposed this difference into a rhetorical resource for constructing her own scientific authority: "—of these different views, it is extremely difficult for a novice in the profession to decide which to adopt—But, in a country like ours, where liberty of conscience and freedom of thought, is granted to all, we are not bound to adopt the opinions of our preceptors or wear their yokes, further than accords with our own judgment, and comports with our own views."[79] The very uncertainty of the case, with its multiple authorities and conflicting information, supports Richardson, the "novice," in adopting whatever view she thinks best. Historical and national values—American freedom of conscience, linked to Enlightenment free thought—sanction her authority. Such a linkage was coherent with nineteenth-century physicians' hope to form an "American" medicine and with early women physicians' view of their entry into the profession as an expression of republican values.[80] Richardson's use of these topics is nicely localized by her equivocating term *preceptors*, which is synonymous with *teachers* and designates her own preceptor, Joseph Longshore, the probable first reader of her thesis. Like Angenette Hunt, Richardson portrayed the medical community as divided and used those divisions to create an authoritative voice for herself.

Other theses from the Woman's Medical College in the register of medicine offer a range of therapeutic perspectives drawn from scientific medicine, traditional modes of treatment, or Eclectic remedies. Hannah Longshore's thesis carried two titles: the formal title page gives the simple title "A Disquisition on Neuralgia, its Treatments" and her thesis is listed in college announcements as "Neuralgia, its Treatments." But on the first page of the text, a sort of internal or hidden title reads "Neuralgia: its treatment by water."[81] Other texts, particularly in the first graduating class, offer general discussions of physiological topics and diseases, referring to the lectures given in the curriculum. We might include in this group Susanna Ellis's thesis discussion of the effects of the nervous system on respiration and digestion and the thesis on wounds by Phebe Way, which closely follows the account in her textbook.[82] Frances Mitchell's thesis on chlorosis is, similarly, an elementary discussion.

Martha Sawin's thesis on anemia, although very general in its medical content, offers a striking instance of tacit adoption of standpoint science by an early woman physician. Sawin asserted that anemia is an underdiagnosed disease of women; her discussion is unwavering in its focus on female physiology. In her discussion of anemia's causes, Sawin quoted from the analysis of the constituents of blood by Carpenter, author of the recommended physiology text at the Woman's Medical College of Pennsylvania: "Carpenters analysis of the blood in females is this. For 100 parts Water 7.91. Fibrin 2. Red corpuscles 1.27. Albumen 70. Extractive matter and salts .7 Fatty matter-6. It may be summed up thus Water 7.91. Solid or coagulable matter 2.9."[83] Turning to Carpenter, we find substantially the same information, differing only in details of presentation, presented as a footnote to the text's main discussion of the constituents of the blood in males.[84] Sawin took authority from the prevalence of the disease in women to use women's bodies, women's experience, and women's biochemistry as the norm, contradicting not only Carpenter's practice but also that of any medical writer she was likely to have read.[85] Conventionally, gender appeared, along with age, diet, and constitution, as a factor that can vary the proportions of blood constituents: "An appreciable difference exists between the blood of the two Sexes; that of the male being richer in solid contents, and especially in corpuscles, than that of the female."[86] Carpenter did not imply that being a woman was pathological, but for him the masculine is the theme and the feminine, a variation. That disjunction is especially powerful within the strong evolutionary framework of Carpenter's *Physiology*, which began with comparisons of the extremities and skeletons of humans and orangutans and compared human blood with that of frogs and "higher animals." While female physiology is not sick, it is clearly different; in Carpenter, "different" often means "less developed." All of this, Sawin silently sets aside. She does not say why women are especially subject to anemia or why their blood differs from men's. She does not even say that it differs from men's. Insisting on taking women as a norm, Sawin's thesis anticipates the project of a standpoint feminist science.

We do not know much about what happened to many of these members of the first graduating class. In the next chapter I will discuss Hannah Longshore and Anna Longshore (later Anna Longshore-Potts), whose family left a rich record, but Sawin, Mitchell, and Way are obscure. Gulielma Fell Alsop, author of the official *History of The Woman's Medical College, Philadelphia, Pennsylvania (1850–1950)*, wrote that Sawin returned to Massachusetts and that Phebe Way practiced in Pennsylvania.[87] Harriot Hunt mentions meeting Sawin and visiting Phebe Way in Baltimore.[88] I find no record of medical practice by Dr. Susanna Ellis or Dr. Frances Mitchell; they may have practiced in their families or under married names. Except for the record of their final exams, none of these students appears in the faculty minutes of the Woman's Medical College, save for a terse note recording that on November 18, 1850, the faculty passed two motions, that "the Dean have an interview with Mis Mitchell in regard to Graduating &c," and also interview her preceptor, Dr. F. X. McCloskey, "in regard to his absence from lectures &c."[89] Whatever lay behind these reticent minutes, Mitchell did indeed graduate without dispute and, according to Alsop, practiced medicine in England; McCloskey left the Woman's Medical College faculty in the purge of irregulars and died in Philadelphia in 1859.[90]

The members of the second graduating class of the Woman's Medical College of Pennsylvania were less timid in their theses; few of them simply repeated their textbooks. Charlotte G. Adams wrote her thesis, a short discussion of nursing, in Latin; like the other theses, hers was routinely passed. But Hannah Ellis's, "A Disquisition on Labor," gave her examiners pause. When the thesis was first evaluated by the faculty, three of the seven voted against it. Ellis's thesis espoused a theory that some of the faculty might have seen as irregular; she argued that the onset of labor is caused by the ovaries irritating the uterus and that the normal period of gestation is in fact ten months. While her preceptor, Joseph Longshore, was a great advocate of ovarian theories, Ellis based her argument on women's experiences.[91] Like Sawin, she was an early standpoint theorist. She wrote of "those, often, perplexing, and discouraging circumstances of prolonged pregnancies, which, irregularities are regarded, by the friends of the patient as the results of a miscount; but which cannot be so readily disposed of by the patient herself; she has the best right to know whether the fault is in the count or not—."[92]

Longshore moved for a reconsideration of Ellis's thesis at the next faculty meeting. The faculty minutes show that she finally received five white balls and two black and was accepted for graduation, although no preceptor's name appears on her title page.[93] Within six weeks of her graduation, Joseph Longshore had resigned from the Woman's Medical College, forced out in the early struggle for regularization. Ellis's essay had no secure institutional support in those bitter controversies; her insistence on the experience of the female patient as a source of knowledge and authority is all the more remarkable.

Henrietta Johnson's thesis on the skin follows the main lines of Carpenter's textbook, analyzing the components of the skin and describing its physiological function. Johnson, however, moves from physiology to politics, extending her topic to an essay on race. Since the causes of skin color are trivial, Johnson argued, there was no medical justification for considering Africans as substantially different from Europeans. And Johnson used that medical argument to support criticism of college policies:

> Three millions of God's children are groaning under a worse than Austrian despotism, because these minute cells are developed in their cuticle. They exclude their possessor from the councils of the nation; they closed the doors of our scientific institutions and crust the aspirations of a soul, which is no less

106

immortal than its earthly tenement, is not of fairest hue. Minute atoms of a human being, yet, how powerful their influence on the prejudices of mankind. A sister asks for a draught, from the crystal fountain of knowledge where we, are daily supplied, when a conservative mind would deny the boon she craves, because our heavenly Father has made her of darker hue.[94]

I have not found any record of the Woman's Medical College refusing admission to an African American woman in 1852 or 1853, but Johnson's thesis suggests a specific controversy that may not have been recorded. Like Angenette Hunt, Johnson undertook to criticize the body that would certify her competence—an audacious and unusual move. Johnson drew her authority from scientific knowledge; to discriminate on the basis of race is to give weight to a distinction not supported by medical knowledge of the body.

The construction of medical authority was never a simple matter for a student, male or female. Male medical students writing in the register of medicine also faced the tasks of establishing authority, representing the body, and explaining disease. John Sale's 1850 thesis, "An Essay on Haemoptysis," contrasts nicely with Margaret Richardson's discussion of phthisis and allows us to trace gender differences between men and women students. *Hemoptysis* was used especially to denote coughing blood from the lungs, although the term could denote any spitting of blood. For Richardson, hemoptysis marked the course of phthisis; it was not an "affection," a term that denoted both diseases and conditions produced by diseases, but an event in the body that could bring on disease or serve as its sign.

Sale, however, discussed hemoptysis as quite simply a disease in itself. He admitted that phthisis commonly caused it, and phthisis, as we have seen, was itself an assemblage of conditions. But hemoptysis could also be "vicarious," caused by suppressed bleeding at some other point in the body. Sale wondered whether the hemoptysis associated with phthisis is a cause or effect of the formation of tubercles:

> It is not the Hemorrhage that brings on the morbid affection, they are both the offspring of a previously diseased state of body. The hemorrhage could only produce the tendency to tubercles, by the depression of system it might induce from the loss of blood, and the feelings of the patient, though it sometimes precedes tubercles yet in the majority of cases it is subsequent. It may depend on the general habit of the body, but its great frequency would lead to the belief that tubercles was in some manner the exciting cause—acting by producing irritation or congestion of the lung from the space they occupy in its substance.[95]

Just as Richardson could not use her knowledge of tubercles diagnostically, Sale could not distinguish whether bleeding from the lungs was a cause or an effect of the tubercular lesion; in fact, the question did not much interest him. Instead, he invoked the "previously diseased state of the body" and claimed that since hemoptysis was itself a disease, one disease caused another. Sale found in hemoptysis exactly the kind of well-formed narrative that Richardson, dealing with the whole uncertain and intractable course of phthisis, was unable to shape. Limiting his discussion to a crisis and bracketing the question of its causes, Sale was able to offer a satisfying story in which clear symptoms prompted the responsive care of the physician. In a vivid narrative, Sale recounted the onset of hemoptysis, described the blood, and discussed treatment, specified as "bold and determined."[96] Sale's initial recommendations were uncontroversial, even quietist: the head and chest should be elevated, clothing loosened, and fresh air supplied in a clean room. A teaspoonful of salt was then administered. Sale discussed bloodletting, a logically depletive therapy within organicist medicine, which understood hemorrhage as the body's attempt to rid itself of superfluous blood.[97] Sale's regimen included cups, cold applications, blisters, sedatives, and astringents, including ergot, turpentine, and opium, leeches to the anus or uterus, and an easily digestible diet of oysters, boiled eggs, jellies, wine, porter. Moderate exercise and the avoidance of excitement were recommended. Indeed, such a course of treatment would provide enough excitement for any one life; it offered both quietist and heroic interventions in an alternating series. Sale's authority for both cautious bleeding and dramatic doses of ergot and turpentine is Dr. Wood, surely the Dr. George B. Wood, distinguished University of Pennsylvania faculty member, who taught twenty-three "office students" in 1850,[98] and whose lectures Sale would have attended. (Thirteen years later, Margaret Richardson's son Thomas would quote Wood with admiration in his thesis on enteric fever, one of the specialties of his mother's practice.[99]) In the absence of a controlling or even a consistent theory of disease, Sale's thesis offers compelling narrative and a single efficacious invocation of institutional authority. Not only does he tell a good story; he offers it on good authority.

S. Wylie Crawford's "Essay on Hypertrophy and Atrophy" demonstrates that, even for male medical students, institutional authority could be difficult to negotiate. Crawford (1827–92) was twenty-three when he wrote his thesis.[100] The son of the Reverend Dr. Samuel Wylie Crawford, principal of the Academy of the University of Pennsylvania, Wylie Crawford had received both a B.A. and an M.A. from the university. Immediately after graduating, he enlisted in the Army Medical Department, becoming an assistant surgeon in 1851. He worked on the Pacific Railroad surveys, fought against the Sioux, and served in Texas and during the Civil War, retiring as brigadier general in 1873 "for disability on account of a wound."[101] In acknowledgment of his industry as a collector of animal specimens, a species of Texas shrew was named after him in 1877. The introductory section of Crawford's thesis shows him in the usual medical student's quandary: what can he write with any authority?

> Destitute entirely of experience, his mind filled with the Theory of Medicine, the student must, upon contemplation, feel his deficiency, as regards practical observation or experience. In surveying the wide field over which he has just passed, he feels *he* can add no new gems to ground enriched with the experience of years; or add new luster to those already there. He is to pursue a beaten tract, to follow, not to lead, and to place his confidence implicitly in those pioneers who have preceded him, till research, or experience, have testified to the correctness of their views, or convinced him of their errors. As a medium course we have chosen the field of Pathology, as the more fitting province for the speculations of the tyro in Medicine, and among all the varied and interesting subjects which it unfolds to us, none have appeared to us more important than those disorders attendant upon the great Physiological process of Nutrition.[102]

This "tyro" economically summarized the choices available to him as a writer: he could write a thesis in the register of health, "one bearing upon the *Practice* of the profession," but with little hope of adding to the gems of therapeutic knowledge, since such knowledge was seen as almost exclusively the product of experience. The field of practice was too full, but *his* field was so empty. Crawford therefore located himself as a willing apprentice who differed from his preceptors only when time and experience convinced him that they were in error. Of course, the same rule also rendered his agreement provisional and temporary; Crawford affirmed confidence in his preceptors but made no promises for the future. Crawford translated his position at the threshold of the institution into a rhetorical resource; he is the credible neophyte whose speculations are entirely based on his institutional membership.

University of Pennsylvania students had other strategies for constructing medical authority. When dealing with a disease that utterly resisted treatment, like diabetes, the apprentice doctor could declare that the physician faced unalterable limits: "Of the many processes going on within the living body he knows little & he can only speculate concerning them. Of the principle of life he knows nothing & it is probable that the secret springs which give vitality to the organized being will be forever hidden from him."[103] Or the writer could establish his membership in the profession through a display of technical knowledge. Jesse Rivins's thesis, "An Essay on Auscultation in the Diagnosis of Pulmonary Disease," described minute variations in sounds audible only to the physician and only when the physician had drawn all his attention to the sounds. Phrases such as *analogous to the sound of throwing salt on burning coals* articulate experiences available only to physicians and establish Rivins's membership in the profession.[104] The thesis does not present new information but argues, through precise description, that the writer experienced the same things as the reader and so belonged in the reader's professional community.

The relation of the student to the medical community differed markedly between the University of Pennsylvania and the Woman's Medical College of Pennsylvania. Both male and female doctors writing in the register of medicine described the tissues and organs of the body quite precisely; both of them gave accounts of diagnostic tests, chemical and pathological. Both male and female students negotiated the differences between scientific medicine and organicist medicine, often borrowing liberally from both schools. They both oriented their theses toward therapy and constructed authority from the therapeutic interventions they prescribed. Both male and female students, not surprisingly, quoted from the lectures they were given and spoke modestly of their own experience. But for male medical students, however marginal or avant-garde the content of the thesis, the relation between the profession of medicine and their own education is transparent. Women students were skeptical of medicine, and medicine was hostile to them. Some women solved this difficulty by historicizing themselves, seeing themselves as new women physicians. Others invoked the faculty of the Woman's Medical College as the true core of the healing profession. But the unbroken chain of sponsorship—from student to medical school to medical profession—that supported the writing of University of Pennsylvania students was never as strong for Woman's Medical College of Pennsylvania graduates. For male graduates, that chain was unproblematic and therefore flexible. The authority of teachers sutured gaps in students' medical discourse or supported positions considered controversial within the profession. Given the marginality of the institution, the Woman's Medical College could not support its graduates in medically innovative or risky positions, although its connection to reform movements offered an alternate resource to students writing in the register of health. Students writing in the register of medicine repeated the information presented in their lectures, as Phebe Way did in her thesis on wounds, producing relatively conventional writing. Students who made innovations in medical discourse, like Martha Sawin or Hannah Ellis, with their woman-centered discussions of anemia and labor, did so tacitly, without argument.

Women students also, as a group, wrote shorter theses in the registers of both health and medicine. Of the eleven theses in the register of medicine written in the first two graduating classes of the Woman's Medical College, four are under fifteen pages long; except for Margaret Richardson's, none is over twenty-nine pages. A group of fourteen theses from the University of

Pennsylvania graduating class of 1850 shows two theses under fifteen pages and four over twenty-five, although fifteen to twenty pages is the most common length at both institutions. In student writing, length is never inconsequential. While this difference does not speak to distinct medical or social orientations, it may indicate that the women graduates were less comfortable in composition and that they were inventing the forms of their texts while they produced them. A second difference between theses produced at the two institutions is also brutally material: corrections and additions in another hand are much more common in the theses produced by women. In the etymological discussion that introduces almost all theses on diseases, the Greek words are painstakingly penned in another hand at the Woman's Medical College but never at the University of Pennsylvania. Many students had spelling problems, improvising both common and technical terms; both men and women varied in their use of conventional punctuation. Many a thesis from both of these institutions handles transitions with a dashing "&c." But corrections are very seldom penciled into the theses written at the University of Pennsylvania; they were very common at the Woman's Medical College, especially in the first class. Frances Mitchell's thesis, in particular, is heavily marked, with punctuation added in almost every sentence. And, to our eyes, the changes are not always for the better. To no particular advantage, McCloskey changes *condition* to *situation* and *assumes* to *resumes*, demonstrating that the urge to tamper with students' prose is among the strongest of pedagogical impulses. (See figure 4.) It may be that, with a relatively small class, the faculty was willing to undertake the labor of marking up these papers. And it may also be that the writing of women was assumed to be less correct, more in need of amendment.

The thesis was, for almost all students, a problematic performance. For a woman who, unlike her male counterpart, wrote the thesis after half a lifetime of experience, including the usual labors of nursing family members, such an apprentice's document must have been even more contradictory. The Woman's Medical College of Pennsylvania, the institution that might have supported that labor, was itself marginal and reflected the insecurity of its students. Whether the women graduates were writing conventional theses or being innovative, they had to construct the authority for their discourse from found materials. Their solutions were often unorthodox; we read in these theses forms that are very unusual for academic writing, including satire and critique. We also see an unusual willingness to cite lay opinion, particularly the opinion of women, and sometimes an unwillingness to accept the male body as a physiological norm. For African American women physicians writing later in the century, both the problem of establishing their authority and the institutional resources supporting them had ramified.

111

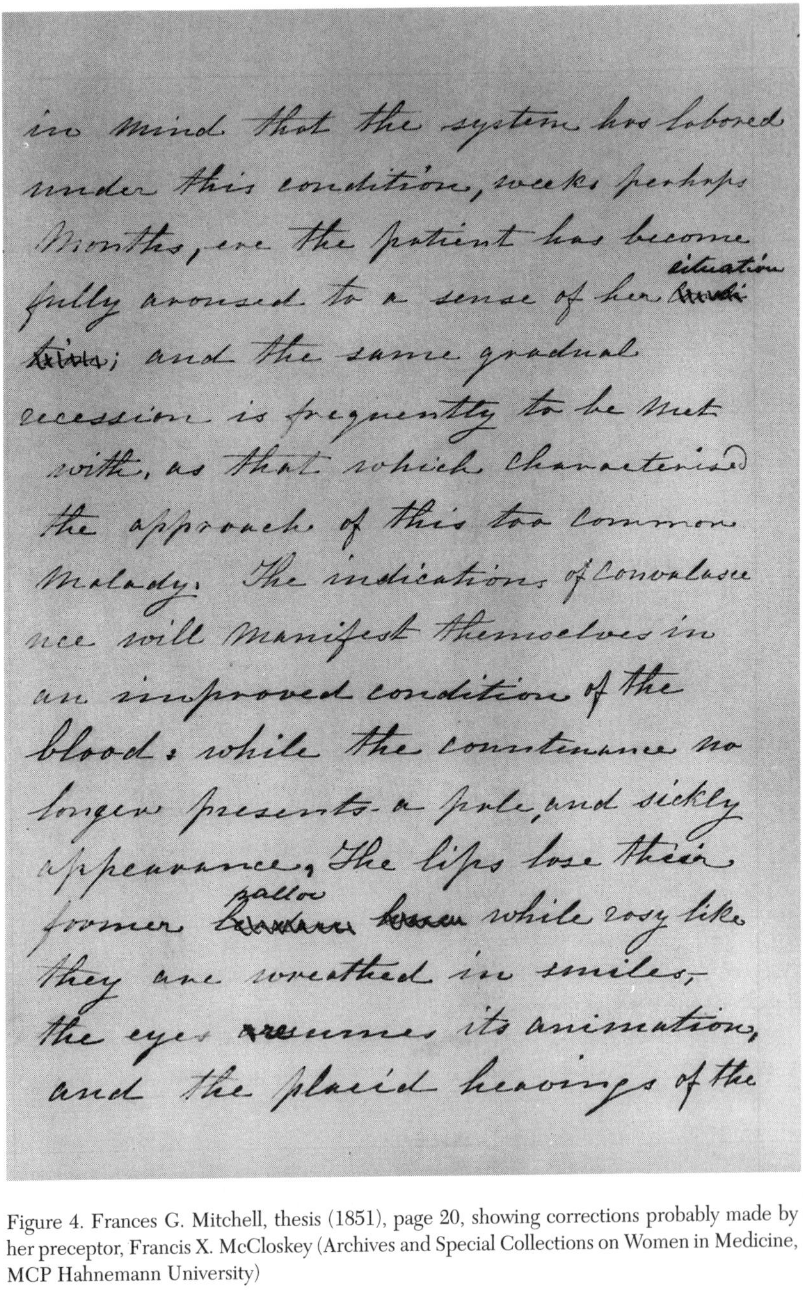

in mind that the system has labored
under this condition, weeks perhaps
Months, ere the patient has become
fully aroused to a sense of her ~~conditi~~ situation
~~tions~~; and the same gradual
recession is frequently to be met
with, as that which characterised
the approach of this too common
Malady. The indications of Convalesce
nce will Manifest themselves in
an improved condition of the
blood; while the countenance no
longer presents a pale, and sickly
appearance, The lips lose their
former ~~sallow~~ sallow ~~hue~~ while rosy like
they are wreathed in smiles,
the eyes ~~assumes~~ its animation,
and the placid heavings of the

Figure 4. Frances G. Mitchell, thesis (1851), page 20, showing corrections probably made by
her preceptor, Francis X. McCloskey (Archives and Special Collections on Women in Medicine,
MCP Hahnemann University)

AFRICAN AMERICAN WOMEN PHYSICIANS
AND MEDICAL AUTHORITY

African American graduates of the Woman's Medical College entered a more prestigious institution than that of the graduates of the 1850s: seven of the twelve known nineteenth-century African American graduates dated from the 1890s, when the women's college was an established institution; its graduates were admitted to the Philadelphia County Medical Society; and its students had access to the medical institutions of the city. Earlier graduates, beginning with Rebecca Cole (1867), were often members of the established African American middle class of Philadelphia; they brought to their medical study the prestige of broadly recognized political and educational connections. Taken as a group, however, nineteenth-century African American graduates of the Woman's Medical College demonstrated a dizzying range of experiences and medical interests.

Consider for example the contrasting careers of Caroline Still Wiley Anderson (1848–1919) and Eliza Grier (18??–1902). (See figures 5 and 6.) Anderson graduated in 1878; she was the daughter of the prominent Philadelphia abolitionist William Still, had been educated in local Quaker institutions, and graduated from Oberlin in 1868. Although she responded to a later Oberlin alumnae survey by saying that she had no academic degrees, as a college graduate, she would have been among the best-educated Woman's Medical College students.[105] Before entering the women's college, she taught for a year at Howard University and entered the medical school there, studying with Isabel Barrows, 1868 graduate of the Woman's Medical College of the New York Infirmary and specialist in ophthalmology. Anderson wrote her own thesis on fibromata.[106] She married the prominent minister Matthew Anderson and with him managed the extensive activities of the Berean Presbyterian Church. She ran the Berean Dispensary, which offered medical care to Philadelphia's African American community, was vice-principal of the Berean Manual Training and Industrial School, where she also taught elocution, physiology, and hygiene, and she managed the Berean Cottage at the seashore, "a place of rest for the hard working and honest toilers of the race."[107] She founded a YMCA for African Americans and was active in the Woman's Christian Temperance Union.[108] Anderson helped build the Berean school into an important Philadelphia institution, one that offered the African American community job training, an education for public life, and diverse cultural opportunities. And she maintained both an active medical practice and her scientific interests, giving a talk, "Popliteal Aneurism," to the Woman's Medical College of Pennsylvania Alumnae Association in 1888.[109] Her death was mourned throughout the city.

Eliza Grier's 1898 graduation from the Woman's Medical College was

113

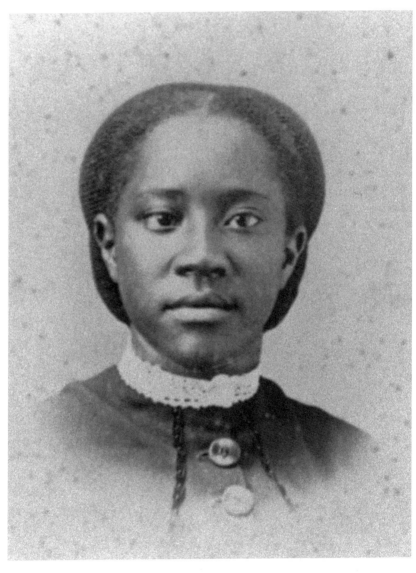

Figure 5. Caroline Still Wiley Anderson, 1868 (Oberlin College Archives)

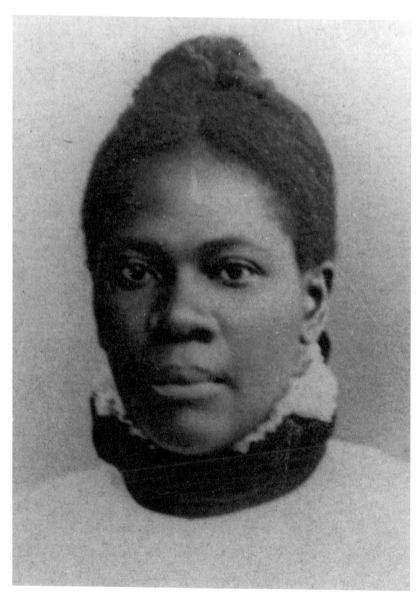

Figure 6. Eliza Grier, from her 1898 class picture (Archives and Special Collections on Women in Medicine, MCP Hahnemann University)

greeted with an article in the *North American Medical Review* entitled "Coal Black Woman Doctor," which gives her first name as "Clizo."[110] Dean Ruth Lathrop wrote a reference for the new graduate, describing her as having "'respectable standing' as a student of medicine; how much better work she would have done had she not been constantly harassed by want of adequate means of support it is difficult to say."[111] And it does not seem as if that question was ever answered. Grier, who described herself as an emancipated slave, studied at Fisk University from 1884 to 1891, taught at Payne Normal School in Augusta for a year, and came to the women's college in 1893. One account describes her going south to pick cotton after a year of school.[112] She practiced in Greenville, South Carolina. In a letter to Susan B. Anthony, she described herself as having "a pretty good practice, but mostly among the very poor and in neglected districts," and explained that illness had exhausted her resources: "There are a great many forces operating against the success of a Negro in business. These, however, I hope someday will be overcome. The only thing that impedes my progress is that I am trying hard to carry on my art and am illy prepared, in a financial way to continue when hardship and want come on." She asked for help, invoking "the blessed Master" to ask for Anthony's aid.[113] Anthony was sympathetic but declared herself unable to help, forwarding the letter to the dean of the Woman's Medical College. A year later, on April 14, 1902, Grier was dead.

While white students at the Woman's Medical College came from a variety of family backgrounds and entered the college with a range of life experiences, it would be difficult to find among them circumstances so starkly contrasting. And the complexities of the sisterhood offered to African American women by the college are illustrated by the experience of Sarah Marinda Loguen, an 1876 Syracuse graduate who came to the Woman's Hospital for her internship. The clinic superintendent was struck by Loguen's resemblance to one Dr. Loughune, a white woman from Nashville, Tennessee, commenting, "Thee might be twin sisters." A hasty consultation determined that the two women were related, and Dr. Loughune resigned her internship.[114]

Caroline Wiley Anderson's "Thesis on Fibromata" demonstrates how African American women physicians negotiated these complex relationships. "Fibromata" is an extensive and assured work; this thesis by the former president of the Oberlin Ladies' Literary Society ran to forty-five orthographically irreproachable pages. Unlike the vast majority of theses by either male or female students, Anderson's argued a point, that the "extirpation of said tumors has been proved a necessity by the results, and the successful performance thereof entitles surgical operations upon such growths to greater favor, and consideration."[115] And, for Anderson, that point was located within an ongoing medical conversation about what caused fibromata, their effect on health, and their efficacious treatment. Her opening page reported:

"Some suppose tumors generally to be due to an accidental, local irritation, and limited to certain parts of the system, among the supporters of this view are Virchow, Fleisch and O. Weber." But she tempered this avant-garde position with an acknowledgment that "there are largely inherited tendencies and innate predisposition to the development of such growths," as shown by "clinical experience, and the views of able writers."[116] Anderson quotes freely from able writers in the pages that follow, discussing the nomenclature of the tumors, the history of their investigations, and their appearance under a microscope. She reported three pages of controversy about the correct name for such growths, concluding, "In these cases there seems no reason why both prefix, and affix might not be retained thus: myo-fibro-cartilaginous etc., and an important portion of the structure thus kept prominent."[117] Anderson, fully conversant with the literature, felt confident to intervene in an ongoing dispute. Writing twenty-seven years after Angenette Hunt, Caroline Anderson had become fluent in a medical discourse that combined the registers of health and of medicine seamlessly, if not consistently.

The thesis continues through the usual topics of appearance, location, differential diagnosis, treatment, and dissection. She records approvingly entirely traditional quietist treatments, like that of Dr. Warren, who prescribed eighteen months of "confinement, and solitude, and strict compliance with his orders" to a young man who developed a tumor from overexertion.[118] The last fifteen pages of the thesis summarize an article by "Dr. Atlee" on the surgical treatment of fibroids; Anderson's citation of the article is distinctive in giving it a date and a place of publication: 1876, at the International Medical Congress. Atlee's article repeats the main categories of the thesis—classification, location, and treatment. But his focus is on surgery, particularly heroic surgery, even when the surgeon is mistaken:

> In another case, "a rough, irregular, tumor-like mass presented in the vagina upon what seemed an inverted uterus," it was removed and found to be the body of the uterus. Whereupon the following query suggested itself to Dr. A, "though an error of diagnosis, will not the amputation of the body or entire removal of such a diseased organ be the best mode of treatment, keeping in view the comfort, and life of the patient"? We can conceive of circumstances which would seem to warrant even such heroic treatment as this, suggested and favored by Dr. A.[119]

Anderson aligns herself with a surgical, if not a medical, avant-garde. And her experience as a medical student supported that identification. Anderson describes two surgeries that she herself witnessed: the removal of a fibroid tumor from the breast, and the removal of a fibroid from a forearm, both at the Woman's Hospital.[120] Anderson gives detailed accounts of both surgeries, including the operative procedures, closing sutures, and subsequent management of the patients. The more developed facilities of the Woman's Medical College allowed Anderson to claim the authority of direct knowledge, to establish her own "clinical experience," that talisman of traditional medicine, while advocating advanced modes of treatment.

But the college could not offer Anderson any credible answer to the question of how fibromata were related to race. "One of the usually admitted predisposing causes of fibroids is Race, the African being peculiarly liable it is said, but no statistics at our command throw any light upon this subject, nor are any reasons offered to account for this statement."[121] Anderson was not the only African American graduate plagued by a lack of information about race and health. Halle Tanner Johnson, acting as infirmarian at the Tuskegee Institute, described six phthisic patients in a letter to the Woman's Medical College Alumnae Association: "I have had no experience worth speaking of, and, therefore, am somewhat timid about expressing myself; but I would simply say that I am exceedingly interested in this question [of treatment for phthisis] and would like to get all the important information upon the subject that I possibly can, as I regard it as an important race question."[122] Tanner's frustration is clear: nothing in her education explains why this illness appeared so frequently in "very black persons,"[123] and she could not see how that question would be answered if not by her own work, the work of a very young graduate. Like Anderson, Tanner felt authorized to intervene in a scientific debate; like Anderson, she realized that nothing in her education was a reliable support when that debate turned to "an important race question."

A very different set of constraints motivated the work of Georgiana Young, whose thesis on opium was written in the same year as Caroline Wiley Anderson's.[124] Georgiana Young, in the words of her grand-nephew, "did not divulge her race while a student" at the women's college.[125] And there is, in fact, no mention of her race in her student records, in the account of her graduation, or in the subsequent records of the alumnae association. Young's thesis is equally disguised; it offers a thoroughgoing performance of cross-dressing. Young presents opium as a source of excitement, an exotic Asian artifact, and a terrifying blight. Although the thesis concludes that opium "may be the source by its judicious employment of more happiness, and by its abuse of more misery, then any other drug employed by mankind," it is much more vivid in its pictures of opium-induced happiness than in its warning against opium abuse.[126] After describing the manufacture of opium and specifying chemical tests for its presence, Young offers the following account of its operation: "It increases the force and frequency of the pulse, augments the temperature of the skin, invigorates the muscular system, animates the spirits. It intensifies all the capacities for thought and gives new energy to the intellectual faculties. . . . a delightful placidity of mind succeeds, insensible to painful impressions, forgetting all sources of care and anxiety."[127] A considerably less compelling account of the bad effects of large doses of opium follows. In describing how opium is taken in the "flowery kingdom" of China, Young becomes lyrical:

> In the mansions of the rich, there is usually found fitted up for the accommodation of friends, a private boudoir, richly ceiled and garnished with superb adornments, such as only art can achieve, and wealth procure, and here rich paintings, with choice scraps from Confucius adorn the walls, and carvings in ivory, with other articles of vertu grace the tables. Here also is provided in chief, the gilded Opium-pipe, with all its appurtences and there host and guests unrestrained by curious eyes, deliver themselves up without concern to the inebriating Chandoo and its beatific transports.[128]

Meigs would have been proud of this interior. Young is certainly presenting the smoking of opium (as against its administration in other forms) as a degenerate oriental practice, but she has made that practice luxurious, artistic, enticing. A page later, she offers an account of the Chinese adoption of the "vice" of opium as if she were beginning a new topic. And indeed, Young simply wrote two stories of opium: one in which it was a source of pleasure, indeed happiness; another in which it was a vice to be avoided. It is the first story that controls the thesis; the second offers a cross-dressed disguise.

Juan Bennett's "Sanitary Chemistry" (1888) took up the topics of public health that had been associated with African American women physicians since Rebecca Cole's service as a sanitary visitor in 1868, but it refunctioned them in light of the chemistry Bennett had learned at the women's college.[129] "Sanitary Chemistry" was organized by the traditional issues of air, water, and food, but it treated them as chemical questions. It detailed tests for the adulteration of sugar, tea, vinegar, and milk, and ways of measuring the contamination of water and air. Bennett thereby transformed the sanitary worker from a teacher who would offer instruction to an authority who could constrain action. Elizabeth Blackwell had praised Rebecca Cole for her tact and care in giving "simple, practical instruction to poor mothers."[130] But Bennett saw herself as joining the "sanitary authorities," monitoring the quality of air and water to prevent epidemics. Their authority would be broad: "The public control in the public interest, must extend to the sanitary condition of every household, not among the poor alone, at least equally among the rich."[131] Every house, every source of water, would fall under their supervision: "During epidemics it is best to condemn all waters containing more than .015 gram of chlorine per litre."[132] But the sanitary chemist retained the moral authority of the sanitary visitor, the medical warrant for judging customs and habits according to the laws of health: "A depraved taste has led to the demand for bright green pickles."[133]

These three theses demonstrate a range of strategies used by African American students for constructing medical authority: borrowing the emergent institutional authority of the institution; translating science into a source of socially sanctioned knowledge; and disguising the race, position, and even the opinion of the cross-dressed writer. None of these strategies organized a productive medical discussion about race, a problem which, as we have seen, was still unresolved when W. E. B. DuBois surveyed health conditions in 1898 for *The Philadelphia Negro*. But in Anderson's and Bennett's theses, scientific knowledge is joined with the student's experience, mediated through her medical education, to offer a way of speaking as a doctor, whether as a practitioner of what Bennett called "the great medicine of the future, Preventive Medicine,"[134] or as Anderson's cool, heroic surgeon.

Did the graduates of the Woman's Medical College, then, write science differently from the graduates of the University of Pennsylvania? Yes and no. The two registers of health and of medicine construct two kinds of bodies, two accounts of medical practice. The differences between these two registers are as marked as the differences between the most distinct male and female performances within each of them. Very many passages in very many theses are not at all marked by gender differences, and these passages often work out the serious intellectual problems of the essay, negotiating incompatible understandings of the body in more or less consistent ways. In their approach to therapy, women did not differ from men, a finding that has been stable in studies of women physicians since Morantz-Sanchez's pioneering work.[135]

Although doing medicine was quite similar for men and for women, being a doctor was not, particularly when the doctor was African American. In particular, the marginalization of the struggling Woman's Medical College set rhetorical problems for its graduates and deprived them of a rhetorical support that was quite commonly used in the theses written at the University of Pennsylvania. While a male medical student could present himself comfortably as a "tyro" or an "apprentice," a new woman graduate could not. If women were to be doctors at all, they must be heroic doctors, inheritors and inaugurators of an honored tradition. Such a stance, of course, placed an impossible strain on the decorum of the student essay, not to mention the obligatory modesty of a woman moving from her separate sphere. It is not a small part of their achievement that women students found solutions to the problem of authority that were not self-abnegating.

This chapter has been a long argument for local knowledge, an argument against seeing women's perceptions or scientific interests as necessarily connected to a feminine cooperative nature or an inherent disposition toward disclosure rather than objectification. In these texts, we hear singular voices, those of women who believed that electricity flowed in the ground like water and that the ovaries prompted labor; I want to take them seriously as scientists, working on the scientific issues that faced medicine in the middle of the nineteenth century. Their performance of these discourses was never simple; medical discourse, after all, represents women's bodies as objects of a particular kind of knowledge. These writers were among the first to answer that representation as subjects; we misunderstand them if we forget either their commitments as scientists or their experiences as women.

5

Invisible Writing II
Hannah Longshore and
the Borders of Regularity

Hannah Longshore (1819–1901) is at once more obscure and more available to us than Ann Preston. She maintained a careful distance from the Woman's Medical College and its alumnae association and never identified herself exclusively with any institution. But unlike Martha Sawin and Phebe Way, she did not vanish from the public record. Although Hannah Longshore's career was grounded in active clinical practice—forty patients a day, by her husband's account—she also wrote and spoke in public. And her large, vocal, active family connected her to reform circles. Her brother-in-law Joseph Longshore (1809–79) was a well-known radical, active in the Underground Railroad and women's rights movements and also in temperance, spiritualist, and vegetarian circles; he was among the founders of the Woman's Medical College of Pennsylvania.[1] Her sisters, Jane Myers and Mary Frame Myers Thomas, also became physicians, graduating from Penn Medical University, an Eclectic school founded by Joseph Longshore after he left the Woman's Medical College. Mary Frame Myers moved to Indiana, where she collected supplies for the Union during the Civil War and worked on the suffrage papers *The Lily* and *The Mayflower*.[2] Anna Longshore-Potts, her sister-in-law, was also among the first graduates of the Woman's Medical College, traveled to Australia and New Zealand as a lecturer, and published both her lectures and a book, *Love, Marriage, and Courtship*.[3] Her obituary also mentions travels to India, Britain, and Ceylon; she died in San Diego in 1912.[4] Hannah Longshore's daughter Lucretia, later Lucretia Blankenburg, was the wife of a Philadelphia reform mayor and herself a proponent of public health measures; she popularized a version of her mother's biography in which the daughter's girlhood sufferings were prominent.[5] Hannah's husband, Thomas Longshore, kept her notes, wrote her lectures, and wrote extensively, ostensibly on religious topics. This chatty and opinionated family surrounded Hannah Longshore with a web of stories; we can know things about her that we can never know about Ann Preston—what she ate for breakfast, what she was like as a mother. And, just as the early theses of Woman's Medical

College students speak to their location within the school and the institutions of medicine, Hannah Longshore's writing can be placed, with that of her family, in the social world of reform, where science and health were intimately connected with religion and politics. These texts supplied Hannah Longshore with characteristic tropes; looking at her writing in the context of the discourses that circulated around her, we can understand better her performance of the anomalous role of the woman physician.

Hannah Longshore's favored strategy for that performance was travesty, a characteristic trope of the Longshore family. When they seemed most conventional in their reproduction of received forms and genres, the Longshores were often using them against their grain. Particularly in the case of Hannah Longshore's gender performance, travesty supported complex and doubled positions: admiration was overlaid with pointed criticism. Travesty's attitude toward its objects has often been contradictory. The medieval *Second Shepherds' Play*, with its parody of the nativity, is a deeply reverent (and very funny) retelling of the Christmas story; Scarron's *Virgile Travesti* (1648–52) was an elaborate tribute to the *Aeneid*. But travesty, burlesque, and "taking off" have also organized devastating satirical attacks. (Oddly, all three terms are associated with clothing; *burlesque* and *taking off* are associated with stripping, while *travesty* is etymologically identical to cross-dressing.) And the contemporary common use of *travesty*—"travesty of justice"—suggests that such attacks have serious consequences.

Longshore was a parodist in her use of medical forms; she took them on as disguises, but subtly overturned them. In her most extended performance, her response to a toast delivered at the annual banquet of the Woman's Medical College Alumnae Association, she travestied institutional identifications, medical regularity, and medical biography as practiced in nineteenth-century Philadelphia.

THE FIRST CASE: HANNAH AND HER SISTERS

Hannah Longshore spoke often in public, but her only surviving speech is a narrative of her life delivered to an audience of medical women. Longshore replied to a toast at an annual supper of the alumnae association of the Woman's Medical College of Pennsylvania, probably in 1895. At least on the surface, Longshore performed the role of an exemplary scientific professional, but she also used her personal narrative to refuse affiliation with her audience and to suggest alternates to the scientific regularity of her alma mater. The speech is therefore a disguised attack on the solidarity that it celebrates. Since we have her speech in both its final version and a number of rough drafts, we can reconstruct Longshore's work of composition and understand both what her toast said and what it did not say.

The toast was a specific speech genre, staged in a complex site. The Woman's Medical College Alumnae Association was a professional home for women doctors in Philadelphia, barred as they were from the Philadelphia County Medical Society. The alumnae supper was carefully orchestrated, held after a day of scientific papers and clinical reports. New, old, and returning members wore distinctive ribbons. It was not easy to organize a supper that all members could enjoy; arrangements about wine were especially vexing, since many members were abstainers, and some refused even to enter an establishment that served alcohol. An early president of the association, Mary Putnam Jacobi, commented:

> I do not see that the fact that two ladies were so extremely squeamish as not to come to the Hotel Bellevue for the reason alleged, ought to influence the Association. Nothing could be more free from alcohol than our own supper last night. If anything could have been added to make the table look prettier, it would have been some sparkling wine. It is not necessary to drink, but it is always pretty to look at.[6]

Toasts, taken with water or other nonalcoholic beverages, were the high point of the evening; usually given by an officer of the alumnae association or a member of the faculty, they honored groups of female physicians and their supporters. The toasts addressed groups in the audience, such as "the New Graduates" or "Our Forerunners." A representative of the toasted group would "reply" with another short speech.[7] Although the members of the alumnae association were educated women, members of a respected profession, they found this ritual daunting. When the association debated inviting men to the banquet, its members demurred; they preferred to have their first efforts at toasts and replies remain unwitnessed by the "specially dinner-giving and speech-making sex."[8] The toasts and replies ring the changes of the epideictic, from the sentimental through the humorous to the heroic. In 1892, Mary Putnam Jacobi toasted the corporators; "Mrs. Mumford responded in a witty speech"; and Jacobi responded with the joke (it must have been old, even then) that "to look at me, of course, you will not realize how completely that period belongs to ancient history."[9] On other occasions, dead alumnae or the sacrifices of medical missionaries were honored. Similar after-dinner toasts at University of Pennsylvania alumni events included both serious policy speeches and humorous or sentimental performances. At the 1875 University of Pennsylvania alumni dinner, for example, the toasts were followed by "several songs," and the "company did not separate until a late hour."[10] As a speech genre, the toast was linked to males, and expressed a professional urbanity alien to women physicians, even those used to lecturing and public address. The woman physician who rose to make a toast or to reply to one, then, was undertaking a gender-marked performance, one that she and her spectators understood as male.

Though new at making toasts, Hannah Longshore had extensive experience in communities which accepted women in public speech roles. Like Ann Preston, Hannah Longshore was a Quaker, associated with the Hicksite group and familiar with their practice of plain-spoken female preaching. Quakers did not generally accept women as congregational overseers or as rule-givers but did value them as intuitive, inspired preachers.[11] In Longshore's connections with the spiritualist Harmonial Circle, she would have encountered women as authorized speakers, skilled negotiators of the borders of life and death.[12] Finally, as a close friend of Lucretia Coffin Mott and a participant in the midcentury reform movements, Longshore would have heard effective women speakers in a variety of styles and situations.[13]

At the time of her speech, Hannah Longshore was nearly eighty years old, veteran of forty years of medical practice. Her four teams of horses and her house in fashionable Logan Square spoke of her professional success; her simple dress, Grahamite diet, total abstentionism, and spiritualism linked her to the diverse medical reform movements of midcentury; her suffragism, abolitionism, and membership in international peace societies connected her to Philadelphia Quaker activism. The speech she gave was an autobiographical narrative, an account of her experiences as a medical pioneer. Longshore's career intersected with the increasing professionalization of medicine and with the entry of women into "regular" medical practice; her speech organizes these complex events as a simple dramatic narrative.

In its final version, Longshore's talk is a story of triumph over opposition.[14] Longshore recalled that "the first women physicians in Phila. did not find their paths strewed with flowers nor their advent welcomed by the general public or by the profession." She remembered the threatened disruption of the first graduation by male medical students and the rude comments that greeted the sign "Hannah Longshore, M.D." on her window shutter. And she remembered early triumphs: her cure of a patient who had been given up, her growing practice. Since pharmacists refused to fill Dr. Longshore's prescriptions, she began to compound drugs herself and to carry them in an emergency case. Longshore's struggle to prescribe and administer drugs figured in the climactic episode of the speech:

> A little later the following incident occurred; I went to one of the leading pharmacist to purchase an ounce of Sulphate cinchona, placing my business card on the counter, the proprietor looked at it and then at me and said "I will not sell this cinchona to you" you are out of your sphere "go home and darn your husbands stockings! Housekeeping is the business for women" I informed him that the stockings were darned, my house was probably as well kept as his, and

as a graduate of the Female Medical College, chartered by the Legislature of Penna. I proposed to practice medicine as long as the women of Philadelphia saw fit to employ me, and I have the strength to work. And laying my emergency case open on the counter told him it had kept dollars out of his business and would keep more. Bystanders listening to the episode indulged in such flippant remarks as "strong minded woman" and "go it while you are young" and made the scene more annoying by their vulgar epithets, I turned to leave the store when near the door the proprietor called to me, and said you can have the cinchona for two dollars," I observed that $1.50 is the price to physicians when he consented to take that sum.[15]

This is, of course, a very good story, a story that has been honed and rehearsed. In three of the four versions of the speech, it is the centerpiece of her performance, written with few corrections, in words virtually identical to those used for the final version. Hannah Longshore's is a straightforward account of plucky self-assertion, professional confidence, and economic self-interest victorious over prejudice—a triumph of liberal feminism.

Longshore's story also negotiates quite complex relations with both her immediate audience and the profession in which she had prospered. It bid for her inclusion in the institutional memory of the Woman's Medical College, a history from which she and her family had been virtually erased; without mentioning her family, this speech reinscribed them into the history of the institution. From the 1860s until the end of the century, the role played by Hannah's brother-in-law Joseph Longshore in founding the Woman's Medical College of Pennsylvania went unmentioned in its official documents, which treated the college's first ten years with elegant vagueness. Only in the twentieth century—after this speech and Lucretia Blankenburg's promotional efforts—do we read references to darned socks and medicine cases in the publications of the institution. Hannah's was a good story that had been in danger of being lost; the Woman's Medical College had to forget its initial conflict with the Longshore family before it could afford to remember Hannah Longshore. But instead of going quietly into the institutional pantheon, Hannah inscribed in her story an indelible reminder of that conflict.

The Woman's Medical College had taken advantage of the relative openness of professional medicine in the mid-nineteenth century and of the Jacksonian willingness of legislatures to charter new schools.[16] Given the exuberance of medical styles and the wealth of irregular schools,[17] a female medical college was one transgression among many, and we can see in Longshore's claim that she had graduated from a school "chartered by the Legislature of Penna" an assertion of her relative respectability, of the regularity of her education. Ann Preston would have been proud of such a compliant speech performance.

The path of the early graduates was not "strewed with flowers," but neither was that of its founding teachers, recruited from various corners of the profession. Many of the physicians came to the women's school from reform circles; like other reform-minded people, they were interested in alternatives to regular medicine—dress reform (to avoid restrictive corsets), the water cure, and mesmerism. The first classes at the Woman's Medical College heard lectures from the homeopathist Livezy and from Seth Pancoast, author of several works on light therapy. These physicians taught for derisory sums. While medical school professorships were never expected to support a professional career, pay was especially scanty at the Woman's Medical College. The faculty minutes for February 7, 1863, report that twenty-seven dollars in student lecture fees would be divided among the seven faculty members—physicians who had cut themselves off from the Philadelphia County Medical Society and from consultation with its members. Not all the faculty, and least of all Joseph Longshore, were willing to comply with the regular medicine that had rejected them. The early minutes of the Woman's Medical College faculty, especially those from 1850 to 1860, show a constant struggle, seldom explicit, to limit professorships to regular rather than Eclectic doctors, leading to a complete turnover of the faculty during the first ten years of the institution, many chairs being filled by recent graduates of the college. By 1860, the Woman's Medical College was no longer a hotbed of political activism and free thought. Reform energies were focused on the war, and the faculty—now mostly women—presided over a medical school that was struggling and controversial but in every other way conventional.

Joseph Longshore, a founder of the Woman's Medical College, resigned during those struggles; a militant total abstentionist and a believer in the water cure, the use of electricity, and mesmerism, he was apparently reluctant to limit his instruction to regular medical topics. Even his gynecological theories were controversial; Longshore's emphasis on the ovaries placed him at odds with a physiology that still focused on the uterus.[18] Thomas Longshore, Hannah's husband, tells the story of Joseph Longshore's exclusion in his unpublished "History of the College":

> I was present on one occasion when Dr. Johnson (the Dean) openly attacked Dr. Longshore, charging him with his unfitness, and severely criticizing him and denouncing him for his defects in style and manner in which he illustrated and expounded the theory and practice of obstetrics. He made things too plain and full for the fastidious sense of propriety and false modesty of Dr. Johnson, when speaking to a class of ladies. Dr. Longshore was interested in what was then called Woman's Rights, Total Abstinence from intoxicants, in mesmerism and the phenomena of Modern Spiritualism, and would use the arguments, the facts, and what appeared as the natural forces, influences or principles developed by these and the nerve theories of occult Sciences, in connection with the

practice of medicine. He had seen a marvelous power exerted by mesmerism in his own practice, and would refer to it in his public lectures before the class.[19]

Joseph Longshore resigned from the Woman's Medical College in March 1853 to found the coeducational Penn Medical University, an Eclectic school that welcomed faculty of various medical persuasions and offered an innovatively organized medical training to both men and women in separate departments.

Not surprisingly, Joseph Longshore's disputes with the Woman's Medical College affected Hannah Longshore's relations with her alma mater. After graduation, Hannah took up a faculty position as Demonstrator of Anatomy at the Woman's Medical College. She resigned that post at the end of 1853 to become Demonstrator of Anatomy at the Penn Medical College. And Hannah must have been affected by the general purge of sectarians; her "hidden" thesis title, "Neuralgia: Its Cure by Water," inscribed, not on the title page, but on the first page of the text, was only one sign of her irregular tendencies. She gave a course in "psychiatry" to the Harmonial Circle, a spiritualist group, which, for that audience, meant the study of spirits. In her own practice she was "not governed by any routine, nor limited to one school of medicine, but considers that she is at liberty to avail herself of any means which her experience has proved useful or the peculiarities of the case suggest."[20] Often, the peculiarities of the case suggested homeopathic remedies. Unlike Joseph Longshore, who enjoyed and sought controversy, Hannah generally abstained from conflict. One of her letters discussing the Hicksite controversy, dated May 1850, laments, "Who are 'friends' nowadays which way do Lisbon friends go—How do those at Salem and Beighton? How *hateful* is *sectarianism* the more of it the less humanity the less goodness."[21]

After the exclusion of the irregulars, Hannah Longshore kept aloof from the Woman's Medical College of Pennsylvania, never joining the alumnae association. She did not visit the college unless she was specifically called, never consulted with the faculty, and devoted herself to her practice and her family.[22] Although she was one of the preeminent women physicians in Philadelphia, seeing many patients and supporting her household at increasingly fashionable addresses, within the Woman's Medical College she was never mentioned as a model, invited to address the college, or even listed among prominent graduates during the first forty years of the school's history.

At the alumnae dinner of 1895, then, Hannah Longshore encountered an institution from which she had been separated and which she had avoided for forty years. In her assertion that she was a competent physician because she was "a graduate of the Female Medical College," Longshore replaced herself in the history of the institution, asserted the legitimacy of her own "memories of olden days," and joined her own early struggles to those of the institution and its more regular graduates. By 1895, after all, Joseph Long-shore was dead, and the battles between homeopaths and regulars were dim memories. The adventure of the medicine case would be incorporated into the public narrative of the institution.[23]

Hannah Longshore's reply, then, took up the cover of regularity and drew it decently over a past scandal. But covering something is also a way of draw-ing attention to it, and Longshore's adoption of the language of regularity is also a travesty, a shifting of apparel that makes the normal seem strange, even ridiculous. Longshore was speaking to an audience of "co-workers" to whom she remained an unorthodox figure. For them, the drug Longshore ordered, sulphate cinchona, would have been significant. Longshore named cinchona only in the final version of the speech; in the two early versions of this story, she simply referred to "some ounces of drugs." Derived from the same plant that produces quinine, cinchona was one of the few items in the mid-nineteenth-century pharmacopoeia that was really effective; it was a specific for intermittent fevers, although it was probably less effective for scarlatina, rubeola, or typhoid, for which it was also prescribed. The drug was also associated with the history of women's medical work; in the words of Ella Upham, author of "Women in Medicine": "A Spanish lady, the Count-ess de Cinchona, wife of a Viceroy of Peru, was attacked by the fever of the country. She insisted upon trying the Indian remedy of Peruvian bark, which had not then attracted the attention of any European. She was speedily cured, and on her return to Europe in 1632 she made a great effort to spread the knowledge of the new medicine."[24] In asserting her right to cinchona at the physicians's rate, Hannah Longshore was claiming her professional inheritance. But not only that.

Cinchona evoked, tacitly, the conflict that had led to the Longshores' rup-ture with the Woman's Medical College and asserted Hannah Longshore's continued separation from the tradition of regular medicine. "Women in Medicine" was, after all, published in the *North American Journal of Home-opathy;* there, cinchona appeared as the paradigmatic homeopathic remedy: "It was in the use of a preparation of Peruvian bark that Hahnemann ob-served that if administered to those in health it produced a fever similar to the one it was given to cure; from this was evolved our law of similia. Thus we are indebted to the discoveries of this woman, supplemented by the wis-dom of Hahnemann."[25] Cinchona signified not only the resources of women in medicine but the "wisdom" of homeopathic methods. No homeopathist would have used cinchona as a sulphate; cinchonida sulfate, a cheap form of quinine, began to be very commonly prescribed by regular physicians in the 1870s.[26] But *cinchona* was a resonant word in both the homeopathic and the regular vocabularies.

That resonance would have been difficult for Longshore's audience to contain, because so many of them might have remembered, and suffered from, women patients' interest in homeopathy as an alternative to harsher regular therapies. Hannah Longshore had studied homeopathy after her graduation; like many other women physicians, she found that patients disliked large doses of strong and disagreeable medicines, which were, in any case, falling from favor under the influence of French clinical medicine. In the words of Thomas Longshore, "Many intelligent women had become tinctured with the heresy of Homeopathy."[27] Longshore's mention of cinchona tacitly questioned the central strategic choice for regularity that characterized the Woman's Medical College in general and Ann Preston in particular. Longshore at once claimed and refused membership in the discourse community of female physicians. Like them, she was heir to the tradition of women's medical work; unlike them, she did not exclude homeopathy from that tradition. She is a part of the group she speaks to and apart from them.

Hannah Longshore's reply to the toast repeated the central action of her story, the defiant display of the medicine case from which she had dispensed throughout her career. She metaphorically opened that case upon the banquet table and told her audience that it had taken dollars from them and would take more. The moral would not have been lost on them: Hannah Longshore was a wealthy woman, preparing to fulfill her lifelong dream of traveling to Europe. Her audience was asked to identify with her victory but also to be chastened by it. Her doubled evocation of contradictory relationships, relationships of admiring affiliation and distanced criticism, is contained by Longshore's entirely conventional performance of a deeply conventional genre. The toast has been travestied: it is not that Longshore's performance was contemptuous of her audience but that she enacted both her connection with them and her distance from them.

We can hear in Hannah Longshore's 1895 speech the echoes of her brother-in-law Joseph Longshore's 1851 valedictory address to the first graduates of the Woman's Medical College. Joseph Longshore claimed for the new women's college equality with celebrated Philadelphia medical schools, the University of Pennsylvania School of Medicine and Jefferson Medical School:

> By an act of incorporation, by the legislature of the commonwealth of Pennsylvania, your Alma Mater has been placed on an *equality*, in chartered immunities, with that colossal Institution of our city, around which the names of Kuhne, Wistar, Rush, Godman, Physic, James, and Dewees cast a halo of unfading glory; or her proud and successful rival, with the history of which are identified the imperishable names of Eberle, McClellan and Revere.[28]

But those institutions were known for their irreproachable regularity, a regularity that Longshore steadily undercut in the rest of his speech. The authority of these schools was passed through an unbroken line of male ancestors; Longshore satirized their opposition to women physicians: "Many there are who will make it a matter of conscience, believing that woman is sadly wandering from her legitimate sphere, when she attempts, scientifically, to administer to the necessities of the sick and suffering—though to do it ignorantly and empyrically, would seem to be within her appropriate province."[29] Against common regular practice, he urged graduates to avoid prescriptions based on alcohol. Longshore even cast doubt on the scientific value of regular medicine: "While we regard the system of medicine in which you have been instructed, technically called Allopathy, as embracing within its expansive range, more of truth and philosophy, than is possessed by any other claiming the attention of the Medical Student, we are very far from viewing it as the embodiment of perfection."[30] Longshore's "technical" term for the school's curriculum violated a shibboleth of regularity; *allopathy* was a term used by homeopaths and other irregulars, never by regular physicians themselves. Longshore urged graduates to investigate alternatives and hoped for "a more perfect and beautiful system." He was promoting the Eclecticism that would lead to his resignation, blandly asserting it as the policy of the school. Longshore's valedictory, then, established his doubled relation to regular medicine and to the school whose success he celebrated; he borrowed their authority but distrusted their practices.

Hannah Longshore's speech, like Joseph Longshore's valedictory, can be located within a genre of ceremonial academic performances; in this context, travesty is directed at institutional membership and scientific regularity. But Hannah Longshore's performance of membership and distance is organized as a life story and so also responds to the generic exigencies of autobiography. She told the traditional story of the isolated, triumphant subject, in its middle-class inflection—the narrative of professional success. Within the growing scholarship on women's autobiography, such narratives are seen as typically male, and women's autobiographies are described as episodic, closer to the journal or diary than the triumphant unitary narrative, and shaped by issues of relationship and personal connection.[31]

Longshore's narrative of solitary success against odds is just the sort of story women are not supposed to write, even though such stories are not difficult to find; we might remember Ann Preston's escape with a disguised fugitive slave. Stories of individual assertion figured in the most retired lives. The early graduate Rebecca Fussell never practiced medicine or was heard of in any public way, but, sitting on the speaker's platform during an abolitionist meeting in Ohio, she thrust her infant son between Frederick Douglass and a club-wielding proslavery thug.[32] Neither Fussell nor Preston told her own story publicly, leaving them to their families or colleagues. And these are stories in which a woman saves others rather than claiming her

131

own rights. To tell a heroic story about herself, with no invocation of divine succor or any other external support, was an unusual, if not a singular, performance for a woman of Hannah Longshore's generation. Hannah's life story violated the Quaker stricture against self-promotion, a convention so strong that one eighteenth-century writer revised his autobiographical journal three times to eliminate as many instances of the pronoun *I* as possible.[33] Especially since her story established Longshore's distance from the regular community of the Woman's Medical College—she has entered a professional community but not exactly *their* professional community—her speech forbids any easy connection of the feminine with the relational (dare we say, with what is nice?). There was no easy negotiation between Hannah's connections to her professional community and those to her family. *Connection* could not be, in this singular life, a univocal goal or state; rather, Longshore's connections, as she would have called them, were formed around issues of both professional practice and familial relationship, around both intellectual and financial investments. Her narrative does not resolve those contradictions and antagonisms; it represents them, performs them.

While Longshore's narrative is not a conventional feminine autobiography, it also travesties the specific conventions of late nineteenth-century medical biography. Longshore would have encountered such biographies as part of her professional reading; she subscribed to medical journals and could have read memorial notices such as those published in the transactions of the College of Physicians of Philadelphia. William Osler's biographical essays, originally delivered as addresses to various medical schools and institutions, can serve as an example of this form.[34] In his biography of Philadelphia physician William Pepper (could he, perhaps, have been *the* Doctor Pepper?), Osler described a relentlessly coherent career. We hear of Pepper's education and early practice, of his service as provost of the University of Pennsylvania, and of his mature work (divided into three phases, treated seriatim). Osler ends with Pepper's death in Hawaii with *Treasure Island* in his hand. This is an unbroken story of success, uninterrupted by personal singularities, by any incursion of corporeality. In Osler's account, Pepper had a father but no mother and certainly no wife or children. Hannah Longshore's speech, too, presents her as emerging, solitary and heroic, battling against the odds, effecting cures impossible for other physicians. But Longshore deploys these topics in remarkably demystifying ways; Pepper never had to account for undarned socks. And her discomfited druggist, finally relenting on his price by degrees, is a ridiculous opponent rather than a dangerous enemy. Longshore's life story, then, performed her doubly negated travesty: Longshore was not a woman, not a doctor, but a woman doctor.[35]

Hannah Longshore's speech also travestied the Quaker genre of biographical testimony; she used its associative structures but refused its modest self-presentation. Examples of Quaker biographies can be found in *The Journal*, a short-lived Hicksite paper which also published many of Thomas Longshore's religious essays, and in the orthodox *Friends' Intelligencer*. A typical memorial notice presented the subject's life as biographical testimony.[36] It represented a life directed toward serious ends but also offered a sense of the singularity of the subject; we read of family relations, hobbies, and talents. While the memorial conventionally moved from the subject's birth to death, its central sections were associative in their organization. The writer focused on the "testimony" or "witness" of the subject's life, particularly in the face of suffering, told as a series of loosely linked episodes. These texts are quite similar to the memoirs of British clergymen's wives described by Linda Peterson: discontinuous and fragmentary documents that originated in private circumstances and are published for purposes of edification.[37] Longshore's speech, like these memorial narratives, offered her life as a witness, but its edifying message diverged from Quaker formulas; this was a prominent public life, presented as a quite worldly success.

Hannah's husband, Thomas, wrote much more extended narratives that refunction the genre of memorial biography to present an unorthodox religion of science. The most sustained, if not the most finished, of these documents is Thomas Longshore's "Autobiography," a manuscript in which he tells the story of Hannah Longshore, investing her life with heroic and transgressive significance while maintaining the genre decorum of testimony. Handwritten in a ledger, "Autobiography" is well over a hundred pages long and still carries the marks of its composition: small pieces of paper with notes and drafts are inserted into the notebook, and the narrative breaks off once to describe what Hannah is doing as her husband writes and again to record what he believed were her dying words. Although it begins in the first person, with an account of Thomas and Hannah's first meeting, the text rapidly becomes a memoir of Hannah's life. (The title "Autobiography" was assigned to the text after Thomas Longshore wrote it, probably because of its opening words: "On the 2th of February 1835 the writer left the paternal roof . . ."). The text cannot have been written before 1882; while internal evidence dates one section of the manuscript at 1892, it does not mention Hannah's retirement that year or her tour of Europe soon after.

This text of Thomas Longshore's evokes the discontinuous, episodic structures we associate with women's autobiographies. And Thomas Longshore's authorial presence was as complicated as that of an anonymous woman writer; many of his publications were uncredited or signed with various initials. But especially when contrasted with the hagiographic pallor of our picture of Ann Preston, Hannah Longshore emerges in this account as energetic, singular, difficult, and massively interesting. Thomas Longshore speaks of her habit of standing out in thunderstorms, of her sewing all the family's underwear, of her falling asleep whenever she took time to sit down, of her breakneck carriage rides through the city, and of her "toleration for a large liberty" among her friends and family.[38]

Thomas Longshore's published biography, *George Fox Interpreted* (1881), casts light on the fascinating morass of his "Autobiography" and on what was at stake in the Longshore family trope of travesty. In *George Fox Interpreted*, Longshore subordinated biographical narrative to the exigency named in his subtitle: to interpret Fox ". . . *in the Light of the Nineteenth Century and Applied to the Present Condition of the Church.*" Fox was, for Longshore, a scientific rationalist disguised as a Christian. *George Fox Interpreted* travesties the Quaker witness story, transposing the story of the original Quaker into a criticism of religion in general. The canonic episodes of Fox's life are interpreted as exempla of his scientific spirit, so that Fox's plain dress made of leather was motivated solely by reason and economy. Fox renounced oaths, incurring heavy penalties, because prudence prompted him to reject superstitious ceremonies from pagan sources.[39] Using etymological arguments, Longshore interpreted *god* as synonymous with *the good*, arguing that Fox personalized the good only to accommodate superstition. Longshore himself was deeply skeptical of any stable distinction between good and evil: ". . . what is called good and evil by finite, fallible men, in what is transpiring in the outer world, are so inseparably blended, and necessary to constitute the whole, that the good could not exist without the evil, nor the evil without the good; and our distinction of them is entirely arbitrary and determined by the way we are affected by them."[40] Etymologically, *Holy Ghost* became "benign gasses"; and *inspiration,* the breath. Fox was a scientific savant, not to mention a health reformer, *avant la lettre.*

Longshore's biography of Fox is reflexive and self-replicating. If Fox was a reform-minded "scientific spirit"[41] whose religious statements were canny adaptations to a society under the sway of religious myth, what are we to make of the biographer Thomas Longshore, a public-spirited believer in science, who writes as a Christian (to an audience concerned with doctrinal orthodoxy) while rejecting belief in a personal god or an afterlife, let alone the divinity of Christ? Longshore fashioned himself to represent the ascetically "scientific spirit" he found in Fox. If his "Autobiography" is actually a memoir of his wife, Thomas Longshore's real autobiography is perhaps to be found in *George Fox Interpreted*, the story of a master of disguise, a travesty of the Quaker witness story of suffering and consolation. When Thomas Longshore and his family wrote about science, they could well mean religion; when they wrote about religion, they could well mean science.

Thomas's biography of Hannah Longshore, therefore, is a celebration of her scientific spirit and desire for reform. The stories we read as demonstra-

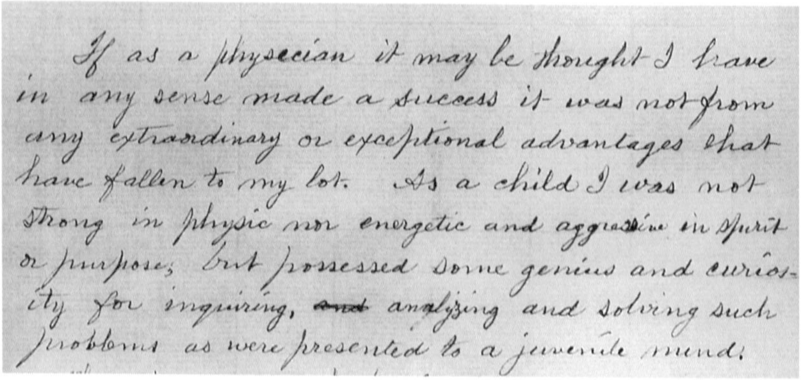

Figure 7. Hannah E. Longshore, autobiographical speech, first version (Archives and Special Collections on Women in Medicine, MCP Hahnemann University)

tions of her singularity actually serve as evidence of Hannah's rationality, economy, or devotion to the scientific "laws of life." Hannah "all her life . . . believed it best to sleep in rooms winter and summer with windows and doors wide open. For forty years this has been her constant practice with the full belief that she did it to her great advantage."[42] For us, this habit speaks of Hannah as a flinty pioneer, her bedroom ventilated by midwinter gales. But in both *George Fox Interpreted* and in *The Higher Criticism in Theology and Religion*, Thomas Longshore argued that the Holy Ghost is the benign gas that inspires men with reason and benevolence as against the evil spirits of alcohol and opium. In this light, Hannah's relentless pursuit of fresh air aligns her with the forces of godlike, but essentially scientific, inspiration.

While Preston's invisible writing was inscribed anonymously in the documents of the Woman's Medical College of Pennsylvania, Longshore's invisible writing was fugitive and displaced. Her words were tied to particular occasions of utterance, so deeply situated in familial and social contexts that they are almost unintelligible to us. When we hear her voice, the voice that "is not afraid to die," that is "possessed of some genius and curiosity for inquiring," it reverberates with other discourses, taking them on and translating itself into their alien forms.[43] Such a performance did not come easily to Hannah; it was painstakingly composed, thought through, and revised. In three early drafts of her speech, Longshore experimented with alternatives to the story of success against the odds. The first two versions of the speech tell stories of pleasure and community. (See figures 7, 8, 9.) Only in its final version do we read Hannah Longshore's masculine story of triumph over difficulties:

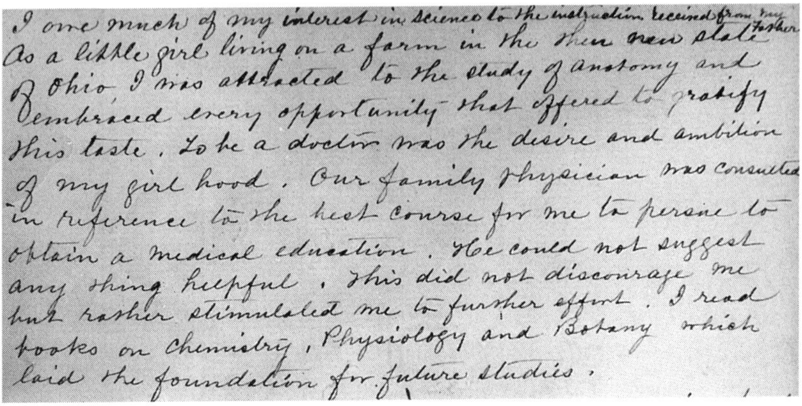
I owe much of my interest in science to the instruction received from my father
As a little girl living on a farm in the then new state
of Ohio I was attracted to the study of anatomy and
embraced every opportunity that offered to gratify
this taste. To be a doctor was the desire and ambition
of my girl hood. Our family physician was consulted
in reference to the best course for me to persue to
obtain a medical education. He could not suggest
any thing helpful. This did not discourage me
but rather stimulated me to further effort. I read
books on Chemistry, Physiology and Botany which
laid the foundation for future studies.

Figure 8. Hannah E. Longshore, autobiographical speech, second version (Archives and Special Collections on Women in Medicine, MCP Hahnemann University)

> The first women physicians in Phila. did not find their paths strewed with flowers nor their advent welcomed by the general public or by the profession. They encountered no little bitterness, opposition, and persecution.

In the second draft, however, medicine was a source of childhood pleasure:

> If as a physician it may be thought I have in any sense made a success it was not from any extraordinary or exceptional advantages that have fallen to my lot. As a child I was not strong in physic nor energetic and aggressive in spirit or purpose, but possessed some genius and curiosity for inquiring, analyzing and solving such problems as were presented to a juvenile mind.
>
> The structure of the bodies of insects, rodents and domestic animals enlisted my attention, and to satisfy my inquisitiveness, I ventured to attempt the experiment of dissecting some parts of these as at times convenient they fell into my hands, perhaps merely to indulge a freak.

And in the first draft, medicine is Longshore's patrimony:

> I owe much of my interest in science to the instruction received from my father. As a little girl living on a farm in the then new state of Ohio, I was attracted to the study of anatomy and embraced every opportunity that offered to satisfy this taste. To be a doctor was the desire and ambition of my girlhood.

These early drafts do not tell a story of unremitting effort against the odds. Longshore described her choice of a medical vocation as a matter of attraction, almost seduction:

> Science applied to life to lessen human misery and multiply human comforts had in the thought a charm and enchantment that could not be relinquished, so

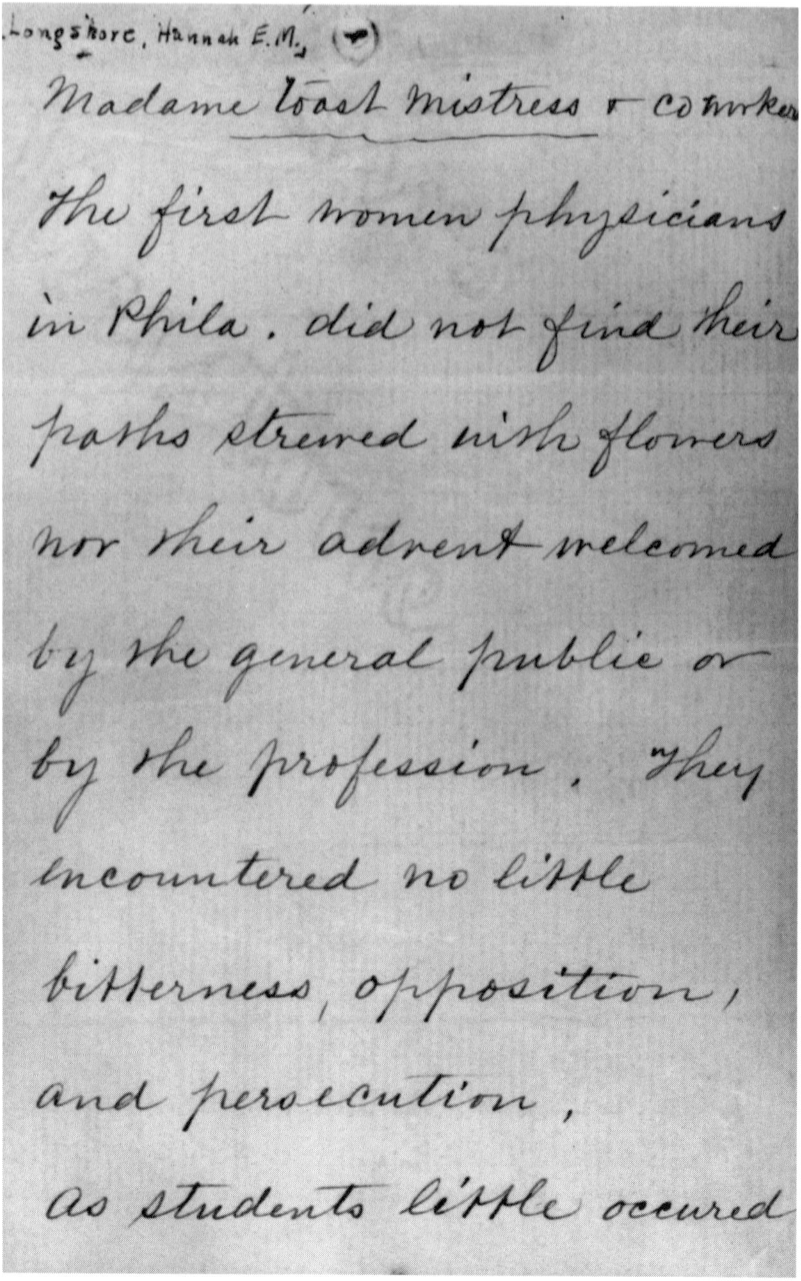
Longshore, Hannah E.M.

Madame toast mistress & coworkers

The first women physicians
in Phila. did not find their
paths strewed with flowers
nor their advent welcomed
by the general public or
by the profession. They
encountered no little
bitterness, opposition,
and persecution,
As students little occured

Figure 9. Hannah E. Longshore, autobiographical speech, final version (Archives and Special Collections on Women in Medicine, MCP Hahnemann University)

long as it was possible for any way to open where it could be in some measure realized. (second draft)

She spoke of reform politics, of her close relation to her husband, of her reliance on the support and encouragement of her family. None of this material appeared in the final draft of the speech; all these expressions of pleasure, of delight in science, of political commitment, of family connection were omitted from Hannah Longshore's memoir of "early years." But precisely these topics—wayward and independent scientific research, politics, the Longshore family—were the points of tension between Hannah Longshore and the Woman's Medical College. In order to produce one narrative of pleasure and difficulty, Hannah Longshore has re-created exactly the silences and exclusions that made her narrative necessary. Her story of pleasure, knowledge, and connection was elided, and appeared in the final text as a bitter taste of cinchona.

Such revisions suggest that the strategy of travesty was a solution, and perhaps not an entirely satisfactory solution, to the rhetorical problems Longshore faced as she took up the urbane masculine form "replying to a toast." One of the stories she might have told—the story of family connection and support—would have brought her close to an explicit mention of her brother-in-law's role in founding the school. Other stories of pleasure, delight in seeing the interior of the body, "perhaps as a freak," may have seemed insufficiently edifying. In the end, she took up the contradictory stories of solitary success against all odds, of the faithful disciple witnessing her calling, and turned them to her own purposes. Her speech demonstrates the demanding possibilities of travesty; she disputes the easy regularity to which the received forms of medical discourse aspired. Longshore's narrative of personal success reminds us that scientific arguments can, and often do, encode personal stories.[44] Her cordial and aggressive claim and refusal of membership remind us that *connection* is not the special province of women but has been part of the ongoing work of science since Boyle staged his first experiments with the vacuum as spectacles and bids for patronage.[45]

THE SECOND CASE: HANNAH LONGSHORE
WRITES REGULAR MEDICINE

Eleven years before her autobiographical speech, Hannah Longshore had published her sole written intervention into medical controversy. Her "Case of Conception Without Intromission" appeared in the *Medical and Surgical Reporter*, published in Philadelphia, in 1884; it responded to a contemporary debate about conception.[46] The correspondence columns of the *Medical and Surgical Reporter* were lively and central to the journal; they included letters from other journals and were themselves often reprinted. Longshore's letter resembles what we might think of as the "masculine" texts of nineteenth-century medicine: the body is described meticulously and objectively. The letter can be quoted in its entirety:

> A Case of Conception Without Intromission.
> EDS. MED. AND SURGICAL REPORTER:
> Mrs. A—, aged nineteen, a native of Ireland, called on me for an examination. She had menstruated regularly and comfortably until after her marriage, some three months previously. As coition was out of the question, her condition seemed to her a mystery. On examination, I found the hymen closing the os externum.
> After a long and diligent search, found a foramen close under the urethra, where I depressed the hymen half an inch, and introduced a number eleven bougie, and with my finger in the rectum, succeeded in penetrating a distance of nearly two inches through the firm, inelastic hymen, when the point plunged into the vagina. This condition was undoubtedly congenital.
> All of her symptoms indicated pregnancy. Dilation was tried without success, then I operated with director and scalpel.
> In six months after, I attended the lady in confinement, which was normal, and she had a good recovery. In this case the spermatozoa were abandoned in the depression of the hymen, and traveled through the narrow channel two inches long into the vagina, and continued their journey to the uterus to fecundate the ova.
> This fact, with others of the same kind, demonstrate not only the possibility, but the actual accomplishment of impregnation, where the spermatozoa were abandoned a long distance from the uterus.
> H. E. Longshore, M.D., Philadelphia, Pa

This letter directly violated one of Joseph Longshore's rules for professional practice, promulgated in the 1851 valedictory: "Never publish, or consent to have published, any of your professional acts, however meritorious or laudable they may be." Such publication was for Joseph Longshore a form of advertisement, a "means of gaining notoriety . . . beneath the dignity of your position."[47] Joseph Longshore had been five years dead when Hannah published "A Case of Conception Without Intromission," but her presence in the text, her bid for "notoriety," is palpable. The letter is signed, although the signature does not foreground the writer's gender. Hannah places herself in nearly half the sentences of the letter, usually as the subject: *I found; I succeeded; I operated;* and *I attended the lady*. The letter does not tell the story of a pregnancy but rather tells the story of a doctor investigating pregnancy.

The topic of pregnancy was actively debated in nineteenth-century medicine in ways that remind us that, although any theory of gender is also a gendered theory, few performances of gender are univocal.[48] We might think that Longshore's letter, with its foregrounding of the investigator, its relentless objectification of the female body, would have been indistinguishable from essays written by male physicians during this controversy; it followed the conventions of objective medical reporting of an anatomical case. Hannah Longshore presented herself, in her only appearance in print, as the ultimate phallic physician: she probed, sounded, and ultimately ruptured the hymen of the patient. Her impassive account of these interventions suggests that it is not masculinity but science, particularly the scientific ability to trace anatomical structures, that resolves the "mystery" of conception and opens the female body.

Received medical opinion, however, held that conception took place only when the sperm was propelled directly through the cervix; instances of conception without intercourse, therefore, contradicted medical common knowledge. And Hannah Longshore's impassivity was not at all the rule in writing on this issue. For many nineteenth-century physicians, impregnation was not a physiological process like any other but a defining instance of masculinity. The debate on conception organized unruly energies; it became a matter of pride, of national identity. In the same issue of the *Medical and Surgical Reporter*, the letter of Ohio physician Edward Cass refuted the "European opinion" that semen is "thrown into the uterine cavity during intercourse." Recounting a case similar to Longshore's, Cass concluded:

> Here is a fact—a truth. Here is an accidentally discovered theorem that demonstrates the possibility that the uterus may be impregnated when the "spermatozoa have been abandoned only in the vagina." The American medical professors, in their docility to European speculative teachings, are peculiarly credulous. Since I have made this narrated discovery, I have doubt that the seminal fluid is almost never thrown into the uterine cavity. . . . It may be that Pallen, Fraer, and Kolbert, et.al., would take this case to be an exceptional one to the rule, that the spermatozoa in the Americans are possessed of greater energy to surmount difficulties than those of other countries—and take into consideration that this occurred in *Ohio, too,* where we find the most determined, enterprising, and aggressive of the race. If this could be copied into every European journal, it might be a cause for them to reflect, and revolutionize a little speculative theory.[49]

Compared with Cass's triumphant (and self-parodic) story of discovery and energy, in which the writer identifies overtly with the sperm, Longshore's case enforces the clearest of boundaries between subject and object. Although many feminist rhetoricians would describe Longshore's rhetoric as masculine, it puts into play a professional performance of gender quite different from Cass's. Cass writes of *impregnation,* for example, and Longshore, of *conception.* Longshore's credibility is not ratified by the energy of Ohio sperm or put into the service of an emerging American medicine. Her letter travesties objectification to cover her own phallic performance and give an account of reproduction that stands outside of, and by implication against, masculine triumphalism.

Both Longshore's speech and her letter to the Philadelphia *Medical and Surgical Reporter* speak to our understanding of the relation of gender and science. Both texts require contextualization in a comprehensive account of nineteenth-century medical genres, a project that is both long overdue and beyond the scope of this book. To skim the surface: Nineteenth-century medical writing included many narrative forms. Both male and female physicians published clinical studies, descriptions of patients and their treatment, presented with varying specificity and narrative presence, usually as arguments for new forms of treatment, as illustrations of problems with conventional methods, or as puzzling anomalies. Many were "singular" cases, usually patients with anomalous bodies, especially anomalous reproductive organs. Mid-nineteenth-century medical journals included a limited number of empirical studies of physiology, pathology, and the effects of drugs. Those studies increased in frequency toward the end of the century and included comparative results of pathological examinations, of experiments, of surveys. The discourse of health led a vigorous life long after the medical school thesis; both inside and outside professional publications, a great deal of physician's writing, for both men and women, addressed broad public health issues: How did diseases spread? Which hygienic practices were effective? How should infants be fed? Should prostitutes be regulated? Then as now, physicians wrote books of general medical advice and told (often heroic) stories of medical careers addressed to a general audience; the borders between these forms and the professional discourse of medicine were much more permeable than they are now. Nineteenth-century medical writing recalls Darwin and Freud as much as it anticipates the *New England Journal of Medicine*.[50]

Feminist critics of science have sometimes characterized scientific thinking as male in its valuation of dichotomy and hierarchy and opposed it to a women's discourse governed by a logic of connection and relationship. In many feminist theories, science exemplifies masculine objectification; women's discursive forms are seen as more fluid and associative.[51] This characterization is not fanciful; scientific professions consistently underrepresent women and have done so from their inception. It would be remarkable if the discourse of medicine were not gendered male, concerned as it is with necessarily gendered bodies, elaborated in contexts that were until recently almost entirely male. But Hannah Longshore's writing calls this characterization of the feminine voice into question. Nothing that she wrote resembles our understanding of a feminine prose register. And her writing suggests that medicine, as a scientific practice, was not a simple discourse of patriarchy but one in which women physicians could intervene. This bare presence of women is significant; Harding has taught us to be generous in assessing the significance of both the remembered and the forgotten writing by early women scientists.[52] Even the unadorned fact of women's participation in scientific work subverts its claim to a universalism that is actually masculine.

But women did not simply take up received forms and use them without elaboration. In Hannah Longshore's hands, the discourse of masculine objectification became a way of containing unruly medical discussions of reproduction, of making present the specific activity of the female bodies of doctor and patient. Longshore's life story also included contradictory and transgressive forms of membership, displaced performances of self-sufficiency. The subtlety of Longshore's travesty becomes apparent when we place her writing in the context of specific genres as they were performed for specific audiences. Like Ann Preston's cross-dressed texts, Longshore's travesties suggest that as medicine was forming, women were participants in its discourses, articulating a relation to the body and to professional authority that was quite different from the hegemonic story now told in canonic medical discourse.

Many stories of illness and cure circulated in the nineteenth century; one of them survived, in various versions, to become the happy story of modern medicine, the story of "miracles" touted on *Chicago Hope* and *ER*.[53] Women physicians and patients also told other kinds of stories: of generational repetition, of an obscurely speaking body, of the doctor as repository of family secrets. We can recover those stories, place them, hear them in some of their complexity. Ann Preston's and Hannah Longshore's versions of these stories come to us only after interruption. Preston's enacted the forms of decorous male scientific discourse with a vengeance; as an institutional writer, she established a rhetoric for the Woman's Medical College that insisted on its exact congruence with the norms of established, male-dominated institutions. But Longshore appropriated such masculine forms as the autobiography or the case study, subverted them to her own rather singular purposes, and offered them as conventional performances. Her very substantial embodiment as she stood to reply to the toast established her speech as a woman's appropriation of a genre associated with men. (See figure 10.)

The gender of medical discourse is never simple or binary; and it has always included women's voices, whether or not they were pitched in "feminine" tones. Speaking in a form associated with men, speaking to an audience of women, Longshore used the tropes of distance, objectification, and professional success, tropes often seen as masculine, to claim connection and to express distance, to affiliate with her unnamed family and to assert her standing as its chief breadwinner. Taking up the genres and speech acts most ex-

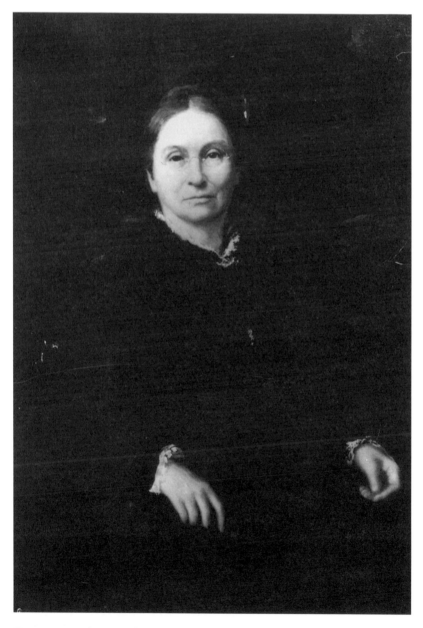

Figure 10. Hannah E. Longshore, portrait, 1897 (Archives and Special Collections on Women in Medicine, MCP Hahnemann University)

plicitly associated with masculinity, Longshore enlisted them to speak for the female body in its singularities, for the woman practitioner and her necessities. Her challenge, the display of the medicine case, made both the officious, relenting druggist and the hyper-regular woman physician seem ridiculous. She did not speak *as* a man; still less, *as if* she were a man; she acceded to the definition of science as a particularly male discursive form and then contradicted that definition by performing "male" science as a woman. Read as a rhetorical performance, a speech given to a very particular audience, Longshore's narrative in all its intertextuality offers a deeply determined representation of contradictory social relations. Hers was no polite performance of affiliation and membership; it was at once an act of aggression, specifically intellectual and professional aggression, a refusal to tell a feminine story of life lived in the family, and a symbolic invocation of family relations. Longshore's relatively simple text, therefore, bears the impress of complex personal, intellectual, and institutional histories; remarkable on its face, it becomes more remarkable read in its generic context.

READING INVISIBLE WRITING

What is at stake for us in these stories? Biography, both individual and collective, has been the site for formulating contemporary feminist theories of science from Evelyn Fox Keller to Donna Haraway. Feminist scholars have engaged in primitive accumulation of the simplest information about women scientists: they existed; they wrote; they did the work of science. This work, which one important anthology calls the recovery of "lost and buried women heroes of science," is critically important.[54]

That mission animates *Out of the Dead House*. I am deeply grateful to the nineteenth-century women physicians who have given me such a good story to tell. They are worth remembering, worth celebrating. But, as Evelyn Fox Keller and Donna Haraway suggest, historical retrieval is not, and should not be, a pretheoretical enterprise; the celebration of a particular woman scientist suggests a model for "how some women do science," or "how women do science," or perhaps "how women should do science." My own impulse is to argue against essentialism; it is no accident that I have mounted this argument in a historical study of nineteenth-century medicine, with its unsettled habitus, focusing on women who varied widely in their scientific beliefs, politics, and styles of gender performance. These lives speak to me of the "large liberty" they claimed for themselves and urge that claim anew; they call into question any unitary understandings of scientific practice or of gender. The articulation of these two claims—agency and pluralism—

144

offers us an alternative to the same old bad choice between essentialism and exclusion.

The reader—I and perhaps you—arrives at the text as desiring, specifically as desiring images of possibility, openings in the texture of what can be known. The nineteenth-century woman physician, in her different guises, offers a practice of knowing the body under conditions of extreme gender differentiation, a practice that acknowledges the social constraints of gender but refuses to accept them as they have been given to her. She practices a science that both investigates and preserves the body; medicine sponsors her deserved reputation for benevolence and her right to see what is normally forbidden, to go where she would normally be excluded, to know people who would normally be outside her sphere; in the words of the "Autobiography": "A doctor she says is introduced to all phases and conditions of human life and can learn more of it than those in any occupation."[55] Both Longshore and Preston were sustained and preserved by their profession; they felt that they had been saved from lives of marginal inconsequence. I have no defenses against such a story.

Just as the woman scientist's choice to write about medicine is not innocent, neither is my choice to write about women scientists (rather than their patients, or nurses, or women who hated scientists). Such writing inscribes a wish that scientific practice, an expert and differentiated system, could become more porous and accessible; it enacts a desire to cut through the knotty questions posed by identity politics without painfully working through them—wishes and desires that could become parasitic on the lives of the nineteenth-century women physicians, reducing them (yet again) to the status of edifying examples. Such a project itself necessarily risks travesty, taking up heroic figures as disguises that authorize ideas that they would have found transgressive. I approach these texts with desires to disclose a surprising past and to reconstruct a usable past. I want to remember them, to place them among the crowded nineteenth-century pantheon of tireless women writers; I also want them to speak to us, to make our work less inevitable in its trajectories, less enclosed in the boundaries that our choices and theirs have created. This Hannah, my Hannah, probing and gesturing, standing in the lightning or falling asleep in her chair, offers us an image of scientific practice that is no longer possible to us. But it is for us, reading these quotidian and singular texts, to reflect on our own implication in projects of recovery and reconstruction—and on our strategies for joining or distancing ourselves from them.

6

Mary Putnam Jacobi
Medicine as Will and Idea

My interest in contemplation persisted, and even increased, but I acquired an increasing reluctance to effort and voluntary mental exertion. I appreciated Schopenhauer's "Condemnation of the Will," and felt confirmed in my view that his entire theory sprang from a deep inner consciousness of personal weakness of volition.

This impressed me the more from its sharp contrast with the vivacity and strength of volition which had been a leading characteristic with me all my life.

—Mary Putnam Jacobi, "Description of the Early Symptoms of the Meningeal Tumor Compressing the Cerebellum. From Which the Writer Died. Written by Herself"

"Description of Early Symptoms of the Meningeal Tumor" was a self-report of Mary Putnam Jacobi's final illness, circulated to her physician friends to confirm that her case was not treatable.[1] Nothing less than a brain tumor brought Mary Putnam Jacobi (1842–1906) to the limits of her will; to her, only a terminal illness could have explained an unwillingness to plan and project. Unlike Ann Preston or Hannah Longshore, Mary Putnam Jacobi inhabited a world close to ours, but the life she lived, vividly expressed in her writing, is not one we can easily imagine. The medicine that she studied and practiced was a mature science, and she wrote medical texts that are recognizable as scientific discourse; they are located within disciplinary controversies, discuss issues that have been constructed during those controversies, and foreground relatively modern methods of drawing conclusions from evidence. True, we do find her, as a medical student in Paris, repeating conventional refutations of Lister and refusing to admit the specificity of Bright's disease.[2] But she would never write—we could never imagine her writing—like Ann Preston, who commiserated with a friend upset by a visit to the Woman's Medical College dissecting room: "How glad I am that thee had Chandler to mesmerize and soothe thee."[3] Still less can we imagine Putnam Jacobi, a lifelong positivist, dispensing homeopathic remedies from a satchel or attending meetings of the spiritualist Harmonial Circle. *Homeopath* was for her a lifelong term of contempt.

146

Even in bare outline, Mary Putnam Jacobi's life speaks of her energy, decision, discursive force. She invented her own medical education, traveled to Union-occupied New Orleans during the Civil War, remained in Paris during the Commune, and married a German Jewish physician who had been prosecuted in the Cologne Communist trial and would later become the founder of American pediatrics. She carried on a thriving practice, treating C. P. Gilman for neurasthenia. She taught medicine and published some 149 articles on medical topics, besides fiction in her youth and political writings at intervals throughout her career. She won the prestigious Boylston Prize for Medical Writing from Harvard in 1876 for her *Question of Rest for Women during Menstruation,* a refutation of George Clarke's dire warnings against educating women.[4] If Ann Preston and Hannah Longshore ventured into territories of language closed to women, Mary Putnam Jacobi laid claim to vast tracts of forbidden ground: menstruation, hysteria, nervous disease, the interior of the uterus. Other nineteenth-century women physicians were active scientists or prolific popular writers; few combined both genres, and none as productively as Mary Putnam Jacobi.

If Ann Preston's strategy for managing the gender of scientific writing was a marked and nontransgressive cross-dressing, and if Hannah Longshore's gender strategy can be described as travesty, then Mary Putnam Jacobi's writing is a series of experiments in gender performance. She attempted, at different points in her career, all the available styles for enacting the oxymoron *woman doctor.* Sometimes her performance insisted on her gender; other times, she emphasized traits that, for a nineteenth-century audience, were strongly marked as male: cool-headed courage under fire, readiness in emergencies.[5] Putnam Jacobi also wrote anonymously, sometimes in contexts which would lead her audience to read her writing as that of a male; this rhetorical cross-dressing is unmarked, since its quality as performance was lost on the original audience. In her student years, she often elided her gender, writing anonymously and only occasionally, although always provocatively, examining gender in her writing. Later, she would experiment with various styles of gender performance: she collaborated with her husband, Abraham Jacobi, blurring the gender of the author. Her medical texts are insistent in their regularity and scientific rigor, and very often gender is salient in them; Putnam Jacobi could pretend to write as a male, using that pretense subversively. Like Preston and Longshore, she presented her writing of medicine as totally compliant and conventional; however, she was both rigorously attentive to what counted as a medical proof and creative in devising new means of argument. Rhetorically, Putnam Jacobi was virtually immune to the sentimentalism that was characteristic of nineteenth-century northeastern progressive circles.[6] Her distinctive voice—dry, self-aware, analytic, sometimes passionate—is audible from her first writings. Her first

147

publication was an adolescent short story, "Found and Lost."[7] The narrator is a physician who has settled down to read next to a corpse on a dark and stormy night. Not many sixteen-year-old girls, now or then, imagine a physician's life as a chance to stay up late, reading cozily next to a dead body.

TELLING A MEDICAL LIFE

Putnam Jacobi's writings include an autobiographical manuscript in the Schlesinger Library, Radcliffe College, dated 1902 and privately circulated.[8] This sketch seems to have been Ruth Putnam's source for most of the information about Putnam Jacobi's early life in her *Life and Letters of Mary Putnam Jacobi*, the standard biography. Putnam Jacobi's autobiography is cognate to Hannah Longshore's toast: late in her life, she decided to tell a version of her story. Putnam Jacobi's is a story of childhood, of childhood regrets and childhood triumphs. The very young Mary Corrine Putnam tormented a sickly fellow passenger on her voyage from England to America by dangling her doll out the window into the waves. A slightly older Mary Putnam refused to believe her cousin's warning that she was out of her depth in the Long Island Sound and thought as she sank, "Tomorrow I shall be thrown up on the shore just like the drowned kittens that are always being thrown up here."[9] The nine-year-old Mary found a dead rat in the stable and planned to dissect it to find the heart, which she "greatly longed to see."[10] Her nerve failed her; she told her mother about her plan and was relieved when she was forbidden to touch the rat. She proved her desire for social reform by sliding in the snow "belly guts" instead of sitting up like the other girls. When she was twelve and the family had moved to Yonkers, Mary walked ten miles on nutting expeditions or climbed twenty feet up the Croton Aqueduct and sat high on a ledge, playing cards.

After her father, founder of Putnam's publishing house, went bankrupt in 1857, Putnam Jacobi's haphazard education suddenly became serious because she would have to support herself. The family moved to New York City, and Mary entered a public school. Mary Putnam, as she told her story, was a girl unwilling to take anything on faith or to bow to custom, a girl suffused with strength and vitality if not wisdom or generosity, an inquirer rather than an intellectual. That is not the only story Mary Putnam Jacobi could have told. Her correspondence shows vexing religious doubt and turmoil in the early teens; her letters to her grandmother are filled with a sense of sin and loss, and she continued as a church member until she was twenty-one.[11] On her twelfth birthday, she wrote a note mourning that "I am not two years younger, so I need not enter the artificial world which the stupid ingenuity of man has created."[12] Later, Mary and her family fought an ongoing war of position about her medical career and future prospects, although her family had introduced Mary to the Blackwell sisters and admired them.[13] Both Mary Putnam's father and her mother, however, doubted the wisdom of her following a medical career.[14] When she began her medical studies in Paris, Mary Putnam thanked her father for the "large liberty" he had always left her; that liberty was not constructed without the labor of both father and daughter.[15]

As a writer, Mary Putnam Jacobi helped to shape the emerging discourse of scientific medicine at the end of the nineteenth century. She published in the full range of medical genres: While she taught materia medica at the Blackwells' school, the Woman's Medical College of the New York Infirmary, she published articles on specific drugs and their activity. She gave a total of fifty-nine presentations to the New York Pathological Society and was also active in the New York County Medical Society, the Medical Library and Journal Association of New York, the Neurological Society, the Therapeutic Society, and the Academy of Sciences. In 1900, she was seeking admission to the Obstetrical Society of New York. She attended meetings of the alumnae association of the Woman's Medical College, insisting that they include presentations of medical papers; she served as its president from 1888 to 1891 and again in 1894–95.[16] These presentations were written up and reported, as was customary, in the active medical press; the proceedings of the New York Pathological Society were regularly reported in the *Medical Record,* including the twenty-eight presentations Mary Putnam gave during the 1880s and the subsequent discussion.

Nor did Mary Putnam Jacobi limit her research to conventional genres. She was avidly interested in the technologies developing in the 1880s and 1890s for tracing bodily functions, devising experiments in which they could be used and publishing her findings. Putnam Jacobi collated and recorded the results of therapeutic interventions, often using the patient populations at the New York Infirmary for Women and Children or those of Mount Sinai, where she had established a children's dispensary and pediatric ward in the style of French clinical medicine. She also used information gathered from patients in a survey—a device that was not at all in the French clinical style. Putnam Jacobi wrote thirteen articles on therapies during the 1880s and 1890s, reporting on the results of cold baths, surgical drains, electricity, and, in one of her last-published essays, hypnotism. Especially after her career was established, Putnam Jacobi wrote on women's rights, including essays on the right to medical education, producing (like Ann Preston) the usual round of inaugural and commencement addresses and also bracing essays on political topics for the *Medical Record.* She addressed the New York State Constitutional Convention on woman's suffrage and wrote a long chapter entitled "Women in Medicine" for a volume on women's work in America.[17] Because of the Boylston Prize essay, Mary Putnam Jacobi is remembered for her work in gynecology; those studies began with clinical investigations of the effects of treating anemia with cold water and massage and culminated in a series of essays on hysteria, both published in book form.[18]

In sheer volume and range, Putnam Jacobi's work is more substantial, more central to her profession, and more sustained than that of any other nineteenth-century woman physician. And nineteenth-century women physicians could be active writers. Elizabeth Blackwell wrote a number of books, most of them intended for popular audiences, but was generally silent on medical controversies as medical writers debated them.[19] Other graduates of the Woman's Medical College wrote regularly, but none published in so many medical genres or sustained their writing over thirty years.[20]

Putnam Jacobi enjoyed a distinguished reputation. Just as Ann Preston exemplified the self-effacing and dignified woman physician, just as Hannah Longshore was captured by her husband as a saint of science, Mary Putnam Jacobi was, for regular physicians, the exceptional example; she proved that a woman physician, if sufficiently scientific and regular, could succeed. Presentations that she gave in the 1890s were received with enthusiasm. In 1892, after she read her paper "Urethral Irritation" to the Philadelphia County Medical Society, a group legendary for its hostility to women, discussants vied with each other to praise it. The first respondent, Dr. Frederick P. Henry, had agreed to speak, not only because it was an honor to reply to Dr. Putnam Jacobi, but also because, as he explained, "I felt confident that the subject would be so exhaustively treated that my part in the matter would be simply nominal." Dr. Henry's praise was seconded by Dr. Tyson, who could "add nothing to what has already been said," and by Dr. Roberts, who held that "a paper of this importance should not be allowed to fall entirely into the hands of the specialists."[21]

How did Mary Putnam learn to write, and especially to write medicine? What intellectual problems did she address, and what tools did she bring to bear on them? And finally, how did this writer perform gender (or refuse to perform it) in her medical writing?

APPRENTICESHIP OF A WRITER

Mary Putnam attended the New York College of Pharmacy in 1861; her father had requested that she suspend any plans for medical studies away from home for two years.[22] Putnam Jacobi planned to attend the Woman's Medical College of Philadelphia after graduating from the pharmacy school, but in 1862 she traveled to New Orleans, then occupied by the Union Army, to nurse her brother, Haven; years later, Haven told of her preaching "right powerful" at a service for escaped slaves.[23]

In 1863, Mary Putnam traveled to the Woman's Medical College of Pennsylvania. Her arrival may well have seemed a mixed blessing to the faculty: she was a brilliant and hard-working, but incorrigibly unprocedural, student. Unlike those young women who extended their studies for up to three years, hearing the same lectures each year, Mary Putnam felt quite ready to graduate after one round. When asked to supply evidence of two years of study, she proffered lecture tickets from the New York College of Pharmacy. Her thesis, a Latin discussion of the spleen,[24] seems to have taxed the faculty's classicism; Professor Coates agreed to read it on February 3, 1864, but no report from him was available when they next met. In response to faculty requests, Mary Putnam offered assorted additional lecture tickets but admitted that she had stopped attending some of the weaker College of Pharmacy lectures and that her tickets for the course in the practice of medicine were just plain lost. In fact, she had never been matriculated at the College of Pharmacy. The faculty were not pleased with Putnam's casual attitude toward academic procedure, but Ann Preston moved to admit her to examination on the grounds that she had studied medicine for three years and completed the other requirements. Coates finally read half of Putnam's thesis and reported that it "seemed to be a fair expose of what is at present known concerning the spleen and to be of satisfactory latinity though containing some errors of grammatical construction."[25] Inquiries to Elizabeth Blackwell and to the dean of the New York Medical College were pronounced inconclusive; after weeks of debate, Mary Putnam was admitted to examinations. Dean Edwin Fussell resigned in protest after her graduation, convinced that Putnam had deceived the faculty and that their standards had been fatally relaxed. Ann Preston succeeded him, becoming the first woman dean of any medical school.[26]

Mary Putnam was as dissatisfied with her education as her teachers had been with her. Connected throughout much of her professional career with the Blackwell sisters' institution, the Woman's Medical College of the New York Infirmary, she seldom spoke about her early experiences at the Philadelphia school outside its alumnae association. But thirty years later, in her essay "Woman in Medicine" for Annie Nathan Meyer's collection *Woman's Work in America,* she characterized the school's "knowledge and pecuniary resources" as "both inadequate," with "rambling lectures, given by gentlemen of good intentions but imperfect fitness, to women whose previous education left them utterly unprepared to enter a learned profession, and many of whom were really, and in the ordinary sense, illiterate."[27] She quoted without dispute Elizabeth Blackwell's opinion that the physicians graduated by women's colleges before 1859 were inadequately trained, and she characterized Preston, ungenerously, as one who believed that "if the moral behavior of the new physicians were kept irreproachable, intellectual difficulties would take care of themselves, or be solved by an over-ruling Providence."[28] In the story of women's medical education that Putnam Jacobi wrote in 1891, the Woman's Medical College of Pennsylvania was the problem; the Woman's Medical College of the New York Infirmary, her own institution, was the solution.

After graduation Mary cast about, even proposing to manage the Putnam family housekeeping "on scientific principles."[29] She established a small practice, studied chemistry, and traveled to Port Royal, South Carolina, to nurse her ailing sister Edith, a Reconstruction teacher. She was briefly engaged to her chemistry teacher, Professor Mayer. Her mother announced the engagement with some surprise to a family friend and also reported that "Minnie" did not enjoy the practice of medicine but was absorbed in chemical study; "*Dr. Putnam* is laid upon the shelf."[30] She broke off the engagement and returned to New Orleans to earn money as a tutor. With those savings, she traveled to France, arriving in 1866, at the age of twenty-two.

Although Mary had published some short stories during her teens and had published regular correspondence from New Orleans, it was in Paris that she began to write on medical subjects for medical audiences, to take up serious political issues, and to write compelling fiction. Mary Putnam wrote to gather information, shape for herself a professional register, and earn a living. She produced regular columns for the New York *Evening Post* and the *New Orleans Sunday Times;* she summarized French medical news for the New York *Medical Record.*[31] The columns for the *Evening Post* and the *Sunday Times,* on such topics as the new Parisian bonbon boxes, were simply a source of income, but the *Medical Record* correspondence was substantial and extended; it led to a lifelong association with the journal and provided the twenty-two-year-old medical student with sustained practice in the writing of medicine, a practice facilitated by anonymity.[32]

When problems developed with her newspaper correspondence, Mary Putnam looked for other literary work. She needed the money. Her father invited her to submit something to the new *Putnam's Monthly,* and her letters in 1867 outline a dizzying range of writing projects: a scientific account of the miracles of the Bible; a critique of Tuckerman's popular guide to Paris; an essay on pain; a brochure on facial expression as a means of diagnosis;[33] popular scientific articles; essays on the French intellect, on proof, on the duties of intellectuals; a romance; a translation for the Putnam's series of "railroad books";[34] and an essay on heaven as pure thought, conceived as a refutation of Elizabeth Stuart Phelps's resolutely material paradise, *The Gates Ajar.*[35] What Mary Putnam actually wrote was both more and less interesting: essays entitled "Imagination and Language" and "A Study of Still-Life, Paris," published in *Putnam's Monthly;* the short stories "A Sermon at Notre-Dame," "A Martyr to Science," and the novella *Concerning Charlotte,* also published in *Putnam's Monthly;* and two political sketches, extracts from an unfinished account of the siege of Paris and the Commune, "The Clubs of Paris" and "Some of the French Leaders," both published in *Scribner's Monthly.*[36] Putnam therefore wrote, during her five years in Paris, some 170 pages of medical journalism, 300 pages of essays, stories, and commentary, and an undetermined amount of popular journalism, while maintaining an active family correspondence. Even by the standards of the overachieving nineteenth century, this is a lot of writing. Mary Putnam established the cadences of her medical style and invented the logical figures that would shape her writing. In one of her family letters from Paris, Mary Putnam described herself as "quite innocent of grace, but expressing a certain force and vitality . . . ; with no pretensions to dignity, but not deficient, I believe, in self possession and repose."[37] (See figure 11.) Except for repose (nobody ever described her as quiet), these adjectives characterize Mary Putnam's prose quite aptly.

We might begin with her letters, records of a vivid mind, disposed to learn everything, encountering with exhilaration a metropolitan culture. Putnam studied French, immersed herself in art, and walked all over Paris. She made what arrangements she could for medical study but wavered, in those first months, between medicine and chemistry, settling on medicine so that she could earn her own living. She found that she suddenly had "the most vivid admiration for dress."[38] After she had arranged for admission to hospitals and clinics, she embarked on a daily routine (at least as far as her letters home were concerned) that began with two hours of reading at five o'clock in the morning. Then she might walk to the Lariboisière hospital or to one of the others to which she was admitted, including the Salpêtrière, a hospital for the insane. She would hear lectures, attend an autopsy, have breakfast, hear a histology lecture, work in the microscope lab, and write a letter to the New York *Evening Post.* At night, finished with her work, she would walk to the Madeleine, "whence one could look down to the Rue Royale lined by a hundred lamps, to the obelisk of Luxor on the Place de Concorde, and up, among the beautiful columns that supported the roof, to the perfectly stainless summer sky." "Some day," she wrote to her sister Edith, "we must stand together on that porch."[39]

Later, after a long struggle, she gained admittance to the École de Médecine. She attended its clinics and lectures and put herself into training for the series of four oral examinations which she faced (her Woman's Medical College degree had exempted her from the first three exams in the degree program). And she became friendly with a group of "real French reformers and red-hot republicans"[40] centered on the Réclus family. Mary, who could be prudish about student balls and masquerades (especially in letters to her

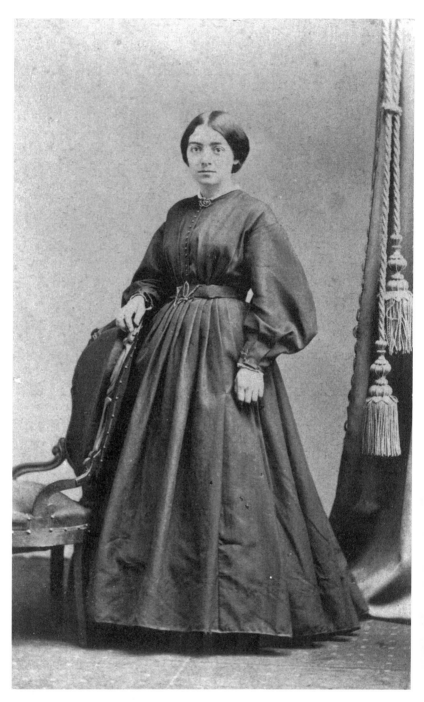

Figure 11. Mary Putnam Jacobi, 1860–65 (The Schlesinger Library, Radcliffe College)

worried mother), was palpably surprised when Mme. Réclus herself left to wash up the dishes after a dinner party, but found this circle "strange and fresh and vivid."[41]

In Paris, then, while continuing her connection to the Blackwells, Mary Putnam worked in settings remote from the middle-class literary and reform circles she was accustomed to; she made her way into social settings which required new strategies for the performance of gender: the relentlessly male world of the medical schools and hospitals, and the plebeian, experimental social relations of anarchist circles. The stories that Mary Putnam wrote during this period, almost against her better judgment, investigate precisely the issues of gender performance and of female agency that would be central to her medical writing. Consumed by a dread "of becoming a 'literary physician,'" she asked her parents to keep her authorship of the stories secret, not to mention her writing "to anybody."[42] And although Putnam circulated drafts to some Parisian friends, she felt that it would damage her reputation as a serious student to be known as the writer of such frivolities; above all, she did not want her friends "dissecting" them to see whether they were about her life.[43] After she began medical practice, she renounced any further literary work. (Silas Weir Mitchell followed Oliver Wendell Holmes's advice and delayed literary publication until he was established as a physician; the mere figure of Holmes was sufficiently monitory to end Putnam's literary career.[44]) These essays work seriously at the problem of what it meant to be a politically engaged and scientifically absorbed nineteenth-century woman, a problem that Putnam continued to encounter and resolve provisionally throughout her career. Sometimes her solution was a version of professional cross-dressing. In her "Study of Still-Life, Paris," originally published in *Putnam's Monthly*, Putnam described the public reading room where she studied medicine before she was admitted to the library of the École de Médecine. We see the room, and we look from its windows into the street, but we are not told what it was like to be a woman occupying that space, perhaps the only woman in it. The decision to elide her gender was implied in the decision to write anonymously; Mary Putnam could no more have published an anonymous account of her experience as a woman medical student in Paris than Chelsea Clinton could write anonymously as someone who had lived in the White House as a teenager.

A quite different performance of the scientific persona is offered in "A Martyr to Science," narrated by a fanatic physician who has devoted his life to preparing for his own vivisection so that his beating heart can be studied. The incision would be made over several days with caustics, and doses of woorara (a drug which always fascinated Putnam Jacobi) would allow the motion of the normal heartbeat to be studied for the first time.[45] The narrator trained an apprentice for precisely this grisly task. Putnam showed an early draft of the story to M. Réclus, who declared it "impossible"; she re-wrote, consigning the narrator to Charenton. Another reader urged her to rewrite the ending "with a scalpel"; she lost patience and sent it out as it was.[46] Putnam had read her Edgar Allen Poe, and "A Martyr to Science" connects his gruesome fantasies to the intense, very widespread desire of scientifically inclined nineteenth-century Americans to see the interior of the living body. We might remember—and we will remember again, in the next chapter—the old Mary Putnam Jacobi's story of the young Mary Put-nam's great desire to find the heart of the dead rat. The narrator of "A Martyr to Science" occupies the full range of gender positions; he is absorbed in speculation, a being beyond gender whose "mind becomes hopelessly fasci-nated, and continues to pirouette about an invisible point, that is neither a thought nor a material phenomenon."[47] He is consumed by masculine activ-ity as he advances his career in Paris, and he identifies with a feminized subject as he fantasizes his own luxuriously passive dissection. This vagrant gender performance is stabilized, for a time, when the narrator and his pupil Guy begin their collaboration, a project which is homoerotically charged:

> "You love me then, Guy?"
> "Love you!" He rose from the table, and coming to the sofa, kneeled and kissed my forehead without shame, as in France men *can* kiss each other.
> "My master, my friend!" he said; and I felt that he was mine, bound to me by a love passing the love of women. I drew him before me, and ran my fingers through his clustering hair.[48]

But this stability is not secure; in a moment, the narrator dismisses his af-fection for Guy as "a feminine desire" and puts his experiment in train. In "A Martyr to Science," Mary Putnam connected the desire to see the interior of the body with both masculine ambition and feminine desire to be seen, organizing those desires in two bodies of the same sex.

A similar strategy marks the longest of these early stories, *Concerning Charlotte*. The novella is extremely episodic, as befits a story published in installments and never meant for consecutive reading. In the most remark-able and transgressive episode in the story, Charlotte, a passionate heiress, impersonates her rival, Margaret, the reserved, virtuous, and mistreated gov-erness beloved by a magnanimous republican refugee named Ethelbert. Charlotte longed to "intercept the one pleasure of Ethelbert's first words, and drain their sweetness, even though nothing but husks should be left for the person for whom they were intended";[49] she disguised herself as Marga-ret at (of course) a masquerade.

Concerning Charlotte investigates, again, the desire to see a living, beat-ing, human heart: Charlotte, like Guy, wants to see what should not be seen and herself remain invisible. Margaret, understandably, is not mollified by

Charlotte's protest that she has faithfully reported Ethelbert's declaration, and her indignation leaves Charlotte feeling "miserably small and inadequate."[50] Charlotte resorts to the time-honored romantic strategies of renunciation, political adventure, and erotic triumph. She undertakes a dangerous mission for Ethelbert, returns in triumph, and an indeterminate passion sweeps them both away. This story, ostensibly remote from any medical issue, is also a representation of the gender choices arrayed before the young Mary Putnam. The virtuous and boring Margaret offers one version of the *habitus* of the female physician: the impersonal, benevolent reserve exemplified, in different ways, by Elizabeth Blackwell and Ann Preston. Charlotte's willingness to risk action, to stake her life on the republican cause, offers another version of a feminine medical *habitus*, one that might remind us of the young Zakrzewska setting off for North America after she heard that there women were allowed to become doctors. Charlotte's desire to enact her philosophical commitments—she runs a school on Rousseau's principles—recalls Putnam Jacobi's own explanation of the particular attraction of medicine: its close connection between theoretical knowledge and practical activity:

> Hence in the most abstract reasoning—if the physician be capable of such—he must always keep his mind intently focused upon the practical purpose toward which it must converge. . . . He must see that his antiseptic fluids actually reach the infected surfaces; he must see that his hot baths are of a given temperature, and that his cold applications are renewed as often as they grow warm; he must know whether the medicine prescribed has been vomited, whether the food has been given at the stated intervals, whether the pulse has responded to the stimulant.[51]

What drew Putnam Jacobi to medicine, what held her in medical practice, teaching, and research, was the possibility of simultaneously engaging difficult intellectual problems and acting on the most quotidian level of the real; it was exactly this conjuncture that nineteenth-century culture found very difficult to gender as female, preferring to contain female agency as housekeeping, hygiene, prevention. The problem Putnam faced as a young student—and by 1880, she had not entirely solved it—was that of imagining such activity performed by a woman who was recognizably feminine. Much later, in 1895, Mary Putnam Jacobi would write, "Too much attention is paid to women as objects, while yet they remain in too many cases insufficiently prepared to act as independent subjects."[52] Mary Putnam's fiction rings the changes on women as objects and as subjects, as self-forming, active, and independent subjects; these issues are particularly pressing in *Concerning Charlotte.* Charlotte, who has no trouble acting as a subject or having ideas, who can be erotic or appetitive, is also dauntingly amoral, damaging, and cruel to Margaret. Charlotte and Margaret split the representational work of agency: Charlotte offers activity; Margaret, responsibility and self-possession.

Mary Putnam was not alone in organizing the dichotomy between agency and feminine subjectivity in a pair of split characters. Many nineteenth-century images of the medical woman organize all the benevolence and propriety in one character and all the pleasure and action in the other, as if it were impossible to imagine a female character "prepared to act as independent subject" without unchecked narcissism. Charles Reade's *The Woman-Hater*, a novel that mentions "Miss Mary Putnam at Paris," includes both the active and eccentric Rhoda Gale and the passionate, womanly Ina.[53] Rhoda's obsession with Ina, like Charlotte's with Margaret, is presented as a desire to merge with a passivity seen as both deeply attractive and intrinsically feminine. Underneath the sanctioned ideological fantasy of the good woman (maternal, energetic, and prudent) was the dream of passive indulgence (Ann Preston's fantasy of plentiful strawberries and a drifting boat). For medical women and those who wrote about them, horror could invest either the pole of prudent activity or that of passive repose; images of cranks, of destructive enthusiasms, alternate with nightmares of parasitic invalidism and dependency. The middle ground, an agency that allowed itself periodic repose, seemed uninhabitable, attainable only through borrowing, disguise, and subversion. Throughout her time in Paris, Mary Putnam experimented with these strategies, combining them in new ways, testing their limits.

Although Mary Putnam published her short stories anonymously to preserve her professional credibility, her letters on French medicine for the *Medical Record*, equally anonymous, would have been proof against more damning evidence of frivolity. Signed "P. C. M.," a reversal of her initials, they offer a detailed and circumstantial account of French medicine—its institutions, public events, clinical practices, and lines of research. These letters, written weekly from June 1867 to July 1869, each running about five thousand words, were her apprenticeship as a medical writer. In topic, style, and attitude, they were modeled on the correspondence in French medical gazettes.[54] Through them, we follow Mary Putnam's circulation through the French hospital system; we see such events as the elections to the academy, the opening of the academic year, the sessions of the International Medical Congress, the elections of interns. Mary Putnam reported these ceremonies with a skeptical eye; before the congress opened, she expected great things, but after attending its sessions, she wrote that it was "ill-organized, the programme arranged without sufficient tact, and the legitimate aims of the discussions almost entirely lost sight of."[55] She was particularly disappointed that neither Virchow nor Graefe spoke. Covered by the veil of anonymity, she took positions that would have been difficult for a woman medical student to defend publicly: she was sympathetic to the public registration and examination of prostitutes; she described the experiments performed on the bodies of criminals immediately after their executions.[56] When she gained admission to a surgical clinic, her letters were all of operations; when she studied skin diseases, she celebrated the wards of the Hôpital St. Louis, where "the most repulsive forms of disease . . . are stripped of a large share of their deformity."[57] These letters give us a young woman in the middle of the nineteenth century learning to write a medicine more advanced than that available to women in the United States. They repay close study and analysis.

We might begin by placing a paragraph of Mary Putnam's against cognate passages written by men and women medical students in Philadelphia, students at a comparable level of medical education—the writers of the theses analyzed in chapter 4. Tuberculosis, or phthisis, sadly enough required frequent discussion, both in medical school theses and in Mary Putnam's correspondence. In her account of the International Medical Congress, Putnam summarized one phase of the discussion of tuberculosis, a controversy on the specificity of the disease. Everyone at the congress thought that tubercles themselves displayed no anatomical specificity, but various theories about the secretions of the tubercle as defining the phthisis were advanced. Putnam briefly summarized several talks, concluding:

> In the granulations, these leucocytes are distinguished by pus, chiefly by the absence of intercellular substance; are small, because bathed by no liquid, and have only a single nucleus, on account of their low vitality. These leucocytes arise from the epithelial cells, or those of the connective tissue, and submit ultimately to fatty degenerations, etc.[58]

Let us compare, first, a passage from Margaret Richardson's 1852 thesis, "A Disquisition on Phthisis Pulmonalis," which also takes up the question of the "specificity of the tubercular deposit":

> But in a truly genuine pulmonary affection, tubercles, more or less numerous present themselves in some of their varied forms and stages. In some parts of the lungs, very minute particles, scarcely distinguishable by the naked eye, are discovered while in other parts, larger bodies, varying in size form and colour, are scattered throughout their structure. Other appearances also present themselves. Abscesses of various sizes and secreting a brownish or blackish pus, are more or less numerous and denote the advanced stage of the disease. Cartilaginous bodies indicating the cicatrization of the ulcerous cavities are also manifest.[59]

And we can read a passage on the same topic in John Sale's 1850 University of Pennsylvania thesis, "An Essay on Haemoptysis":

> The appearance of the mucous membrane upon dissection is various, sometimes red, and congested, and all the appearances of inflammation, in others exactly

the opposite pale, and transparent, Bichat although examining carefully with the microscope the mucous membrane of those dying of this disease, could never discover the slightest erosion, from his and numberless other investigations, death is supposed to occur from exhalation from the mucous membrane—The blood issuing from a small breach, too small to be perceived, may sometimes produce death.[60]

Some of the differences in these accounts are the results of the nearly twenty years of research between the writing of the theses in the 1850s and Putnam's 1867 letter. All three accounts are marked by close, detailed descriptions of tissues, but they differ in their use of mediating tools. Mary Putnam summarizes what various speakers said they saw through a microscope. Both Richardson and Sale would have had access to microscopes, and Sale reports Bichat's microscopic discoveries, but these tools were not in routine use in the 1850s; the chair of microscopy was not established at the University of Pennsylvania until 1869 or at the Woman's Medical College until 1872.[61] The apparatus supports Putnam's talk of leucocytes, intercellular substances, and cellular nuclei; for her, the cell is salient, just as the tissue was salient to Richardson and Sale.

But not all the differences in these passages are accounted for by developments in technology. Putnam's argument is framed by the rhetorical exigency of reporting on the International Medical Congress. Her description of the tubercles turns on details that had already been deployed to support the congress's arguments about phthisis. Putnam arranges them to support her own claim that "tuberculization is by no means a specific disease . . . but an affection of the same order as inflammations."[62] But for both Richardson and Sale, tissue, closely described, tells the story of the patient's illness. No specifically medical argument mediates between the details in their theses (particles, pus, and scarring) and the disease processes they account for. In the student theses, the body speaks directly to medicine; in Mary Putnam's medical letters, specific doctors speak about medicine through their descriptions of the body.

This difference can be illustrated by analogy to the conventions of landscape description, a common source for tropes and schemes of anatomy.[63] These passages recall the quite different landscapes described by Sir Walter Scott and by Ralph Waldo Emerson—two perennial favorites in American reform circles. In the Waverly novels, detailed representations of nature serve as representations of the hero's experience; the landscape rearranges the narrative, offers it to the reader at a glance:

> In one place a crag of huge size presented its gigantic bulk, as if to forbid the passenger's farther progress; and it was not until he approached its very base, that Waverly discerned the sudden and acute turn by which the pathway

wheeled its course around this formidable obstacle. In another spot, the projecting rocks from the opposite side of the chasm had approached so near to each other, that two pine-trees laid across, and covered with turf, formed a rustic bridge at the height of at least one hundred and fifty feet.[64]

Scott's description of the landscape resembles Richardson's and Sale's descriptions of tissues: intense attention to proximity and contiguity, precise accounts of size, conformation, and the relations of objects. The landscape is organized by the path the hero takes through it; crags, chasms, and trees suggest his route, so that the landscape suggests a narrative. Richardson's and Sale's descriptions of tissues also support narratives: for Richardson, the progress of the disease; for Sale, the source of the hemorrhage.

Putnam's descriptions, however, recall the Emerson of "Nature":

My house stands in low land, with limited outlook, and on the skirt of the village. But I go with my friend to the shore of our little river, and with one stroke of the paddle, I leave the village politics and personalities, yes, and the world of villages and personalities behind, and pass into a delicate realm of sunset and moonlight, too bright almost for spotted man to enter without noviciate and probation.[65]

The landscape does not promise adventures; it demands a reader who has learned how to enter it—an education supplied, among other things, by reading Emerson. Mary Putnam's letters record a similar education, a transformation of symptoms and signs into arguments and controversies, medical conversations for which her own texts will be an adequate "noviciate and probation" for both reader and writer.

In discussing mid-nineteenth-century medical school theses, I argued that they were organized in two registers: a register of medicine and a register of health. They discussed what doctors should do to understand and treat the body or what patients should do to prevent or manage illness. In Mary Putnam's *Medical Record* letters, the medical argument, rather than the hygienic conclusion, is central; she describes tissue not to tell the story of the patient but to summarize a medical argument about the "affection" of tuberculosis: "Sometimes the centre is already consistent and elastic, and at this centre the tubercle is gradually formed by exudation, since vascularization and repletion of tissues by matters destined to be exuded, is common to inflammation and tubercular formation."[66] The scientific discourse in which the story of tuberculosis will be organized is one that entertains multiple possibilities, that proceeds by constructing evidence that will rule them out successively, that searches for a unified explanation of the dispersed, contradictory signs and symptoms of illness. For medicine as Putnam Jacobi wrote it, the body was not a landscape but a scene of instruction (or perhaps a

161

crime scene); the story it told was not of suffering but of detection, of patient reflection, of postponed certainty and prolonged argument.

Putnam Jacobi's early medical writing is distinguished by her enthusiastic use of technical language, her attraction to systematic and deductive explanations, and her construction of arguments by ruling out counterfactuals. In her letters on Bright's disease, written at the end of the *Medical Record* series, Putnam offers multiple layers of description, from macroscopic discussions of the range of lesions and granulations to microscopic analyses of the urine taken from various locations in the kidney. These descriptions speak of the course of the disease counterfactually, by ruling out incompatible theories. Arguments are ramified: Putnam began by opening many possible relations between specific states of tissues and disease processes and then ruled them out, citing contradictory features of tissue or fluid. As the argument narrows, possible contradictory explanations are investigated. The story of tissues and lesions is subordinated to the developing medical argument.

Putnam was also interested in systematic theories that explained many disparate phenomena—a style of medical research and scholarship that was deeply at odds with American quietist practice. In her report on Salpêtrière, the Parisian insane asylum, one of the first hospitals that allowed Mary Putnam in its wards, she summarized the theories of the "alienist" Dr. Morel, who proposed a unified theory of the heredity of nervous disorders including "insanity, epilepsy, hysteria, chorea, eccentricities, dypsomania, etc."[67] As Putnam's medical knowledge increased, her sense of what counted as a system became more demanding. She moved from the slight, undertheorized, and facile general theory of mental illness that opened her letters to the exhaustive system for categorizing skin diseases developed at the Hôpital St. Louis, a theory that organized organs in pairs via the vascular glands, a system for classifying aphasia, and a theory that linked rheumatism and chorea as "a widely ramifying constitutional disease."[68]

These early texts are also marked by an apprentice's zeal in the deployment of technical language, including the feature that M. A. K. Halliday describes as grammatical metaphor.[69] The thin vocabulary so marked in the theses of mid-nineteenth-century medical students is hypercorrected, as in this account of a case of rheumatism:

> The complete defervescence, the persistence of great pain and swelling after the redness had disappeared, caused M. Gosselin to fear the formation of a white swelling (*tumeur blanche*) although neither the patient's appearance nor antecedents indicated scrofula. . . . The inflammation finally subsided about three weeks later, but the joint was perfectly ankylosed in extension. Examination then made for the first time discovered a purulent oozing from the urethra, and the patient acknowledged the previous existence of blennorrhagic accidents.

162

> This case is the more interesting because many persons have denied the exis-
> tence of blennorrhagic rheumatism in female patients.[70]

This is the writing of a young woman who was learning a number of new languages simultaneously. It is also a performance that, unlike any of the theses, anticipates the lexicon of the mature scientific register. We find in Mary Putnam's construction *blennorrhagic rheumatism* an instance of M. A. K. Halliday's grammatical metaphor: the text nominalizes a process or relation and then uses that nominalization as the basis for further investigation. Her medical lexicon is also marked by multiple chained nominals; later in the same letter we read of "an oedmatous phlegmon of the left submaxillary region, whose point of departure existed in the inflammation of a lymphatic ganglion at the angle of the jaw,"[71] a compact nesting-box of anatomical nominals. Together with her focus on the development of the medical debate rather than on the specificity of the disease process, these features place Mary Putnam's medical writing, even at this early and hypercorrect stage, in the register of mature scientific prose.

Some features of Putnam's letters can be understood as evidence of her immersion in the world of French clinical medicine. Following the Parisian practice of drawing conclusions from systematically collected records of large numbers of patients, Putnam often analyzed or summarized analyses of a large number of cases or autopsies to support or refute a proposition. This figure emerges in Putnam's account of the International Medical Congress sessions on contagion of cholera and on tuberculosis, in her account of experiments on the inoculability of tuberculosis, and in her discussion of Bright's disease.[72]

But while Mary Putnam had taught herself to write something like the modern register of scientific medicine, her letters also included figures of thought distinctive to nineteenth-century medical writing, including the perennial desire to view the interior of the living body. Ludmilla Jordanova has suggested that the desire to unveil the body was congruent with a gendered unveiling of Nature, seen as a particularly masculine activity.[73] In Mary Putnam's fiction, the woman who saw what she should not have seen and the medical project of seeing the interior of the living body both appear as transgressive, threatening images. In her letters to the *Medical Record,* these desires became less problematic. Putnam offered an account of the somatoscope, an apparatus which was essentially a light bulb: a glass tube containing a platinum coil, connected by copper wires to a battery. The somatoscope was introduced into the stomach, vagina, or rectum of a cadaver and "enabled the observer to see by transparence the walls of the abdomen";[74] Putnam hoped that the device, used on living patients, would be a tool for diagnosing ovarian tumors and calculi and tumors of the bladder. The soma-toscope transformed the walls of the body into screens; rather than opening or severing tissues, it worked through them, so that they were no longer barriers to sight but fields on which interior organs and structures could be displayed. The pleasure with which Putnam reported on this apparatus, "too good, or at least too striking, to be passed over in silence," would accompany many of her assisted explorations of the interior of the body in the decades that were to follow.

MARY PUTNAM AND THE COMMUNE:
TO "GO THE WHOLE HORSE"

On March 11, 1871, Mary Putnam reassured her anxious father that republi-can excitements had not displaced her medical studies.[75] She had passed her third public examination, and her thesis could be presented whenever the École de Médecine reopened. Since she had finished her article on the Ger-man siege, she was now entirely devoted to "natural studies." Daughterly reassurances aside, Mary could not help "believing . . . that I am better able to judge of what goes on in Paris,—than any one can possibly be in New York." Her father should trust her intransigence, her willingness to "go the whole horse," since that intensity had made her a successful medical student.

On March 18 the Republic became the Commune, the first socialist gov-ernment in history and perhaps the most interesting. Mary Putnam had al-ready published an account of the proclamation of the Republic in *Putnam's Monthly* (Sept. 4, 1870). She participated in the political life that led, eventu-ally, to the Commune, undergoing the privations of the German siege from September until January and becoming engaged to a French medical stu-dent who went to the front. After the surrender of the Republican govern-ment in January and the proclamation of the Commune, Mary Putnam's old occupation was gone, since medical lectures were suspended. She was abso-lutely caught up in life in the Commune:

> My interest is immense in the events that are passing, especially since the Re-public, and as far as I myself am concerned, I feel really quite ready to die in its defense, especially if in so doing I could help the Réclus. I probably shall not do so, however, in the first place because I feel that I owe myself as much as pos-sible to you; in the next, because as yet there is no way clear by which I could serve the republic, either living or dying.[76]

She was turned away from the overstaffed ambulance corps, and in mid-December she had replaced a hospital surgeon who had gone into the army, but she resigned in January to protest the chief of surgery's intention to vote for the monarchists. She was often cold and sometimes hungry but always had jam, wine, chocolate, and coffee, "and with that one can not be very miserable."[77] She moved house to avoid bombardment and slept with some five hundred of her neighbors.

And her writing speaks coolly and indirectly of this engagement and commitment. Her long article on the siege of Paris, mentioned in her correspondence but not included in her papers, did not see print intact. An unsigned sketch, "The Clubs of Paris," was published in *Scribner's Monthly*. (The author is listed as "Mary C. Putnam, M.D." in the cumulative table of contents for the bound volume.[78]) Her much longer article, "Some of the French Leaders: The Provisional Government of the Fourth of September," also appeared in *Scribner's* and was reprinted in *Stories and Sketches*.[79] Signed "Miss Mary C. Putnam," it is described as an extract "from a MS. History of the Siege of Paris, written there before the occupation of the capital by the Government of Versailles."[80] The sketch was markedly more sympathetic than other contemporary American reports, which mourned the absence of Parisian gaiety during the Commune. Later, Richard Watson Gilder remarked in his eulogy for Putnam Jacobi that the article "Some of the French Leaders" was "one of the ablest ever printed in an American magazine." This praise would have soothed young Mary Putnam's deep annoyance when *The Nation* suggested that the article must have been imperfectly translated from the French, because no native speaker of English would have written so badly.[81]

These two articles contain none of the avowals of Mary Putnam's letters home. They analyze the collapsing, contradictory positions held by the prominent leaders of the Republic; they report the scenes at workingmen's clubs directly but unsparingly. While engaging, they are also adroit and satirical. "Some of the French Leaders" finds none of the leaders entirely admirable; the last days of the Republic are presented as a contest among self-representations. In "The Clubs of Paris," Putnam's satire is directed against the reporters from the *Revue des Deux Mondes* and the *Journal des Débats* who policed the republican working people's clubs for bad grammar and dangerous ideas. Mary Putnam herself came to the clubs as "an impartial bystander"—the position she most enjoyed—and there were times when she detested both the bourgeois and the "people." But Mary Putnam was not actually impartial, only detailed and objective; she saw the talk of the clubs as developing a new form of life, as manifesting more intelligence than the government. The scene is drawn:

> Everything was strange and grotesque. The room where the meetings were held was generally small compared with the audience, filled with wooden benches, and dimly lighted with petroleum lamps. On the benches a motley crowd of

men, women, and children,—of which each individual was inflated with the consciousness of his newly recognized dignity as a sovereign people.[82]

The debates are described rather than summarized; her details of shrill women and sleepy children, of mixtures of sense and nonsense, transpose the stylistic conventions of Putnam's scrupulous, depersonalized medical letters. For her, the scene was impressive:

> . . . peculiarly complex . . . strange, pathetic, absurd, foreboding unknown destinies. Such an impression is made by a human foetus scarcely formed,—with its immense head,—its exaggerated nervous system,—its shapeless, powerless limbs,—its huge uncouthness,—in which, like pearls hidden in a mantle of rough skin, lie concealed unlimited possibilities of power, and beauty, and grace.[83]

Here, Mary Putnam broke her customary narrative reserve and also connected the political republicanism that animated her earlier stories to the scientific interest that brought her to medicine. Just as the physician can see hidden pearls in the uncouth fetus, the republican can see prudent deliberation in the debates of the working people's clubs; the disciplined eye of the physician informs the sensibility of the republican. In the Commune, for the first time, under the pressure of chaotic historical events, the central intellectual concerns of Mary Putnam's life came together. It would be the project of her first decades as a physician to reconstruct that conjuncture. On May 20, government troops recaptured the city and imposed a bloody repression. Mary Putnam's friends the Réclus were jailed; she secured their release. Alienated and shocked, she stayed in France for a few hectic weeks, broke her engagement, and passed her final examination. She visited both Elizabeth Blackwell and Sophie Jex-Blake in England, considered Jex-Blake's invitation to teach but decided to accept Elizabeth Blackwell's long-standing offer of the chair of materia medica at the Woman's Medical College of the New York Infirmary, and returned to New York in September 1871.[84]

UNDER HER OWN NAME: MEDICAL WRITING
AND THE PERFORMANCE OF GENDER, 1871–79

Upon her return to New York, Mary Putnam taught materia medica, established a private practice, worked in the wards of the New York Infirmary, and joined the professional organizations that would accept her. Among them was the New York Pathological Society, where she presented the first of many specimens in February 1872.[85]

No longer an anonymous apprentice, Mary Putnam experimented with other styles of gender performance. Sometimes she foregrounded her gender in remarkable ways. For Ann Preston, cross-dressed masculinity was expressed as medical regularity, but Mary Putnam demonstrated her ability to go where only male doctors had gone. Putnam's presentation to the Medical Library and Journal Association of New York, "Some Details in the Pathogeny of Pyaemia and Septicaemia," was quite probably the first paper presented by a female physician to a mixed medical audience in the United States. (Sadly enough, the paper is a critique of Lister and Pasteur.) She told the association that she had become interested in infected wounds during a "rather prolonged sojourn in the hospitals of a great metropolis."

> I had abundant opportunity for observing this fact [the innocuous effects of gunshot wounds of soft tissues], in the case of numerous shell wounds that came under my observation during the siege of Paris. . . . A curious case of impunity, even though the bone was involved, was that of another woman who had been for four years an inmate of the hospital on account of chronic rheumatism in shoulder, wrist, and knee-joints, all of which were more or less completely ankylose. During the bombardment, a shell exploded in the hospital ward, and carried off this patient's right arm about three inches below the shoulder-joint. It was a very clean amputation, with very slight haemorrhage; and but little trimming of the wound was needed to make a neat stump, which was speedily covered by fleshy granulations.[86]

There is no mention of gender here (except for the unlucky patient's), but this is surely a gendered performance. Mary Putnam Jacobi demonstrated exactly those traits—resolution under fire, surgical sangfroid—which were held to be impossible for women. She refuted the received opinion that women physicians could never be surgeons. Quite likely the only veteran of the siege among the members of the association, she claimed the authority of that status.

The most significant advance in Mary Putnam's career, however, was undoubtedly her election in November 1871 to the New York County Medical Society, five months after the admission of Emily Blackwell. Not only did these women's admission open to them the professional organizations of the city; it also laid the basis for women's admission to the state medical society and eventually, after many years of struggle, to the American Medical Association. The New York society admitted women early; both Philadelphia and Boston bitterly resisted the admission of women until the 1880s. Putnam's name was put in nomination by the president of the society, Abraham Jacobi (1830–1919), who was to become Mary Putnam's husband and, for a time, her collaborator.

Abraham Jacobi had come to the United States as a political refugee; he was among the defendants in the 1852 Cologne Communist trial and had been imprisoned for two years. Upon his release, he traveled to London, showed up on Karl Marx's doorstep, was quickly bundled off to the Engels household, and decided to immigrate to the United States in 1853 with Engels's hearty encouragement. Abraham Jacobi's first home in New York was in the "lower city," as Mary Putnam would have called it, or *Kleindeutschland,* as it was called by its inhabitants. This neighborhood was organized with the full array of German voluntary associations; Jacobi was initially supported by a fund raised by the New York Socialist Gymnastic Association for the Cologne defendants. He continued to correspond with Marx, acted as his agent in the United States, established a busy outdoor practice, wrote, edited, and investigated the neighborhood's high mortality rate for the German Society. For Jacobi, as for other communists of the 1848 movements, scientific discourse was a model of utopian public life: only a democratic culture could organize scientific competition, ensuring that the best work flourished; a scientific culture could support and inform the institutions of democracy, free from patronage and state control. Having been refused membership in the established German Medical Society, Abraham Jacobi and other radical physicians formed a new medical society and established a dispensary in 1856. The German Dispensary was managed by a collective physician's association, with a "self-evolved" organizational form that was never fully fixed. The dispensary was to be a model of scientific, democratic culture, supported by research; Abraham Jacobi established its Department for Diseases of Children, the first systematic pediatric department in the United States.

Abraham Jacobi was also an advocate of German laboratory methods, advanced in the late 1850s as an alternative to French clinical and statistical work. His advocacy of these methods allied him with forward-thinking physicians outside the German community; he wrote a bimonthly report on the European literature for the *Medical Journal* and was admitted to the New York Pathological Society. When doctors sympathetic to German medicine organized the New York Medical College in 1860, Jacobi took the chair in the Department for Diseases of Children, the first pediatric academic appointment in the United States. During the Civil War, his integration into the New York medical community continued; he began to practice at the Jewish hospital and, while continuing his relation to the Communist Club, also joined the new Republican Party.[87]

With his cosmopolitan support for women physicians, his scientific passion, and his political commitment, Abraham Jacobi was a second chance at everything that Mary Putnam had left behind, scattered and ruined, in Paris. For Jacobi, as for Mary Putnam, the connections between medicine and politics were insistent; science was the vehicle for emancipating society from convention and, eventually, from scarcity and oppression. For both doctors, the exigencies and competitive passions of the medical societies were the lifeblood of scientific progress; for both doctors, these exigencies promised a career open to talents rather than one restricted by gender, religion, or social class. Ruth Putnam, in her narration of *Life and Letters of Mary Putnam Jacobi,* paints a picture of Jacobi and Putnam walking home from professional meetings, absorbed in discussions of pathology; Rhoda Truax portrays them as idyllic intellectual partners, like Dashiell Hammett and Lillian Hellman without the alcohol.[88] And who would not be attracted by this picture of two physicians, both animated by political and social desires, whatever the cultural distances between them? Their relationship was always complex and became more somber with time and mutual loss; much of the correspondence that could have given us a clearer sense of how they managed their lives is no longer available.[89]

After Putnam and Jacobi's engagement in the summer of 1872 and their marriage (at a secular ceremony in the New York city hall) on July 22, 1873, Mary Putnam experimented with collaboration as a style of gender performance, linking her medical work to her husband's. Gender performance had never been routine for Mary Putnam. Her anonymous *Medical Record* letters had used the reader's assumption of her masculinity to support a cross-dressed gender performance distinct from the hygienic regularity established by Preston. Her family letters record Mary Putnam's essays on French medicine as experiments in costume design; metaphors of dress and clothing helped her think through the contradictions of being a female physician. She described her entry into the public space of the École de Medécine: "Day before yesterday, for the first time since its foundation several centuries ago, a petticoat might be seen in the August amphitheatre of the *École de Médecine.* That petticoat enrobed the form of your most obedient servant and dutiful daughter!"[90] In an apocryphal story, one of the professors of the *école* offered to admit her to class only if she would consent to dress as a man; she encountered him in the courtyard, remarking, "Why, Monsieur, look at my littleness! Men's clothes would only exaggerate it; I should never be taken for a man, and the objection to mixing with the students would be increased a hundred fold," convincing the professor to admit her in her own clothing.[91]

Later, Mary Putnam Jacobi used her signature as a costume. The name she signed to her publications varied endlessly during her first years in her profession. Before her marriage, she had signed articles either "Dr. Mary C. Putnam" or "Mary C. Putnam, M.D." After her marriage, she experimented briefly with "M. P. Jacobi, M.D." and "M. Putnam-Jacobi, M.D." Eventually, she settled on "Mary Putnam Jacobi, M.D." but also used "Mary Putnam-

Jacobi, M.D."[92] All these versions of her name are inflections of the themes of gender, marriage, and personal agency; the only element that remains constant in all of them is her professional identification as an M.D.

Soon after her marriage, Mary Putnam Jacobi took on the work of revising and augmenting Abraham Jacobi's *Infant Diet;* this editorial work, like her translation of Elié Réclus's essays, was an experiment in coauthorship. The infant diet book was also an attempt to write for popular audiences.[93] The book began as a pamphlet, an extended address by Abraham Jacobi to the Public Health Association of New York; all the information contained in his first pamphlet is intact in the augmented, popular edition that Mary Putnam Jacobi coauthored. Abraham Jacobi had argued for breast-feeding but offered suggestions for supplemental feeding when necessary. The pamphlet included information on how infant saliva affected various formulas, chemical analyses of cow's milk, and advice for avoiding the "summer complaint," the chronic diarrhea that killed so many nineteenth-century infants. In Mary Putnam Jacobi's augmented version, this material is supplemented with discussions of the physiology of nursing, a comparison between digestion in infants and in adults, and a defense of small doses of whiskey as a treatment for the summer complaint. We might expect a popularization to shorten a professional document, lower the density of its information, and focus on practical advice; Mary Putnam Jacobi's popularization doubles the length of the original text and adds vast tracts of physiology.

Around the kernel of Abraham Jacobi's observations and chemical analyses, Mary Putnam Jacobi built up layers of information that might have helped (extremely patient) lay audiences to follow medical arguments as they had been made in professional contexts. Such education was, she considered, no less than her duty:

> What should be the nature of a popular essay? To judge by the multitude of little books that are lavished upon young mothers to help them in the care of their children, one thing is supposed to be fundamental—theory, or an explanation of scientific basis for the precepts laid down, must be rigidly avoided. . . . Now we assume, contrary to this dictum, that the theory of a fact does concern every intelligent person who is interested in its application.[94]

Mary Putnam Jacobi saw her coauthored book with Abraham Jacobi as a translation; scientific information was to be mediated and explained so that it could be absorbed by a new audience. Translation would ensure the more ready acceptance of medical advice; the mother would become

> the intelligent passenger on a vessel, who learns how to read the chart and to foresee the directions and incidents of the voyage, even while submitting to the control of the captain, so the mother may learn the general plan of her child's life, its future course, and the accidents that beset it, and, in regard to the details

to which her attention is called, learn much, if not all, of their scientific relations."[95]

Like Abraham Jacobi, Mary Putnam Jacobi saw scientific democracy as a matter of disseminating knowledge while preserving professional authority. The mother who read *Infant Diet* was no more to be entrusted with directing the medical care of her child than an educated passenger would have been given the wheel of a ship. Husband and wife, both physicians, addressed together the uneducated female reader; the medical wife fashioned a mediating language that stabilized the reader as the receiver of advice. The authority of the profession was established all the more securely, and the female care-giver rendered all the more compliant.

Mary Putnam Jacobi's concessions to her audience in *Infant Diet* were focused and deliberate. She used relatively nontechnical language, scaling down the lexical armamentarium she had developed in Paris. She offered background, and she restricted the text's information to "what is already positively assured to science" rather than including the "new researches or the original criticism which alone constitute the *raison d'être* of a book professing to be scientific."[96] But within these boundaries, Putnam Jacobi connected the popular essays to those directed toward physicians: "What is told should be the same in kind as what is told to the scholar. Few women seem to be aware of the insult implied in the assertion 'that the theory is of no importance to them.' Of whomsoever this assertion may be truthfully made, it must be said that he is destitute of the highest characteristic of an intelligent being—the desire, namely, 'to understand himself and the things around him.'" [97] That was an insult Mary Putnam Jacobi never gave to any of her audiences, happily as they might have tolerated it.

While Mary Putnam Jacobi's collaborative popularization was a complex gender performance, so were her more properly professional publications. In them, she offered a compliance with norms of professional discourse that is dazzling in its rigor. If her popular writing was not technical but discursive, her scientific writing was ruthlessly compressed; if her popular writing offered explanation, her scientific writing refused to provide context for the reader; if her popular writing concerned what was generally accepted, her scientific writing continually pushed the parameters of science. None of the thirty-six scientific articles that Mary Putnam Jacobi wrote during the 1870s refers to her own gender, but she did write an unpublished essay in 1873 on the topic of gender. Her "Reply to Prof. Munsterberg" responded to his argument against the higher education of women, an argument cast in Hegelian terms: Munsterberg had argued that a woman must "be taught to consider as the really best for her, what is in the highest interests of the whole of society, even if be second best for the individual."[98] Mary Putnam Jacobi

objected, "Who is to decide?" and then, fresh from the influence of the Réclus family, she referred to Fourier:

> Fourier, in many respects the most sagacious of modern Socialists—is almost
> alone in perceiving that Nature really varies from the start. That about a third
> of all boys possess the tastes and capacities of girls, and, if left to themselves
> would follow their quiet and sedentary occupations. And correlatively about a
> third of the total number of girls thoroughly hate the restrictions and limitations
> imposed upon their own sex—and crave the energetic turbulence of boys. Fou-
> rier's scheme of society, provides for a minority representation in each case: his
> Little Clans consist of one third of boys, and two thirds of girls: his Little Hordes,
> one third of girls, and two thirds of boys.[99]

If such a plan were followed, Putnam Jacobi claimed, nature would be expanded, capacities encouraged, and individuals made happy. Similarly, in her
early medical writings, it is as if Mary Putnam Jacobi declared: "I, the writer,
am a woman, as you can see (usually) by my name. However, I write medicine like a man; in fact, the form of medicine I am writing, bristling with
laboratory results and stories of combat, is especially masculine." Such a performance differed from Preston's cross-dressing, which proclaimed its masculine regularity but inflected its medical register as feminine by focusing
on prevention and hygiene. Mary Putnam Jacobi insisted on herself as the
female writer of insistently masculine medicine, the girl in the horde,
thereby denaturalizing the conjunction between knowledge and gender. Or,
as she would have put it, encouraging "various social combinations . . . [and]
opportunities for interchange of function between the sexes."[100]

THE ANONYMOUS SUBLIME: *THE QUESTION OF REST FOR WOMEN DURING MENSTRUATION*

Yet another, still more complex, style of gender performance is demonstrated
in Mary Putnam Jacobi's entry in the competition for the 1876 Boylston
Prize, *The Question of Rest for Women during Menstruation*. The general
background to this publication is well-known: Harvard professor of materia
medica Edward H. Clarke had argued in *Sex in Education: Or, A Fair
Chance for Girls* that the establishment of puberty and the demands of the
monthly cycle made higher education dangerous for young women and
girls.[101] Although his theory was widely accepted, many physicians were dissatisfied with the extremely impressionistic cases offered in the book and
with its lack of sustained physiological argument.[102] The Harvard medical
faculty, therefore, included among the topics set in 1874 for the Boylston
Prize essay, "Do women require bodily and mental rest during Menstruation,

and to what extent?"[103] Cambridge feminists, led by C. Alice Baker, met with members of the medical school faculty and asked if an essay by a woman physician on that topic would be eligible.[104] (Feminists did not take the success of women physicians lightly, and Boston feminists in particular, since the days of Harriot Hunt, had used all the means at their disposal to influence the intransigent Harvard Medical School.) Dr. Morrill Hyman assured Baker that such an essay would be welcome; although he was no supporter of women's education, he had been impressed with Mary Putnam Jacobi's previous work. Baker urged Mary Putnam Jacobi to enter the competition; her spadework allowed Putnam Jacobi to write with confidence, assured that she would not simply be ruled ineligible.[105]

The spectacle of open, anonymous competition was integral to nineteenth-century American medical publication. It was quite usual for medical journals, bulletins, and schools to offer prizes, both in general categories, such as therapeutics, and for the solution of pressing problems, such as a cure for cholera. Anonymous prize competition offered women physicians the possibility of eliding their gender, fulfilling Marie Zakrzewska's program for a "science which has no sex."[106] In Philadelphia, for example, Melissa Webster, an 1870 Woman's Medical College of Pennsylvania graduate, had been awarded a prize for an essay in clinical practice; her victory was the sweeter because the journal that sponsored the competition had opposed the education of women physicians. The editor was forced to recognize at least the possibility of exceptions.[107]

The dynamic of the anonymous competition was double-edged: It offered to graduates of the women's medical colleges the possibility, perhaps their only possibility, of being judged on the basis of their medical knowledge without being marginalized. But, since the winner of a competition was by definition exceptional, a woman who triumphed in this setting would never be taken as representative. Many women physicians, however, accepted their status as exceptions; both Preston and Putnam Jacobi expected women to remain a minority in the medical profession. With all its complex inflections of eccentricity and individual destiny, the status of exception, of the girl in the horde, was one that Mary Putnam Jacobi accepted and even sought.

The issues of Clarke's book—menstruation, energy, and intellectual work—were central to Mary Putnam Jacobi's political consciousness and medical research. She took the competition as an opportunity to broaden, perhaps to subvert, the constraints of normal scientific writing and to open the discourse of medicine to women's voices, even though in other texts Putnam Jacobi discounted the significance of lay persons' accounts of sickness and health. *The Question of Rest for Women during Menstruation* is a text which is beside itself in a number of ways: the author is not who [he] seems;

[she] is not writing, entirely, for the reasons that led to her having been solicited; she does not believe, in some important senses, the authorities she will introduce into the text.

The medical issues raised by *The Question of Rest for Women during Menstruation* include the perennial questions of ovulation, the nature of the menstrual fluid, the relation of menstruation to fertility, and the relative importance of the ovaries and the uterus in regulating menstruation. These issues were not at all settled during the 1870s, and Putnam Jacobi had something to say about all of them. She argued, for example, the singular position that it is possible to conceive fourteen days after the start of a menstrual period, the time physicians usually recommended to women as "safe."[108] Putnam Jacobi saw all these questions as related to cellular nutrition, a process which she later defined as central to the understanding of hysteria. Nutrition, for Putnam Jacobi, was no mute assimilative function; it was enmeshed with sexuality, reproduction, sensation, and consciousness. While Thomas Laqueur characterizes Putnam Jacobi's essay as presenting a desexualized understanding of women's physiology,[109] within the context of nineteenth-century gynecology Putnam Jacobi was actually connecting the reproductive crises of women's lives to processes of nutrition that biochemistry was beginning to study. Her analysis deemphasized sexual difference, but it foregrounded a sense of women's agency and consciousness. In the framework of cell nutrition, the menstruating woman was undergoing not a crisis of sexual stimulation or receptivity but a normal event in the growth and death of tissues. Menstruation was not a congestion of the uterus, not an erection of the female organs, and certainly not a hemorrhage; it was not analogous to the mammalian rut. Rather, it was part of the process of forming reserves, a process that Putnam Jacobi was later to connect to the possibility of agency, the ability to organize sensation. Far from constructing a feminine mind "presiding over a passive, nutritive body,"[110] Putnam Jacobi framed women's reproductive cycles within the context of their overall strength and mental energy, or what she called force.

Mary Putnam Jacobi considered herself a positivist, a self-description as common among late nineteenth-century progressives as the belief in the inheritance of acquired characteristics had been in the middle of the century. And one phase of her argument in *The Question of Rest for Women* anticipates the programme of positivist social scientific research. She investigated whether women did in fact feel themselves to be in need of rest during monthly periods and whether menstrual pain and fatigue were more common among educated women than among uneducated. What makes Putnam Jacobi's positivism interesting is the source of her evidence; for Putnam Jacobi, in this text, self-report is a perfectly reliable source of information about women's physiology. To collect information about rest during menstruation, Putnam Jacobi simply circulated a thousand questionnaires and collated the results of the 268 that were returned. The questionnaire was straightforward:

The undersigned, desirous of collecting reliable statistics in regard to the menstruation of women in America, would feel indebted to all who would answer accurately, the following questions.
No signature is necessary.[111]

The questions that follow concern the respondent's education and occupation, habits of exercise, health history, and menstrual history. They ask baldly: "Has it been necessary to rest during period? Strength, as measured by capacity for exercise. How far can you walk? Have you ever been treated for uterine disease? Are you thin or stout, rosy or pale, tall or short? Has any change taken place since twenty in color, flesh, or strength?"[112] It is commonplace in Foucauldian studies of medical practice to see such surveys as a means of policing docile populations; one researcher writes that the mass medical survey is "an instrument of order and control, a technique for managing the distribution of bodies and preventing their potentially dangerous mixings."[113] Certainly surveys can be used in that way; certainly they have been used in that way.

However, Putnam Jacobi's survey is not an allegory of control but a performance that inscribes the relentlessly lay voices of women within the discourses of medicine. The survey was a tactic for reclaiming from medical surveillance the experience of the monthly period, an event which could define a nineteenth-century woman as a perpetual patient. Using mathematical techniques no more sophisticated than taking simple averages, Putnam Jacobi combed through the relations among her questions, established classes of respondents, and determined that pain during menstruation was related neither to educational level nor the habit of taking rest but rather to the respondent's general vigor, habits of exercise, and "steadiness of occupation."[114] Putnam Jacobi's correlations, however, are less compelling than the short quotations from the surveys that are included in her tables. Women's words, rather than the numbers that summarize them, constitute the evidence for Putnam Jacobi's argument. In the table that correlates the respondents' general health with the number of miles that they walked daily, we read in the "General Health" column such remarks as "Very fine," "Good. Sick headache," "Strong in America," "Delicate," "Invalid from 17 to 25, now stronger," and "Robust, not accustomed to walk." Respondents report that they can walk daily "Four miles till after 2nd child," or "All day," or "Not much," or "Long distance."[115] No contemporary survey taker would allow respondents to answer a question about "how much" in time or distance, depending on their preference. But in Putnam Jacobi's essay, these variations record how patients themselves described their own health. The survey is not simply *as* authoritative as Clarke's observations; within the positivist framework assumed in this text, the information gathered from many women becomes *more* authoritative than Clarke's observations could ever be.

Within the history of feminist discussions of women's health, Putnam Jacobi's argument resonates with another survey done twenty years earlier by Catherine Beecher.[116] Beecher demonstrated the general poor health of women in the United States; the hundreds of middle-class women who responded to her survey, listing the health of the ten women they knew best, wrote litanies of disorder: "Milwaukee, Wisc. Mrs. A. frequent sick headaches. Mrs. B. very feeble. Mrs. S. well, except chills. Mrs. L. poor health constantly. Mrs. D. subject to frequent headaches. Mrs. B. very poor health. Mrs. C. consumption. Mrs. A. pelvic displacements and weakness. . . . Do not know one healthy woman in the place."[117] Supporters of the medical education of women had used Beecher's survey to argue the urgent need for improving women's access to health care. But, of course, that argument also rationalized women's status as patients, the restriction of their activities, and their exclusion (for their own good) from demanding professions. Putnam Jacobi's survey portrayed American women as generally vigorous, physiologically uncomplicated, and potentially ready for anything; these ladies with "excellent" health who walked "5–10–20 miles" a day were not likely to be laid low by menstruation.

The Question of Rest during Menstruation used the evidence of women's experience to contradict a (male) physician's prolonged clinical observation. By "working up" that experience in the survey, Putnam Jacobi not only devised a new form of medical research, extending the clinical statistics drawn from Parisian hospitals to new populations, but also smuggled women's voices into the emerging scientific discourse of medicine. *The Question of Rest* destabilized medicine's understanding of the male body as normal and the female body as fragile. The women in Putnam Jacobi's text are not in need of special treatment by women physicians because they are not in need of special treatment at all: neither puberty nor reproduction is a crisis for them; both are normal physiological processes. *The Question of Rest* can be seen, within this context, as an episode in Putnam Jacobi's consistent refusal to join many nineteenth-century feminists in accepting a separate sphere for women, however expanded or redefined.

Putnam Jacobi's argument from her survey information simplified the ramified tree structure that she had developed in her letters to the *Medical Record*. The survey allowed her to construct a body of cases that corresponded to the question set by the Boylston Prize Committee. She advanced enthymematically the proposition that if women require rest during menstruation, then many women will either take such rest or suffer ill effects from neglecting it; the survey collected and collated data disproving the proposition. The basic structure of argument through negation remains, supported by data composed collaboratively by the writer and her respondents.

Paradoxically, Putnam Jacobi rejected the idea that women enjoyed special insight into female physiology. She would have been shocked by Elizabeth Blackwell's advice that women medical students should cultivate skepticism toward their male professors or by her assertion of the "positive fact" that "methods and conclusion formed by one-half of the race only, must necessarily require revision as the other half of humanity rises into conscious responsibility."[118] Instead, Putnam Jacobi urged her students to resist taking any special role as women physicians, to demand access to the whole of clinical medicine, including surgery.[119] In her 1880 inaugural address at the opening of the Woman's Medical College of the New York Infirmary, she sternly warned the apprentice physicians, "What the patient has to tell you constitutes precisely the least important part of what you must learn about him in order to be able to understand his case, and to do him any good."[120] The truly scientific, and therefore truly benevolent, physician saw the patient not as a source of information but as the location of disease that required treatment. While Putnam Jacobi offered women's self-reports as reliable information in the Boylston Prize essay, in other contexts she dismissed them as information that the physician would do well to forget.

The Question of Rest during Menstruation subverts the ideological association between femininity and fragility; it offers distinctly feminine voices a place of authority within the register of scientific medicine. Putnam Jacobi also refused both the benefits and the limits of a separate sphere for women, defining their gender-specific physiology as an extension of general physiological processes and assimilating their life histories to a narrative of maturation, education, and maturity that is not dimorphic. Putnam Jacobi's essay is perhaps a unique instance of standpoint theory used to support a critique of gender differentiation. Given the intricate dialectics of the separate sphere, a physiology that deemphasized the specificity of women's sexual and reproductive experience also offered the possibility of depathologizing feminine physiology.

The Question of Rest, in its initial anonymous presentation, would have been read as the writing of a male physician; in its eventual signed publication, it presents the writer, tacitly but powerfully, as female. The writer's discourse, further, encloses and contains the many female voices of the survey, voices which the writer has herself constructed by excerpting and arranging them. Finally, the force of the text is to assimilate women, as objects and agents of medical care, to the norms of science. The speech act effected by Putnam Jacobi's anonymous entry into the Boylston Prize competition—the demonstration that a woman is just like a man—is repeated in the argument of the essay. But since it was the gender of the writer that rendered this Boylston Prize essay, alone among the many written in the nineteenth century, remarkable to a general audience, the essay undoes its own elision of gender. We read *The Question of Rest* because it was written by a woman; what we read in *The Question of Rest* is a denial of the significance of gender. The text as performance contradicts the text as argument. However much Putnam Jacobi wrote a medicine identical to that written by male physicians, it was not the same for her to be a doctor as it was for a man; her writing was necessarily a performance of the gender that she had worked to elide.

Although *The Question of Rest during Menstruation* was Mary Putnam Jacobi's most visible medical publication during the 1870s, it was by no means her only major work during that decade. Her "Pathogeny of Infantile Paralysis" was the first systematic discussion of that disease. Putnam Jacobi also continued to write essays on pathology, fetal development, children's diseases, and particular drugs.[121] None of these were journey-pieces, although by her tenth presentation to the New York Pathological Society, Mary Putnam Jacobi knew the drill. Her interest in technologies of visualization continued. She wrote two essays on experiments with the sphygmograph, a device which recorded pulsations, usually from the heartbeat, on a rotating cylinder. More dramatically than the somatoscope, the sphygmograph permitted a visualization of the interior of the body without any intrusive opening of its surfaces.[122] The sphygmograph mediated the interior of the body and offered a representation of its actions that was as abstracted and defamiliarized as Mary Putnam's anatomical descriptions were hallucinatorily precise. The apparatus came between the transgressive medical eye or hand and the hidden spaces of the body; instead of producing something that looked like an organ or a tissue, it offered an abstract tracing that required interpretation.

We might define the medical aesthetic of Putnam Jacobi's mature writing, as demonstrated in these essays, as one which valued what is made visible, through detailed explanation, technique, or manipulation, rather than what is apparent. Putnam Jacobi offered proof through negation rather than positive connection; she was much more likely to systematically disprove a series of alternate hypotheses than to directly support one of them. As in the very early *Medical Record* letters, arguments proceed through ramified decision trees, although Putnam Jacobi had become much more flexible in her construction of these arguments. In this mature writing, Putnam Jacobi has virtually abandoned the systematic theorizing that attracted her as an anonymous student, but she continued to locate her arguments in ongoing debates about medical questions, to compose them as intertextual rejoinders to other physicians.

178

WRITING THE LARGER LIBERTY: MARY PUTNAM JACOBI
AS ESTABLISHED MEDICAL WRITER

In the 1880s and 1890s Mary Putnam Jacobi was recognized as a major figure in several fields of medicine; her work with hysteria, anemia, diseases of the uterus, and nervous diseases, including tumors, paralyses, and meningitis, was solicited by professional societies and published in major journals. These topics are at the contested crossroads of nineteenth-century disputes about gender, constitutional strength, mental ability, and social role. Putnam Jacobi's *Essays on Hysteria* intervened in these disputes; elsewhere, as in her magisterial (and massive) "Studies in Endometritis," she addressed them by implication.[123]

In her books on hysteria and anemia and in several of her gynecological works, Mary Putnam Jacobi also took on Silas Weir Mitchell, one of the central figures of late nineteenth-century medicine. Mitchell, the virtual dean of Philadelphia medicine, a novelist, and a translator, was one of those "literary physicians" that the young Mary Putnam dreaded becoming; he wrote a brace of historical novels and novels of manners. He was best known in the nineteenth century for *Fat and Blood: And How to Make Them*, his enormously successful book on the rest cure for nervous diseases; for contemporary readers, he is the prototype of the evil physician in Charlotte Perkins Gilman's "The Yellow Wall-Paper."[124] If Mary Putnam Jacobi entered medical life in the 1870s by experimenting with collaboration, she spent the 1880s in agonistic conflict.

In 1880, three years after the first edition of *Fat and Blood*, Putnam Jacobi copublished *On the Use of the Cold Pack Followed by Massage in the Treatment of Anaemia*, written with Victoria A. White, her associate at the New York Infirmary for Women and Children. Unlike Mitchell's congeries of anemic, hysteric, and generally nervous patients, this modest, clinical book is focused on the treatment of a single disease, anemia, for which Putnam Jacobi devised relatively precise diagnostic tools. The book follows eight cases very closely, tracing the composition of the patients' urine during and after each was wrapped in the wet sheets of the "cold pack." Their heartbeats were traced with the sphygmograph; their temperatures were recorded. From these measurements, Putnam Jacobi concluded that the cold pack had improved excretion and nutrition, so that an improved blood supply corrected the patients' anemia. Weir Mitchell's well-known account of the rest cure as an experience of female submission to an omnipotent physician had offered no systematic discussion of why the cure might work. But Putnam Jacobi specified a working hypothesis, modified during the course of the study, and pointedly began her case histories with a patient for whom the rest cure had failed:

179

The prolonged rest in bed might by some persons be credited with the largest share in the recovery, since the essay of Weir Mitchell has so widely popularized the idea of rest in the treatment of anaemia. I think myself, however, that this rest was of the least consequence in the case. The girl had never been over-worked in any way, hence the etiology of her anaemia was entirely different from those in which rest is so beneficial; moreover, owing to her great debility, this patient had been in a state of nearly complete repose for two or three months before I saw her, from incapacity to do otherwise. Yet her condition steadily deteriorated; she was wasting away from slow starvation.[125]

On the Use of the Cold Pack Followed by Massage in the Treatment of Anae-mia is a systematic argument against "Weir Mitchell's popular little essay," as Putnam Jacobi contemptuously called it.[126] But of course, Weir Mitchell's book was read everywhere and saw at least seven editions, while *On the Use of the Cold Pack* was unread in the developing field of gynecology and en-tirely neglected in the literature on nervous disorders. The very precision with which she set up her clinical trial narrowed her influence; anemia was a topic of limited range and salience. Putnam Jacobi's very compliance with the constraints of mature scientific writing had marginalized her work.

In her *Essays on Hysteria,* Putnam Jacobi relocated her investigations into the main territory of the debate. She confronted a paradox: Hysteria was understood as a nervous disorder and therefore as an expression of tempera-ment or constitutional predisposition. But the symptoms of hysteria, includ-ing vasomotor spasms, and "the special, mental, motor, and sensory phenom-ena of hysteria" often involved the reproductive organs. And hysteria was also implicated with "moral and social conditions."[127] These are exactly the issues which Weir Mitchell's rest cure confounded; for him, nervous disease was a moral failing, and stimulation with electrical current could correct anx-iety.[128] This confusion, Mary Putnam Jacobi undertook to resolve; she would discuss both moral and social issues and properly physiological questions, but each in its own terms.

For Putnam Jacobi, moral issues and physiological questions were medi-ated by "force" as it was stored in the brain; differences in the ability of individuals to store such force determine, through the nutrition of their nerve tissue, how they are affected by sensation. Putnam Jacobi suggested that weakened nerve tissue (whether debilitated by constitutional weakness, illness, or overwork) might be overtaxed by relatively ordinary sensations, failing to store force or to take in nourishment. She therefore sketched out a narrative of the onset of hysteria, a narrative located in the "cortex of the hysterical brain": storage power becomes deficient; centripetal (sensory) im-pressions are stored in sensory centers rather than the cortex; centrifugal activities (voluntary acts) decline; sensory centers fail to discharge stored ma-terials and become hyperexcitable; sensory centers inhibit brain activity.[129]

Or, as a later physician would put it, hysterics suffer from reminiscences. Putnam Jacobi, as a positivist, assumed that consciousness was the accumulation of memory traces; she also assumed a psychic economy in which expenditures must be balanced against stored energetic capital. But Putnam Jacobi's hysteric was not transfixed on her own sensations; hysteria was not self-absorption but the inability to absorb sensations or to forget them once they had been stored. The hysteric was not too selfish but too sensitive, unable to impose her conscious direction on the overwhelming flow of sensations.

Putnam Jacobi, like most nineteenth-century physicians, often connected hysteria with the uterus. But she saw its fundamental origin as nervous and understood hysteria as a kind of mourning, as if the brain withdrew in dismay from its own impaired function. Affections of the reproductive organs could cause this failure of function; the first case history in *Essays on Hysteria* concerns a patient whose "profound consciousness of distress" was traced to a prolapsed uterus, and cured by the cup-pessary.[130] Uterine affections could restrict the flow of blood to the brain, and "the arrest of cerebral activities suggests as irresistibly oppression, defeat, humiliation, disaster in external events; imposes subjectively the depressing emotions of mortification, distrust, and apprehension—the depression of spirits which is unconquerable, even when the patients themselves recognize its objective groundlessness."[131]

"Some Considerations on Hysteria" investigated, in medical terms, the dichotomy that had informed Putnam Jacobi's early novella, *Concerning Charlotte*—the relation between feminine passivity and activity. But while it was the sadistic and active Charlotte who posed a danger to herself, her beloved, and the innocently passive Margaret, here the passive faculties of sensation (Putnam Jacobi's "centrifugal" activities) are dangerous impediments to the active faculties of movement, thought, and action (Putnam Jacobi's "centripetal" activities). Putnam Jacobi saw these faculties traversing the nerves like waves; incoming waves of sensation could break up and disorganize outgoing waves of action. No one would want to argue for such an understanding of sensation and action today, just as no one would argue for Freud's hydraulics of consciousness, but Putnam Jacobi's understanding of hysteria placed the disease in the nervous system and the brain. This theory of hysteria suggested a therapy that was both physical and mental, that respected the hysteric's consciousness and potential strength. The rest cure sought to relax the will of the patient, subjecting her to days of bed rest, tiny feedings of milk, massage, electrical stimulation, daily paternal visits from the doctor and weekly letters from her spouse, but Putnam Jacobi saw the patient's consciousness, beleaguered by a surplus of sensation, suffering from the suppression of its own ideals, as the agent of cure. More broadly, the essays on hysteria represent Putnam Jacobi's most sustained attempt to refunction passive sensation and active thought as complementary processes; the action of the physician, not surprisingly, is to balance or, in Putnam Jacobi's word, "harmonize" the relation between these two poles rather than to suppress one or the other. The hysteria essays suggest an understanding of women's agency, including the agency of the woman physician, which is risky but not dangerous, which seeks a change in the state of the object but is not sadistic, which regulates and "harmonizes" sensation but does not preclude passivity. This understanding led Putnam Jacobi back to the "moral and social" questions that she had avoided for a full decade in her medical writing. In discussing the treatment and prophylaxis of hysteria, she focused on the emotional and mental life of the patient in relation to the physiology of the disease:

> The inference has too often been drawn [from changes in the condition of the hysteric prompted by mental events] that the symptoms were "imaginary" and within the control of the patient, while the fact that the imagination, the consciousness, the very citadel of personal existence, has been invaded by a morbid process, cannot fail to threaten paralysis of volition and self-control.[132]

Putnam Jacobi's clinical practice employed the widest possible range of devices to treat hysteria. We have Charlotte Perkins Gilman's account of what it was like to be treated by Mary Putnam Jacobi for a nervous disorder, an inconclusive series of fragments that contrasts with the passionate aria of "The Yellow Wall-Paper." In her address at the unveiling of the Philadelphia memorial tablet for Mary Putnam Jacobi, Gilman spoke of having met her in New York, of their discovering common interests, and of Putnam Jacobi making Gilman an offer: "She had originated a system of treatment which she desired to try for that ailment [neurasthenia], and nobody would allow her to do so. I said I was perfectly willing to let her try it on me, and we formed a compact." Gilman went on to speak, with maddening vagueness, of Putnam Jacobi putting her "through a course of most remarkable performances" during her daily office visits.[133] Luckily, Gilman's recently published diaries are somewhat more forthcoming: in her entries for 1901, she wrote of being treated with an "electric plat" to the solar plexus; of taking "phosphoglycerates in wine," which she enjoyed; of Putnam Jacobi reading her manuscript and then setting her to work writing in the doctor's office; of reading a book, *The Cell;* and of building kindergarten blocks, all the while playing on a women's basketball team.[134] Putnam Jacobi's scandalous regimen, then, included electrical stimulation (one of her continuing interests and also a part of Weir Mitchell's rest cure), drugs, and a regimen of "moral" interventions that directed the patient toward the external world and activity within it.

Because Putnam Jacobi understood hysteria as a nervous disease, she advocated changes in social conditions as a means of prevention; her emphasis on the nervous, rather than a uterine, origin for the disease allowed her to account for women's susceptibility to hysteria without allegorizing it as intrinsically feminine. The characteristic moral traits of the hysteric, she claimed, were—when they appeared at all—results rather than causes of illness: "The most amiable, unselfish, and affectionate character [can] be not infrequently found among [hysterics]."[135] Putnam Jacobi recognized that the diagnosis of hysteria was applied selectively and judgmentally: "A distinction is often made, based upon the sex and temper for the patient. If this be a female, and notably selfish, the case is pronounced hysteria. If a man, or though a woman, amiable and unselfish, the case is called neurasthenia."[136]

If hysteria was caused by a decreased storage capacity, an inability to screen out or forget sensations, then the moral impressions most useful in preventing hysteria would be those effected by the patient's own activity. Putnam Jacobi quoted approvingly the neurologist Eulenberg, who held that it was social conditions rather than uterine "catarrhs and erosions" that rendered women susceptible to hysteria: arrest of will and independent thought; suppression of the ability to test individual subjectivity against external objects; restraint or supervision of all impulses; and especially opposition to "any attempt at emancipation from the limits of a narrow and trivial existence."[137] As a physician, Jacobi recommended change of scene, change of occupation, and exercise on horseback, rowboat, or the Butler Health-Lift. As a citizen, Putnam Jacobi was active in various attempts at emancipation, including the League for Political Education and the Consumer's League; she met with young working women under the auspices of the Knights of Labor and encouraged unionization.[138]

Throughout the 1880s and 1890s, Putnam Jacobi continued to publish on more conventionally physiological topics. One strand of her work dealt with uterine disorders; among these publications, we can count not only her extensive "Studies in Endometritis," published through the 1885–86 issues of the *American Journal of Obstetrics* and totaling some eighty pages of text, but also her articles on intrauterine medication for the *Medical Record* and the *American Journal of Obstetrics* and a short essay on gynecological uses of electricity in the proceedings of the alumnae association of the Woman's Medical College.[139] Putnam Jacobi wrote up surgeries, especially heroic surgeries of the abdominal cavity, including two articles on "Battey's operation," the removal of ovaries and connected tissue, and an account of trephining the sternum.[140] More and more, Putnam Jacobi was called upon to write on medical politics, especially the medical education of women. Although her bibliography lists only one such publication for the 1870s, there were seven in the 1880s and six in the 1890s. Putnam Jacobi's performance of these registers demonstrates her self-conscious adaptation to professional and lay audiences.

In Putnam Jacobi's writing to physicians, we can trace many of the elements that, according to Halliday, distinguish a mature scientific style. As early as the *Medical Record* letters, Putnam Jacobi's medical writing was marked by the use of grammatical metaphor, heavy chaining of nominals, the elision of personal forms, the use of a technical rather than a colloquial vocabulary, and the organization of the text as a disciplinary argument rather than a story about nature. Putnam Jacobi's prose was from the beginning extremely dynamic—it varied in different contexts. Even when her early writing deployed a specialized vocabulary, it was seldom syntactically simple. The *Medical Record* correspondence, to appropriate Mary Putnam's metaphor for the communard clubs, is like a promising fetus: a median form recalling the undifferentiated medical writing of the mid-nineteenth century, drawing on the conventions of the familiar essay. But turn-of-the-century texts, published in specialist medical journals, were addressed entirely to a medical audience.

By the 1880s and 1890s, the stylistic sampler arrayed in the *Medical Record* correspondence was reorganized into a number of distinct discourses addressed to particular audiences. Putnam Jacobi produced a variety of medical styles at distinct levels of discourse and also found ways to present the dreaded "theory" in writing addressed to lay audiences, to offer a distinct authorial voice in professional texts, and to perform gender in interesting and inventive ways. Putnam Jacobi's essay "The Prophylaxis of Insanity," collected in *Essays on Hysteria,* was originally addressed to sociologists. Putnam Jacobi discussed insanity as a hereditary disease:

> There are as many degrees in the soundness of men's minds as in the soundness of their digestions. Study of the organism of the family, sometimes in several generations, often serves to detect flaws in the individual organization too minute for notice. It is to the family organism that especially applies the doctrine of the blending of apparently opposite elements,—as genius and insanity,—both springing from an unstable equilibrium of the nervous system. These elements sometimes, though rarely, blend in the same person. But far more frequently it is inheritance from the undeveloped side of an organization of genius which results in an organization of imbecility.[141]

This passage is marked by modest use of chained nominals; we read of the *organism of the family* and then of the *family organism*, which functions as a grammatical metaphor. The unstable, undeveloped, and flawed elements of the organism are manifested in successive generations; from this comparison, Putnam Jacobi extrapolates an inheritance that determines, in part, the disposition of individuals. The comparison becomes an explanatory framework, a way of associating propositions elliptically rather than explicitly naming their logical relations. Like the *Medical Record* letters, this paragraph is extremely complex syntactically: modification is heavy and densely layered. But although Putnam Jacobi's syntax is complex, no one would call it conversational. Its particular features require the reader to suspend the thought of the sentence while searching for delayed head-words; the passage is closely connected to a culture of reading printed texts. Mary Putnam Jacobi may have been the first woman physician to write *in* publication rather than simply writing *for* publication.

Whatever syntactic demands the paragraph makes on the reader, it is in other respects remarkably accessible. None of the sentences is strictly tautological—all of them advance the argument—but each repeats some given information, usually at the beginning, so that the reader must absorb only a few new concepts at a time. The ramified arguments of Putnam Jacobi's more properly medical writing, proceeding through a series of negations, are absent. She offered theoretical ideas in carefully calibrated prose, so that theory came to readers—to use a term Putnam Jacobi would have hated—in homeopathic doses.

The writer, then, appears not as an avuncular family counselor but as a teacher. Putnam Jacobi seldom indulged in the hortatory flights that marked Corson's and Preston's theses or Meigs's sermon to Helen Blanque; she warned of dangers by stating them soberly rather than by painting lurid pictures of consequences. And the discourse of health has seldom been elaborated with less domestic detail. Although Putnam Jacobi herself was quite occupied with her household and wrote a detailed book about the education of her daughter (*Physiological Notes on Primary Education and the Study of Language,* 1889), her advice on helping a child establish mental health is very general. The essay constructs its reader as someone who is aware of the complexity of science and the vastness of the world, as someone who understands children and who makes her own provisions for them. The writer grounds the reader's experience in scientific concepts rather than mediating the authority of science over her practice, so that the gender positions of both reader and writer hover indeterminately. Nothing in the essay speaks from the experience of caring directly for a child; nothing speaks to the gendered experience of care-giving. Science and medicine appear not as male provinces but as territories traversed by all enlightened citizens.

Putnam Jacobi's medical writing had, of course, quite different aims. Her "Studies in Endometritis," published in the *American Journal of Obstetrics* in 1885, for example, took up the question of the causes of menstruation. Before the discovery of hormones in the 1930s, menstruation was likely to be understood mechanically, but it raised for Putnam Jacobi the question of how the tissues of the reproductive system, tissues which are periodically destroyed, differ from others which continue to grow and maintain themselves. After reflecting on the functions of menstruation, Putnam Jacobi concluded, "Without fantasy it may therefore be said that there is a certain antagonism between the reproductive forces and the individual forces of the organism, even at their fundamental point of junction, where the muscular force of the uterus touches upon its reproductive capacity."[142] She saw uterine functions as episodes both in the history of the "parent organism" and in the quite distinct narrative of reproduction. Putnam Jacobi's text established an interest in women's health and well-being over an interest in their capacity for reproduction; her argument unsentimentally asserted the "parent organism's" self-interest. So thoroughgoing was Putnam Jacobi's rejection of a separate sphere that she wrote these paragraphs in systematically, and quite awkwardly, gender-neutral language. The cultural fantasy of the pregnant male haunts this passage, as if the "parent organism" were only accidentally female.

Paradoxically, the speaker of "Studies in Endometritis" is much more clearly available in the text than that of "The Prophylaxis of Insanity." There, Putnam Jacobi had asserted impersonal necessities: "study . . . often serves . . . to detect flaws . . . too minute to notice."[143] The endometritis essays, however, are animated by the writer's sense of her authority; she replies confidently to the chorus of established medical opinion. Putnam Jacobi took up the venerable weapon of feminine satire, and the bracing irreverence of her private correspondence emerged (at last) in her medical writing. Putnam Jacobi's review of the literature, a lament for the disorganized, pretheoretical state of gynecology, is especially hard on a writer who asserts that all uterine diseases are surgical and "curable by the knife alone." In a footnote, Putnam Jacobi names names: "Sims' 'Uterine Surgery,' Is this not a singular way to define the nature of a disease by the method used in combating it? On this principle we could as well speak of iodine diseases, or pessary diseases, as of surgical diseases of the uterus."[144] Since the "Sims" named by Putnam Jacobi was James Marion Sims, widely regarded as the founder of the prestigious New York Hospital for Women, it is perhaps not surprising that the Obstetrical Society of New York never got around to admitting Putnam Jacobi. She had located herself in the thick of controversy, satirizing powerful figures who would be among her readers.

Putnam Jacobi's medical writing is enmeshed in her enjoyment of guilty pleasures, of seeing colleagues caught out in error, or of dismissing their "little essay." It fosters distinctly professional pleasures of aggression and combat within a professional community, of carefully staged and orchestrated argument, of settling scores with professional rivals, of shuttling effortlessly from the level of the cell to the level of the species. Putnam Jacobi associated these pleasures with the sight of the interior of the body, with the possibility of opening to view what had been hidden, an act she had associated with pleasure from her childhood. She found ways of realizing this plea-

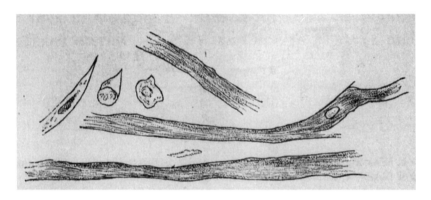

Figure 12. "Ribbon-like fibres with nucleus, from uterus eight days after delivery," woodcut from Mary Putnam Jacobi's "Studies in Endometritis," *American Journal of Obstetrics* 18 (1885), 813 (Photograph courtesy of the Library of the College of Physicians of Philadelphia)

sure in her medical writing. "Studies in Endometritis" was among Putnam Jacobi's first illustrated articles. Medical journals, of course, had long included small inset graphics; from midcentury, woodcuts and other engravings appeared in monthly journals such as the *Archives of Medicine,* although never in the weekly medical bulletins. But by 1879, images began to appear even in the weekly *Medical Record,* and "illustrations" or "cuts" were common in the *American Journal of Obstetrics* throughout the 1880s. These pictures might show a surgical procedure, a design for bandages or other apparatus, a pathological specimen, or cellular structures. "Studies in Endometritis" is profusely illustrated, including a score of woodcuts from microscopic slides. Some illustrations were copied from other texts, but others were apparently produced for this essay.[145] The figures extend Putnam Jacobi's prose argument; they are often arranged in series to facilitate comparison.[146] The text redundantly describes what is visible in the drawings, and the caption often draws our attention to the same features. While Putnam Jacobi characteristically moves her exposition briskly, her use of these new technologies of the visible is less assured; the textual deictic is multiplied and repeated. A drawing of long fibers is captioned, "Ribbon-like fibres";[147] the fibers will be indicated later as "fusiform fibre-cells." (See figure 12.) The text gestures, repeatedly, to the inset image; devices for suturing together these two sources of information had not been conventionalized.

Putnam Jacobi's more immediate response to technologies of visualization is recorded in her remarkable essay "The Practical Study of Biology," originally an address to the Massachusetts Medical Society's annual dinner in 1889. After arguing that a medical student must be changed in "his whole mind" so as to "insensibly . . . blend with the phenomena they can profoundly contemplate,"[148] Putnam Jacobi offers a personal anecdote. So unusual is this gesture for Putnam Jacobi that she is not at all sure how to introduce the story: "I should like, Mr. Chairman, to mention an incident that occurred to myself in the course of a very simple laboratory experiment." She was examining the circulation in a frog's lungs:

> I happened to so focus my lens that all the outlines of the capillaries and blood corpuscles disappeared, leaving visible only the spaces between the epithelial cells. Nevertheless there remained a vision of the streaming movement of the invisible blood through the ramified spaces. The streaming was so rapid, so energetic, so ceaseless, it seemed as if it were pure motion or force divorced from the accidents of matter. The microscopic shred of tissue from the insignificant animal seemed for the moment to give a glimpse of a mighty vision of endless life, streaming with infinite energy into the minutest particles of an infinite universe.[149]

Putnam Jacobi found this perception "indescribably powerful." No wonder. The ghostly image of the hidden, moving, and clearly indicated blood recalled the intellectual energies that had animated her work; an overarching theory (a mighty vision of endless life) joined to detailed, concrete, and precisely located physiological structures (spaces between the epithelial cells), organized in ramifying branches and speaking above all of force, motion, will. She repeatedly reproduced this figure for her students: "Since then I have confronted students with this same impression," offering it deictically as "the horizons towards which they were henceforth to keep their eyes directed."[150]

GENDER PERFORMANCE, GENDER TRAVESTY, AND GENDER MOBILITY

Mary Putnam Jacobi's performance of gender was self-conscious and experimental. If Ann Preston saw her work as a physician as essentially connected to her gender, and if Hannah Longshore continually constructed temporary connections between received ideas of femininity and her shifting scientific commitments, Mary Putnam Jacobi combined a steadfast refusal to essentialize her gender with a steady curiosity about what it meant to write and practice as a woman physician. Judith Butler has advanced an understanding of gender as performative, modeled on "performatives" in speech act theory—sentences which effect the action that they name, such as *I pronounce you man and wife,* or *You are sentenced to be hanged by the neck until dead,* or *I promise I will repay this loan.* In Butler's succinct statement, ". . . *gender* is not a noun, but neither is it a set of free floating attributes, for we have seen that the substantive effect of gender is performatively produced and compelled by the regulatory practices of gender coherence. Hence, within the inherited discourse of the metaphysics of substance, gender proves to be performative—that is, constituting the identity it is purported to be."[151]

Mary Putnam Jacobi's apprentice medical writing was often read as the work of a male author. At this early stage, she avoided tropes associated with women physicians (the importance of prevention and hygiene, opposition to the legalization and medical control of prostitution, interest in maternal and child health) and took up issues that women physicians generally avoided (questions of surgical technique, pathology, and medical theory).[152] In private settings, Mary Putnam Jacobi explored more indeterminate performances of gender. Her Parisian family correspondence is a veritable anthology of gender experiments. Putnam kept her mother posted on the state of her wardrobe; one of the subplots of these letters is the progress of her second silk dress, after many trips to the dye-shop, from garish cherry to decent black with a long stop at dignified maroon. In fact, as we have seen, it was not exactly Mary Putnam but "a petticoat" which arrived at the amphitheater of the École de Médecine. And Putnam also noted with satisfaction every time she was addressed or referred to as *confrère,* the ordinary collegial term among French physicians, a term whose atrophied gender marking was suddenly rendered visible by her presence. She was flattered when one of her teachers, a Dr. Hérard, greeted her by giving her his left hand, "the distinctive salutation of a *confrère!*"[153] This gesture was, for her, floridly gender-marked. After she passed her last exam, she was pleased to be greeted as both *madame* and *confrère,*[154] terms that were both, in certain senses, counterfactual (she was not married, she was not a brother) and in other senses entirely appropriate (she was a mature woman, a professional colleague). And Mary Putnam was not alone in her preoccupation with the indeterminacy of a female *confrère.* She translated the notice of her final examination in the *Figaro:* "Our confrère is among ceux—pardon the word,—celles who define life resolutely."[155] If the noun does not mark gender unambiguously, then the pronoun must; but of course the war between the noun and the pronoun renders the question of gender always salient and never decidable.

For Putnam Jacobi's Boylston Prize essay, *The Question of Rest for Women during Menstruation,* multiple audiences conserved the complexity of her gender performance. The male selection committee who read Putnam Jacobi's anonymous essay were expected to mistake her for a male physician. But, since her entry into the competition had been solicited by Boston feminists and agreed to in principle by members of the Harvard faculty, *The Question of Rest* is, to use cultural theorist Marjorie Garber's terms, a performance of marked transvestism disguised as a performance of unmarked transvestism. Putnam Jacobi pretended to pretend to be a male doctor; some of her initial readers would in fact have read *The Question of Rest during*

Menstruation as a methodologically interesting discussion by an otherwise unremarkable (male) writer, while others might have suspected that a text which drew so extensively from women's self-reports might be the entry that they had themselves encouraged. They might have covertly recognized Putnam Jacobi's essay as a work by a woman presenting itself as an essay by a man; one can only speculate about the feats of pronominal camouflage they must have performed during committee meetings, Putnam Jacobi's contagious gender disassignment having infected them. And the readers of the published essay, for whom the writer's gender is patent, would have read *The Question of Rest during Menstruation* as an instance of the triumphant story of the woman covered by anonymity who had bested men at their own game; for them, the moment in which Putnam Jacobi's transvestism was marked and solicited has been elided. In all these positions of reading, something about the gender of the writer is unknown or untellable. The action of a woman writing medicine, as Putnam Jacobi performed it, is a veiled and ironic action, uncontainable in its valence; no reader can be sure of the presented or concealed gender of the writer or even be sure of whether gender is being presented or concealed.

Even in Putnam Jacobi's collaboration on the *Infant Diet* project, no boundary marks the transition from Abraham Jacobi's text to Mary Putnam Jacobi's adaptation. In fact, the only words that the initial readers could have assigned to a single writer are those of Mary Putnam Jacobi's signed introduction, with its reflections on the centrality of theory to popular writing. Neither the text nor its apparatus allows gender to settle comfortably; no particular passage can be assigned to either writer without consulting Abraham Jacobi's original address. The text continually invites us to errors: Was Mary Putnam Jacobi responsible for the recipes? (No, they were in Abraham Jacobi's initial talk.) And such errors productively reveal what was expected of the medical writer in the middle of the nineteenth century, when medical writing was defining itself as a distinct discursive form.

As her reputation grew, Mary Putnam Jacobi had fewer opportunities to exploit the assumption that the writer of medicine is male, but her own gender performance was never simple. In her "Woman in Medicine," for Annie Nathan Meyer's collection *Woman's Work in America*, Putnam Jacobi presented medicine as a field, where "whatever *is*, invariably seeks to strangle in the birth that which is about to be."[156] She satirized her predecessors in women's medical education, who felt that "co-educational anatomy is more easily swallowed when administered in homeopathic doses"[157]—did she ever resist the opportunity to take a swipe at homeopathy? Seldom has the history of early women physicians been written less hagiographically. Ann Preston was all too pious; the early Eclectic women physicians were all too idiosyncratic. Mary Putnam Jacobi's talent for eliding herself from the scene she describes, marked since her very earliest writing, does some of the work of gender performance in "Woman in Medicine." Since contributors to *Woman's Work in America* were major figures, well known in their fields, even a reader who had never heard of Mary Putnam Jacobi would assume that she was an active woman physician. But she leaves her own role as a medical pioneer out of this account; we read a very detailed summary of the struggles to admit women to the county medical societies of Philadelphia and Boston but nothing of their early and uncontested admission to the New York County Medical Society. Mary Putnam Jacobi mentions herself only twice: as a founder of the Mt. Sinai Hospital dispensary, and as a member of the faculty of a school for postgraduate medical education. With these two exceptions, both of which demonstrate Putnam Jacobi's integration into the upper ranks of male institutions, the history of women in medicine is written from an Olympian height. We would never know that Mary Putnam Jacobi had studied at the Woman's Medical College of Pennsylvania, whose students she dismissed cavalierly as nearly illiterate; we would never know that she felt herself compromised by the weak preparation of early women physicians. The pronouns are telling: for Putnam Jacobi, women physicians are *they* rather than *we* or *I*. Her own early struggles vanish into a general narrative:

> Women students have been cheated of their time and money, by those paid to instruct them: they have been led into fields of promise, to find only a vanishing mirage. At what sacrifices have they struggled to obtain the elusive prize! They have starved on half rations, shivered in cold rooms, or been poisoned in badly ventilated ones; they have often borne a triple load of ignorance, poverty, and ill health; when they were not permitted to walk, they have crept,—where they could not take, they have begged; they have gleaned like Ruth among the harvesters for the scantiest crumbs of knowledge, and been thankful. To work their way through the prescribed term of studies, they have resorted to innumerable devices,—taught school, edited newspapers, nursed sick people, given massage, worked till they could scrape a few dollars together, expended that in study,—then stepped aside for a while to earn more.[158]

Putnam Jacobi's youthful struggles have been silently assimilated to those of Zakrzewska and Blackwell; the poverty of their preparation, their crumbs of knowledge, are transposed into a badge of pride. But the writer of this passage is situated outside their struggle; who would have dared cheat Putnam Jacobi of her time and money? She spoke with authority by constructing a position beyond gender; she is not part of "them."

Putnam Jacobi refused to essentialize women, to compound them into a group contained in a single separate sphere. This refusal could be infuriatingly self-righteous; this most favored of daughters sternly warned medical students not to be swayed by the praise of their partial families: "A woman must accustom herself to dispense with the personal approbation of the people she knows, as a stimulus for exertion" or she will "soon cheapen with praise."[159] But Putnam Jacobi never reduced women to symbolic status or referred them to any transcendent reality beyond the struggle to live in "large liberty":

> Women have in the mass, never been publicly and officially regarded as individuals, with individual rights, tastes, liberties, privileges, duties, and capacities, but rather as symbols, with collective class functions, of which not the least was to embody the ideals of decorum of the existing generation, whatever these might have to be. These ideals once consigned to women, as to crystal vases, it became easier for men to indulge their vagrant liberty, while yet leaving undisturbed the general framework of order and society.[160]

Putnam Jacobi acted in common with other women, especially other women physicians; not only did she continue political activity throughout her life, but also she urged women physicians to act collectively. In her 1883 commencement address at the New York Infirmary, she admitted that she had urged her students to see themselves first as physicians and then as women: "Recently emancipated people are always bores, until they themselves have forgotten all about their emancipation."[161] But, Putnam Jacobi conceded, deliberate amnesia had its limits; women physicians have faced a "bitter," "brutal," "densely organized," "versatile," and "incomprehensible" opposition and should act on the basis of a "close solidarity of interests."[162] For Putnam Jacobi, gender identification was based on a common experience of oppression and enacted in the project of dissolving that experience. It is not surprising that Putnam Jacobi's final advice to these graduates was a gnomic reduction of her own practice of gender performance: "You must, on the one hand, forget that any social prejudices stand in your way as physicians: but on the other hand you must remember that, in virtue of these, you continue to have certain class interests, which can not, with either justice or safety, be ignored."[163] Just so, Mary Putnam Jacobi constructed for herself a world in which the difference between physician and lay person was more salient and pressing than the difference between man and woman; she recognized that hers was a constructed world, one in which, in her phrase, horrors were "overcome or transformed by the potency of the Ideal," whereas in life they could only be "borne unrelieved" or undermined by a skillful and destabilizing rhetoric.[164]

7

Forbidden Sights
Women and the Visual Economy of Medicine

THE CLINICAL LECTURE

On November 6, 1869, a small group of students from the Woman's Medical College quietly entered the new amphitheater of the Pennsylvania Hospital and took seats together.[1] Their entry into these clinical lectures was a welcome turning point in the college's struggle for acceptance. The Philadelphia County Medical Society had recently passed its most punitive resolution against the Woman's Medical College, barring from membership graduates of the women's college, professors at the college, and those who consulted with them. The Woman's Medical College had been declared a pariah institution. Although the women faculty of the Woman's Medical College had repeatedly petitioned for admission to Pennsylvania Hospital's clinical lectures, beginning with a letter from Ann Preston in 1855, the managers only agreed to their request on October 25, 1869.

The institution the women students entered was central to the teaching and practice of medicine in Philadelphia. The Pennsylvania Hospital was the oldest and best known Philadelphia hospital, entrusted particularly with the care of accident victims. Although it was called the Quaker hospital and most of the managers were Quakers, Pennsylvania had no official connection with the Society of Friends. The heroic painting given to the hospital by Benjamin West, *Christ Healing the Sick*, expressed the ideology of the institution: healing is a divine work, undertaken in public for the benefit of the grateful people.[2]

Clinical lectures at the Pennsylvania Hospital were given by the attending staff of the institution. Like the house staff of other American hospitals, they battled for control of the institution for decades; the issues of hospital admissions and releases, of student access to patients, and of free and paying patients were all contested. Managers, responsible for the overall management, solvency, and good repute of the hospital, insisted on the right to screen patients for their moral fitness and desert, to restrict student access, and to control finances. They organized their own work meticulously, fining each other for absences from meetings and providently organizing appeals for funds; they expected the same sober and businesslike behavior from the medical staff. (It is far easier to trace the records of decisions made by the board of managers in 1897 than it would be to trace those of, say, a twentieth-century academic department.) The hospital's attending doctors, however, wanted greater professional control over patient care, particularly hospital admissions, and greater student access to patients; the lay control of the hospital compromised their professional discretion.[3]

Although the Pennsylvania Hospital did not sponsor a medical school, its lectures were eagerly attended by students from Philadelphia's university and proprietary medical schools throughout the early decades of the nineteenth century.[4] Schools required students to show their tickets for hospital lectures, the sole clinical education required of a mid-nineteenth-century physician. Tickets were moderately priced, and the Pennsylvania Hospital donated the proceeds to its medical library, which was open to students. And the purchase of tickets could be a formality. Students were not examined on what they had seen; they might purchase a variety of tickets for different hospitals and attend whichever lectures proved interesting, or none at all. Many students, however, attended lectures regularly, sometimes at more than one institution, and kept careful notes on what they saw. In Philadelphia during the 1860s, clinical lectures would have been offered not only at the Pennsylvania Hospital but also at Jefferson, the Philadelphia Hospital associated with the Philadelphia Almshouse, called the Blockley, and in clinics attached to the University of Pennsylvania School of Medicine. Smaller, specialized hospitals sometimes offered clinical lectures, including, of course, the Woman's Hospital associated with the Woman's Medical College.

Conventionally, lectures in medicine and surgery were scheduled for successive hours; two different lecturers publicly examined patients they considered interesting. In the surgery clinic, operations were performed on a table, often a revolving table, in the center of the amphitheater; at medical clinics, the patient would be treated, given medicine, and sometimes told to return. Students themselves do not seem to have had an opportunity to examine the patient or to ask questions. Notes of clinical lectures show five to ten cases being demonstrated in an hour of medical clinic; surgical clinics would feature as many operations as could be undertaken in the allotted time, with running commentary by the surgeon.

At the Pennsylvania Hospital, the clinical amphitheater was itself a dramatic space. It was at once intimate (any word spoken in the amphitheater could be heard throughout the room) and ceremonial (a newly dedicated, splendid structure, an octagonal room with deeply raked banks of seats, lit by eight double windows and a skylight).[5] The median space of the amphitheater was a freestanding building, connected to the hospital only by a covered corridor. The clinical amphitheater connected the academic, physician-controlled world of the medical school to the institutional, lay-controlled world of the hospital. The hospital managers chose the lecturers, but lecturers chose the clinical "material." The audience included students from many different schools, both regular and irregular: the homeopathic Hahnemann Medical College normally sent students to the Pennsylvania Hospital lectures, and male students came from the Eclectic and coeducational Penn Medical University, founded by the redoubtable Joseph Longshore. (Women students from Penn Medical University petitioned for admission in 1855 and were summarily denied.) But while the audience was varied, it was never lay. As J. Forsyth Meigs put it in his lecture inaugurating the new amphitheater:

> Let it not be forgotten, too, that this demonstration is never made to a promiscuous, or rude, or gaping public audience, who might assist at such a spectacle from mere vulgar curiosity. It is made only to those who belong to the same vocation or guild as that to which belong the surgeons and physicians of the house, and but for whom this Hospital could not exist, and who, themselves, but for like opportunities in the past, could not have had that exact knowledge and experience whereby these very patients now profit.[6]

The clinical amphitheater is constructed as a site for the generational transmission of knowledge; the amphitheater forms the physician, who then filially supports the amphitheater. Such a transmission assumes an identity between the surgeons and physicians of the house and those who belong to the same profession. Since the amphitheater replicates the exact knowledge and experience taught in the past, the physician reproduced through its spectacles must be identical to the physician who presents patients: the male doctor demonstrates his craft to the male medical student.

In 1869, the managers of the Pennsylvania Hospital interrupted that transmission, reasoning that since the Woman's Medical College of Pennsylvania had been chartered by the state, its students met the criteria for admission to the "common benefits of the Hospital clinical instruction."[7] Tickets were duly proffered and purchased, and a group of women medical students, numbering somewhere between thirty and thirty-five, accompanied by a woman from their faculty, came into the amphitheater.[8] Male students stood in the tiers above them, passing remarks, reading aloud from their notes, and, by some accounts, spitting tobacco on their skirts. Although many students told reporters that they had been surprised at the entrance of women students into the amphitheater, the day before someone had passed the medical student Marcus Corson a note reading, "Go tomorrow to the hospital to see the She Doctors."[9] Students hissed the two hospital managers who sat on the amphitheater stage to forestall trouble, the traditional Quaker William Biddle and A. J. Derbyshire, a trustee of the Woman's Medical College of Pennsylvania.[10] When Biddle took the stage with his head covered, students chanted, "Hat! Hat! Hat!" Their mocking chant spoke of the distance between the lay managers and the students, ignorant or disrespectful of the Quaker custom of refusing to bare the head. The arrival of the women medical students demonstrated that the Pennsylvania Hospital was already a divided institution. When the chant subsided, the students settled into the first, medical, hour of clinical lectures, led by Dr. Jacob Da Costa, which went off without incident.[11] The second, surgical, hour was more tumultuous. Dr. William Hunt began his lecture by addressing the "gentlemen," obliquely condoning the male medical students' harassment by ignoring the women in his audience. (Twenty-four years later, another Woman's Medical College student would hear a much older Dr. Da Costa beginning his Pennsylvania Hospital lectures with "gentlemen."[12]) One account, in the Philadelphia *Evening Bulletin,* tells that Hunt tested the eyesight of a patient by pointing toward the women medical students and asking the patient what he saw: "Said the Professor, 'Look up! Look higher, and tell me what you see.' The man strained his almost sightless eye-balls and replied, 'Light! I see light!' and nothing more would he acknowledge." The *Evening Bulletin* found in this remark a recognition that "*light*" was "dawning upon bigotry and oppression."[13]

The incident escalated from jeering harassment to riot, however, when a male patient was exposed to the sight of the women students. The *New York Tribune* gave the fullest account:

> The attendants brought forward a man with a broken thigh. This was a particularly interesting and melancholy case; for the fractured bone had refused to unite. The poor fellow was placed recumbent on the revolving couch, and the young doctors proceeded to pull off his boots. At this, a quick, low stamping, like a growl of dissent, ran round the benches. But "off, off, ye lendings" was the rule, and speedily the natural, unsartorial man lay before us. The Doctor had, however, prepared a blanket for the nonce, with which the patient was draped. But in this chamber the surgeon means business; and at times the decorous conventions must shrivel up before the needs of science and humanity. In this case, while measuring the fractured limb, there was a momentary exposure, which proved the signal for an explosion among the students.[14]

This exposure has been theatrically performed: ornamented with a quote from *King Lear,* set on a revolving couch (a feature of the amphitheater since at least the sixteenth century), and presented in stages (boots, a blanket, nothing). The patient's leg appears as a disembodied "part," fleetingly, in a "momentary" transformation of the patient. At least one observer felt that it was this staging, rather than the exposure itself, that was provocative:

If a blanket accidentally falls off partially during an examination of a fractured thigh, to jerk it back again with an air of embarrassment may cause a painful flow on the cheek of a *very* young gentleman or excite the cachennation of a somewhat older blackguard, when women are present; but its proper removal entire, under the requirements of the case, could never call a blush to the brow of either man or woman worthy to be allowed entry to a sick room.[15]

The women were hooted at; there was a storm of hissing and thrown objects. Again, the lecturer did not notice the women students or attempt to restore order, but continued his presentation and left the stage without comment at the end of the lecture.

As the women prepared to leave the lecture hall, the turmoil of the clinical lecture spilled outside and quickly became public. Because the hospital was centrally located, students exiting from the amphitheater were at once on the street, at midday, in a very busy place. By most accounts, male students formed two rows along the path from the amphitheater to the street and also along the street leading away from the building.[16] The women students had to pass through this gauntlet as they left the amphitheater. The male students jeered at them and perhaps followed them on the street; writing many years later, the Woman's Medical College student Elizabeth Keller said that "we were actually stoned by those so-called gentlemen."[17] Although some male students claimed that they were curious rather than hostile, no eyewitness felt that the scene was peaceful. Widespread press coverage of this event was critical of the male medical students: their conduct was a sign of narrow-minded opposition to women physicians; it continued the medical student rowdiness that had plagued antebellum Philadelphia; it was a simple riot.[18]

Physicians, however, saw the jeering incident differently. The medical faculties at the University of Pennsylvania and at Jefferson virtually endorsed the actions of the male students, claiming that their response to the women students was justified, complaining that all the students were being blamed for the actions of a few hotheads, and supporting the student boycott of future mixed clinical lectures.[19] The medical staff of the Pennsylvania Hospital saw the managers' decision to admit women into the clinical lectures, taken without consulting them, as an abridgment of their prerogatives. When the women students announced their intention to attend further lectures, even the liberal medical press felt they were being provocative.[20] At the next lecture, the only male students in attendance were from the Penn Medical University and the homeopathic Hahnemann.

A petition against the attendance of women at mixed lectures circulated among physicians; its 283 supporters included not only the usual conservatives, Agnew, Gross, and Meigs, but also "scientific" physicians like Leidy and Mitchell, along with Alfred Stillé, who himself lectured to mixed audiences at the Blockley. The Philadelphia College of Physicians passed resolutions supporting the medical staff of the Pennsylvania Hospital, urging that justice and courtesy required that they be consulted in the management of hospitals and opposing any change in "the system, established by long usage and general consent, of giving clinic instructions."[21] The medical staff of the Pennsylvania Hospital asked the managers to accept their delegate as a member of the board.[22]

Dean Ann Preston and the faculty of the Woman's Medical College protested that they had no intention of intruding into inappropriate clinical lectures. The women would attend only one day a week, when cases suitable for demonstration to a mixed group could be chosen.[23] The managers of the Pennsylvania Hospital, meeting on November 13, 1869, declared themselves surprised by the controversy, given the mixed clinics at the Blockley, as well as at Bellevue, Edinburgh, and Zurich. But they appointed a committee of five to plan separate clinical instruction for women. Still, surgeon D. Hayes Agnew was so offended by the thought of lecturing to women, even in segregated clinics, that he resigned and took an appointment at the University of Pennsylvania.[24]

In the short run, the dispute over women students' attendance at the Pennsylvania was resolved in a compromise. The medical staff agreed to admit the women students to one lecture a week. They established an elaborate protocol for cases "deemed by the lecturer indelicate or improper." The women students would be given an opportunity to withdraw; if they did not, the lecturer was allowed to dismiss the class. After discussion, the medical staff agreed that if female modesty did not prompt the women students' withdrawal, class simply would be dismissed.[25] The protocol speaks not only of a need to regulate the presence of women but of a panicked recognition that the normal constraints of polite society would not effect such regulation. Since the simple reproduction of male physicians had been disrupted, the whole economy of the gaze was in question, and the medical staff responded with a fever of regulation.

The controversy dragged on through the spring, when the managers asked the annual meeting of Pennsylvania Hospital contributors for guidance. Pamphlets, widely attributed to members of the medical staff, urged the contributors to set aside the action of the managers and to remove the present members of the board.[26] The contributors agreed, after discussion, that mixed lectures were inappropriate but urged the hospital to "arrange for appropriate, thorough clinical instruction . . . to the students of the Woman's Medical College of this city."[27] Separate lectures began in 1871 and continued for a number of years, although the faculty protested, at least once, that this troublesome obligation should be curtailed. The Woman's Medical College faculty professed themselves content and dissociated themselves from a group of women students, possibly from the Penn Medical University, who entered the amphitheater in 1871.[28] The separate lectures were interrupted for a time but were reestablished in 1875.[29]

In conventional medical history, the jeering incident is an episode in the story of growing professional control of hospitals. Although it is unclear that representation on the board of managers immediately increased the relative power of the medical staff, public controversy over the incident seems to have chastened the lay managers more than it did the staff physicians.[30] In feminist medical history, the Philadelphia jeering incident is an example of the harassment women medical students faced upon their entry into mixed-sex spaces of instruction. The jeering incident is also, I would argue, a demonstration of the place of women in the visual economy of medicine and of the disruption of that economy that women physicians effected.

Feminists writing about science, and particularly about medicine, have often described the scientific gaze as objectifying, reifying, and quintessentially male.[31] In the scientific imaginary, the masculine gaze penetrates an object, such as Nature, Life, or the Body, which has been constructed as female. Since Bacon, sexual conquest has been a powerful figure for that gaze; since the pioneering work of Evelyn Fox Keller, feminist students of science have demystified science's pose of objectivity and gender neutrality by considering how its imaginary structures are gendered. To investigate the story of medicine historically, however, is to encounter another gaze, that of the woman physician, absorbed in the pleasure of doing scientific work and most particularly the pleasure of seeing the exposed, or even dissected, body. That gaze is understood, by women physicians and their supporters, as productive of knowledge, of pleasure, and of a certain kind of care; the representation of the exposed or opened body is, in many ways, a textualization of the body alternate to that produced in medical writing. The medical spectacles that nineteenth-century women sought to witness were demonstrations that the body could be understood and treated; they mapped out a formerly unknown terrain and reduced it to a named and understood territory.

The clinical lecture, as a ceremony of patrilineal succession, was a key site for mapping the body; women seldom entered this space without controversy. Nineteenth-century medicine depended on an economy of the visual in which women were to be seen by physicians. While women saw quite enough of the body and of medical treatment as nurses and sickroom attendants, they were not themselves to see the body as the object of scientific knowledge. Most of all, they could not be seen as seeing; they could not be authorized witnesses of the scientific rationalization of the body.

Any disruption of this economy of the visual was controversial. When the Harvard medical faculty admitted Harriot Hunt to medical lectures in 1851, students protested:

199

Resolved, That no woman of true delicacy would be willing in the presence of men to listen to the discussion of the subjects that necessarily come under the consideration of the student of medicine.

Resolved, That we object to having the company of any female forced upon us, who is disposed to unsex herself, and to sacrifice her modesty, by appearing with men in the medical lecture room.

Resolved, That we are not opposed to allowing woman her rights, but do protest against her appearing in places where her presence is calculated to destroy our respect for the modesty and delicacy of her sex.[32]

After this student resolution, the faculty withdrew its concession to Hunt and explicitly excluded women from the medical school. The Harvard resolution established the themes generally invoked to excuse the harassment or exclusion of women medical students: for a woman to hear what medical students heard would be monstrous; no true women could bear it. The women medical students, then, must be females (rather than ladies) in search of sensation, people with whom medical students should not associate. The Harvard resolution ends with the infuriating concession that women's rights are certainly to be "allowed"; opponents of women's medical education often affirmed their support for women physicians, to be educated, one assumes, on a different planet.

Philadelphia had already seen its share of such events. In 1856, women students entered the surgical lecture of D. Hayes Agnew—the same professor who later resigned from the Pennsylvania Hospital to avoid teaching women—at the Blockley. A nude male patient was brought on stage, and the women students were bitterly harassed. When they persisted, Agnew petitioned the hospital board to bar women from further attendance.[33] Women did not return until 1869, when they were welcomed by Dr. Alfred Stillé. (Stillé later, as president of the American Medical Association, fought the admission of women, but he also served as an examiner at the Woman's Hospital and refused to comply with the Pennsylvania County Medical Society's ban on consultations with women.)

New York City women physicians responded to publicity about the Pennsylvania Hospital jeering incident with accounts of grotesque harassment upon their entry into the clinical lectures at Bellevue.[34] The patients, prisoners from a local jail, were crudely exposed and subjected to surgery without anesthesia. Even when an institution agreed to coeducation, women might be segregated in the clinical lecture. When the University of Michigan admitted women, they attended separate clinical lectures at the request of faculty; in 1881, the separation had diminished to a curtain or even a red line down the classroom floor.[35]

Similar scandals would take place abroad. In Canada, women medical students at Queen's University, Kingston, were put in an adjacent alcove "for awkward lectures"; they were harassed by the physiology professor, and left in protest after one outburst in 1881. The men demanded the expulsion of women, under the threat of a mass transfer to Trinity Medical School in Toronto. The Queen's University administration agreed to stop admitting women medical students, although those already matriculated were allowed to graduate.[36] A similar dispute over the exclusion of women anatomy students from Surgeons' Hall in Edinburgh had led to a riot in 1870. When the five women students, led by Sophie Jex-Blake, arrived at the Surgeons' Hall, they were trapped in the courtyard, jostled, pelted with mud and rotten vegetables, and abused with foul language. Inside the lecture room, there was continued harassment; a sheep was pushed into the amphitheater. Jex-Blake, not the most conciliatory of the early women physicians, accused a professor's assistant of inciting the riot. She was sued for libel, lost, and fined a farthing. But Edinburgh was not to admit women medical students until the First World War.[37]

These events confirm that women's entry into medicine required a realignment of complex economies of medical vision; it was a question not only of women doing the work of medicine but also of women seeing the work of medicine, and especially of women being seen by men to see the work of medicine. Those economies were disrupted by women's own very strong desires to see, particularly to see the interior of the body. We might also remember Mary Putnam Jacobi, in "Practical Study of Biology," rapt before a microscope,[38] and Anna Wharton's 1856 account of one of Ann Preston's popular physiological lectures:

> There were several pictures of the human body in different positions hung up, a skeleton and a figure in the middle, or nearly so, of the platform, covered over with a chintz bag. This was exposed to view after some preliminary remarks from Ann and proved to be one very well calculated to illustrate the ideas she wished to convey. It was soon turned inside out, that is taken to pieces, and exhibited and explained. I liked the lady's manner and ease, and was very much interested in what she communicated, but I knew most of the things she told us about.[39]

The "figure" was probably a papier-mâché model made in Europe. Such models, unlike the prohibitively expensive recumbent wax models, were intended for the use of medical students as low-budget supplements to dissection.[40] The organs were nested and detachable, as in the wax model, but they could withstand heat and handling and were numbered, referring students to a list of anatomical features. The Woman's Medical College announcements boasted that the school was well supplied with papier-mâché models, and Wharton's account demonstrates that they were a novelty. Normally the most fluent of correspondents, Wharton cannot quite find the syntax for a three-dimensional figure with detachable parts; she borrows from sewing, *turned inside out,* and finally settles on the mechanical *taken to pieces.* Unlike the skeleton or the "several pictures of the human body," the three-dimensional model, with its illusion of the body cavity opened to view, is considered sensitive and must be screened with domestic chintz until the audience is properly prepared. The practice of opening implies a decorum of covering.

Such spectacles and others like them—the public dissection of a brain or the display of "a colossal ear, capable of dissection," by the Ladies' Physiological Society of Boston, the microscopic soirées organized by the Woman's Medical College—spoke of the intense interest among nineteenth-century audiences, particularly audiences of women, in seeing what was hidden, and particularly the interior of the body.[41] Women wrote enthusiastic letters about these spectacles, which could be repeated informally at home. Sarah Mapps Douglass wrote to Rebecca White, a member of the Woman's Medical College Board of Lady Corporators, about a woman who took up a skull and a book of lectures on physiology and "hunted for the place where the eyestrings (muscles) where fastened. She then explained several things connected with it quite satisfactorily to me and to the wonder of her companions." Douglass herself earned $3.50 lecturing on the circulation of the blood to "38 deeply interested women" and enjoyed Ann Preston's lectures, exclaiming, "I cannot describe the pure intellect and enjoyment they give me."[42]

Barbara Stafford has brilliantly analyzed the formation of this desire to see what was hidden in the eighteenth century, tracing the connections among new technologies of graphic reproduction, intellectual disciplines of analysis, and such diverse images as caricatures, directions for the reproduction of intaglioed jewels, and Piranesi's etchings of Roman ruins. Conventions of medical illustration such as the opening and folding back of external tissues to reveal interior organs, the multiplication of images of the same feature in order to show it in various stages or conditions, and the practice of sketching specimens from one's own investigations were influential in domains remote from medicine. The medical image—opened, multiplied, bearing the marks of direct investigation—had already trained the vision of generations of the privileged readers with access to anatomies. Disciplines associated with medical display of the body had developed and popularized the central intellectual operations of abstraction and criticism, presenting these forms of mental work as practices productive of moral harmony and aesthetic pleasure. It is no wonder that, for many men and women in the nineteenth century, the display of the body or of models, skeletons, drawings, slides, or wax castings representing the body in the context of instruction was a particularly privileged scene.[43] Physiological instruction was understood as scientific,

moral, and parental; it was not prurient but virtuous to learn about the structures of the body; it did not endanger a woman's purity but informed her
maternal care.[44]

Images of the interior of the body in nineteenth-century culture were not
so widely dispersed as they have become for us. Although popular texts in
anatomy and physiology were cheap, available, and often consulted, such
information was concentrated rather than distributed widely in the culture.
Unlike contemporary news media, laden with cell diagrams and schematics
of bodily organs, nineteenth-century newspapers and illustrated magazines
did not include images of the interior of the body, although specifically physiological textbooks and anatomical atlases could be illustrated with engravings,
lithographs, and mezzotints of dazzling beauty and complexity. Until late in
the century, when new printing processes made illustrations cheaper, even
medical journals were very sparsely illustrated. Though many nineteenth-
century medical students would have learned to draw, they seldom made
their own sketches of the structures they had been shown in lectures or clinics. Medical students never included sketches of organs or structures in their
theses but instead wrote out laborious descriptions, specifying locations, at-
tachments, sizes, orientations, and colors. While medical images were anything but ubiquitous, they were available, and those who were interested in
them found ways to view them, subscribing to health-oriented periodicals
and lay physiological lectures or attending meetings of physiological groups.[45]

But the desired demonstration could easily become the dreaded exposure,
as in the nineteenth-century medical horror story of the exposed maiden.
This story appears in a number of contexts, with greater or lesser realization
of detail. It reemerges in the context of the Philadelphia jeering incident; it
is essentially a story of a disruption in the economy of the gaze. In the midst
of the jeering controversy, a letter to the editor of the New York *Herald
Tribune,* signed "A Mother," told the story of attending a clinic "in one of
the largest hospitals of the country." She described the examination of a
young woman patient with rheumatic fever, remarking on the neatness of
her clothing and bedding.[46] The woman was examined, showed her tongue,
and responded to questions:

> Watching her steadfastly from the very beginning, I had seen no motion nor sign
> of life, no curiosity in her face, no sidelong glance from her eye, nothing but an
> absolutely marble face and eyes fixed on the bed. Judge then what must have
> been my feeling when the Professor, in closing, said, "We will now notice
> whether there may be a fine red rash on the abdomen," and without a word of
> permission or warning, he turned down the clothing of the bed to the middle,
> and raised the entire clothing of the patient toward her neck, while he looked
> closely for the rash which he observed was not there, and which, in the nature

of the case, would not have been visible a single yard off. I did not look at the bared body, nor even scan the faces of the crowd, which latter I should like to have done. My eye was fixed on that pale face, and suddenly I saw waves of crimson sweeping round and round from chin to brow in quick successive flashes, wave after wave until the ordeal was past, and then I saw such a pallor settle on cheek and lip as made my heart stand still with awe.

This long quotation demonstrates a quite intense and remarkable web of identification connecting the spectator in the amphitheater and the patient, the most vividly realized character in this drama and the source of the shame that both writer and reader are invited to share. The writer observed the symptoms of shame just as the physician observed symptoms of illness. At the same time, the letter is itself an act of exposure, not only of the patient, whose case has now been circulated, albeit anonymously, in the press, but also of medical education. The amphitheater, after all, was not exactly a public space; although everyone knew that patients were examined publicly there, only doctors and students were normally admitted to the examination. But the general public enters the amphitheater with "A Mother" to see a medical education that brutally disregards the feelings of patients.[47]

Many writers responding to this letter thought that such an exposure would not have happened if women had been in the audience; others thought that it might still have happened and would have been even more shameful. These speculations are especially remarkable because they assume an exclusively male audience, even though the account is clearly written by a woman, and because it is quite likely that women medical students were actually in attendance at the clinical lecture where this event occurred. The story reorganizes the patient's body from the tableau of sickness, packaged on the cot, immobile and unitary, to a set of segmented parts, each of which displays a sign, the "minute rash" or the hectic blush. The patient is no longer available as an object of identification and care but becomes instead a site of instruction and labor. In the account of "A Mother," this transformation is phrased as a choice between gazing at the face and gazing at the stomach: the mother sees the face but not the stomach; the students see the stomach but not the face. The medical gaze erases female subjectivity, which can be restored only by a gaze that erases the body.

A cognate story was told by Dr. Emily A. Varney-Brownell in her autobiographical case history, "A Case of Hemoptysis."[48] Varney-Brownell argued that her initial attack of hemoptysis (spitting blood) was brought on "by a severe nervous shock, occasioned by insults, and ill treatment, from the male medical students at the Blockley in Philadelphia." She dated the event in 1854 and describes "silence soon broken by hisses and cheers" that greeted the four women students at their first appearance, followed by an escalating series of harassments, ending "in gross insults, such as the holding up to their view, on the end of a walking cane, a rag baby in miniature; and taking an imbecile by the arm and marching him up the aisle in a state of nudity." None of these exhibitions truly disturbed Varney-Brownell until a male student took a seat behind her and placed "his arm across the back of her chair, gradually bringing it nearer until it touched her back." She indignantly asked him, "Will you please move your arm, sir!!" but the "strain upon her nervous system" caused a hemorrhage of the lungs. For Varney-Brownell, harassment was an attempt to disorganize women's sight by offering them spectacles which were (somewhat stupidly) transgressive; the gaze, however, eventually gave way to touch, a violation of boundaries that catastrophically disorganized her body.

Other women responded differently to the exposed body of a patient. Mary Pratt, M.D., refuted "A Mother" in a letter to the *Herald Tribune*. This Woman's Medical College graduate attended the clinic described in the "A Mother" letter; she identified it as the Blockley's.[49] Pratt pointed out that the very affecting details of the patient's neatness and cared-for appearance were signs that she had been treated well, since she could not have done such things for herself. The doctor exposed the patient, Pratt explained, because he had found a symptom of typhoid and therefore was obligated to search for other signs of the disease. But Pratt insisted that "in so doing, *he did not* bare that woman's body to the atmosphere of that room." And she turned the Mother's segmenting gaze back upon her: "The writer says: 'I did not look at the bared body; my eyes were too intently fixed on the pale face.' How then did she *know* that the body was bared?" Pratt later visited the patient herself and found that she did not remember any of the details recounted in "A Mother" but appreciated her doctor's devoted care. Pratt concluded, "So you see the flushing and paling, the sinking and nerving, of which the writer speaks must have had their origin in her own morbid imagination." Pratt criticized the Mother's logic of identification, foregrounding her role in the triangular exchanges of gaze and object. The gaze of the Mother on the face of the patient signified not steadfast and devoted care but a form of inattention, an inability to appreciate the medical questions at issue. A brutal and gratuitous display becomes a disinterested inquiry; the Mother's gaze promises not succor but shame; the morbid imagination of the writer produces exposure. It is as if Stendhal had been rewritten by Flaubert; all the inflamed language of social exposure, the whole presence of the palpitating body, has been transformed into a dry and satiric recitation of symptoms, in which the chief source of infection is found to be the reader.

In this vexed economy, the gaze of a woman was sometimes felt to be a benign corrective. Her powers of sympathy would stabilize the uncertain energies of the medical spectacle. Charles Reade's fictional woman physician, Rhoda Gale, describes a mixed clinic where women medical students

205

hung back during the examinations of male patients but "did crowd round the beds of the female patients, and claimed the inner row: AND SIR, THEY THANKED GOD FOR US OPENLY."[50] In the same spirit, many of the comments on the jeering incident speak of the women medical students' moderating influence on the Blockley lectures and at Zurich.[51] Similar arguments on the edifying effect of women spectators emerged in earlier controversies, such as that over Elizabeth Blackwell's presence at anatomical lectures. She saw her attendance at the more delicate lectures on anatomy as "the real test of the influence of a woman upon the conduct and character of a man in co-education," especially since the professor was

> a rollicking, jovial man, who constantly interspersed his lectures with witty remarks and funny anecdotes. Nor did he study to have his language chaste, or the moral of his stories pure and elevating. In fact, vulgarity and profanity formed a large part of his ordinary lectures; and especially was this true of the lectures on the branch of anatomy above mentioned. On this account, chiefly, he was exceedingly popular with his class; and during his lectures stamping, clapping, and cheering were the principal employments of the students.

Blackwell wrote a note to the professor, arguing that she should attend the anatomical lectures, fearing no impropriety, since the study of medicine could not fail to make all doctors reverent. Professor and students agreed to her attendance, and the lectures on anatomy that followed were unusually comprehensive and thorough.[52]

For other observers, the presence of a woman in the audience at a clinical lecture transposed it from a scientific ritual to a sensational spectacle. For a medical student interviewed by the *Philadelphia Press*, even exposure at the Blockley was too much: "Q. Women are present at the clinics held at the Blockley Almshouse, are they not? A. Yes, sir; the laws of this institution are such that a patient is obliged to expose his person, consequently the effect has been to shame the modesty alike of the surgeons and male students. The women have their own hospital; why not let them attend it?"[53] The Pennsylvania Hospital was a much more respectable civic institution, and students there would be disgusted by the presence of "young women who could gaze at, unmoved, and perhaps handle objects of the most repulsive kind, some of them evidences of disease resulting from vicious and criminal indulgences, and requiring for their exhibition unseemly exposure of the person of the patient."[54] The same visual economy structured the story of the exposed maiden and the jeering incident; to see a patient was, in some sense, to become that patient—in the imagined case, an immoral patient whose disease was his own fault. Identification quickly becomes contagion, and the presence of a woman spectator breached the gender decorum that contained it within the story of professional reproduction.

In its "Remonstrance against Mixed Clinics" the Philadelphia medical establishment implicated itself in this economy. The "Remonstrance" was, in effect, the official medical response to the jeering incident. It was silent on the actions of the male medical students but eloquent in its denunciation of the mixed clinics. Such clinics violated the modesty of male patients: "It cannot be assumed, by any right-minded person, that male patients should be subjected to inspection before a class of females, although this inspection may, without impropriety, be submitted to before those of their own sex." Such exposure would strain and embarrass the lecturer, and instruction would suffer. In cases of surgery, the "Remonstrance" continued, the stakes were even higher:

> In many operations upon male patients, exposure of the body is inevitable, and demonstrations must be made which are unfitted for the observation of students of the opposite sex. These expositions, when made under the eye of such a conjoined assemblage, are shocking to the sense of decency, and entail the risk of unmanning the surgeon—of distracting his mind, and endangering the life of his patient.

The "Remonstrance" ends by warning—appropriately, it seems—that the attendance of women at mixed clinic would break down the "barrier of respect" between men and women.[55]

Here again, the presence of women destabilizes the visual economy of the amphitheater. The mixed audience is referred to as a *conjoined assemblage,* recalling the body as it is presented in surgery, as a layered congeries of parts. The lecturer's demonstration, his "exposition," is also a "shocking" exposure, so that the sense of a dangerous spectacle moves from the lecturer, to the exposed patient, to the listening assemblage. And, with the candor that marked so many nineteenth-century discourses of gender, such exposure is identified as a danger to the manhood of the lecturer, the only security for the life of the patient. Seldom have the relations among gender, knowledge, and control been more baldly stated. Only the identification between the urbane lecturer and his male students contained the suffering patient as object of knowledge. The presence of women students raised the terrifying possibility that the viewers of the spectacle could themselves become objects of a cool, surveying gaze. A woman who could engage in such an action must herself be lost to modesty, or, as one writer put it, the women students "disrobed themselves, on this occasion, of the attractive and even protecting vesture of modesty and shrinking reserve from all needless exposure, and chose to appear in a state of demi-moral nudity."[56] Such exposure excused anything: harassment on the street, jeers, catcalls, even, at other times and places, the sad carnival of naked men paraded into the amphitheater and of sheep among the benches, even the grotesque Bellevue incidents. Once the economy of the gaze had been disrupted, no other boundaries held, not the boundaries of the body or the differences between human and animal, between medicine and torture. The women medical students had themselves become spectacles and took refuge in their status as impassive members of the audience, offering their own professional decorum, a performance of not being on display: "The eyes of half the audience were on the lady students who sat calm and unruffled under this brutal treatment, their looks riveted on the lecturer, as if utterly oblivious of aught else that was transpiring."[57]

For the women medical students, the humiliation of being seen, being gazed at, could be rectified only by a redirection of the spectacle in which the male medical students were themselves exposed and held up to scorn. It is remarkable, but probably not accidental, that three scrapbooks survive in the papers of the Woman's Medical College and of the thirty-odd alumnae who entered the clinical lectures. The college scrapbooks gather clippings from the major Philadelphia and New York dailies, weekly magazines, and smaller local papers. Eliza Wood-Armitage carefully kept a smaller scrapbook of clippings. Sarah Hibbard, one of the more eccentric Woman's Medical College students, wrote out collections of quotations from press accounts of the jeering incident in one of her draft "lectures and sermons." "I will not give particulars," she wrote, "I will quote however a few lines from one of the leading journals upon this subject." One quote leads to another; soon, Hibbard has four pages of extracts, a kind of handwritten scrapbook.[58] The jeering incident was an attempt to shame women medical students out of the first important professional public space they had been allowed to enter. They countered this exposure by collecting, arranging, and preserving public accounts in which their harassers had been exposed and shamed; as in the amphitheater, the gaze of another was much more powerful than one's own. The scrapbooks painstakingly compiled by the students of the Woman's Medical College construct a kind of portable public space, a transposition of the abstract relations of public discourse, in which writers address a general audience, to the domestic form of the album.

The visual economy of the nineteenth-century medical amphitheater is aligned, in many ways, with that of the nineteenth-century theater, which was a central location for forming the relations between representations and spectators. It is perhaps relevant to the jeering incident that the conventions of theatergoing excluded ladies unescorted by men from the theater. Mary Ryan's study of the gender geography of public space records an observation that, in a Broadway theater, "one-quarter of the house is set aside exclusively for the use of [prostitutes] in which they nightly and publicly drive their sickening trade"; her characterization of the theater as a "den of male sociability" tellingly recalls the assumption of male medical students and faculty that unconstrained exposition would be impossible in the presence of women.[59] The medical amphitheater may have realized, for some participants, a fantasy of an entirely male theatrical space, one in which the spectacular body of the patient supports an intense identification between the lecturer and the audience.

And nineteenth-century physicians advised their patients about the theater, just as they pronounced on diet, clothing, and ventilation. In his 1850 thesis, "An Essay on the Moral and Physical Education of Females," University of Pennsylvania medical student Abram Smith compared the Roman matron at the Colosseum to the modern theatergoer; his account of the theater's attractions and dangers becomes all too lively:

> Wherever you see a theater you will find plenty drinking houses, grogshops, and whoever chooses to give them a visit will find them filled with our Chesnut St. mustached dandies with their segar in one hand and a glass of brandy in the other, as speaking of the gentlemen is getting off my subject. I only mention it to show the moral influence a theatre exerts within its neighbourhoods. One great cause which affects the health of our theatre going ladies, is the late hour to which they are exposed. The piece is generally long. Which occupies them until eleven or twelve oclock. Whoever that has been at a theatre knows of kind of persons the audience is composed of. Let the fair "belle" who would not condescend to speak to their servants in the kitchen take a look at the "pit and third tier" and see the company they are in. And if they do not blanch their moral feelings must be refined indeed.[60]

Smith, who later in the thesis apologized for writing such a "nauseous" paragraph,[61] here recorded quite accurately the wandering identification of the spectacle. The lady who goes to the theater comes to resemble the dandy with his segar and his brandy, the bad company of the cheap seats, and especially the performer, who throws "her light fantastic legs above her head, exposing her form to the whole audience."[62] The mere presence of a woman at such a spectacle shows her to be without moral feeling; she has made herself available as an object of the gaze.

And the same D. Hayes Agnew who had resigned from the Pennsylvania Hospital rather than lecture to women was also an active antitheatrical pamphleteer. His memorialist, in fact, connected his "belief that the theatres, against which he once wrote a vigorous philippic, were on the whole both a cause and a symptom of moral deterioration in the community" and his disapproval of "the co-education of the sexes, [and] of the medical education of women under any circumstances, believing that any possible advantages to them were far more than counterbalanced by what he thought would be the inevitable loss of dignity and delicacy resulting from the association of the sexes under such conditions and from the character of their studies." Agnew was willing to suffer for these beliefs: "In accord with the one opinion

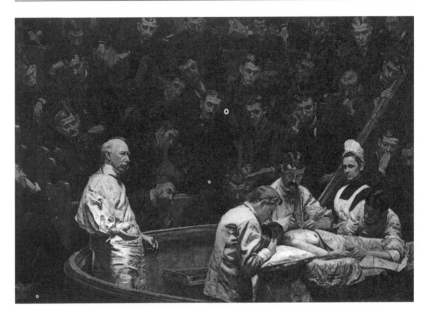

Figure 13. Thomas Eakins's *The Agnew Clinic,* unveiled at the University of Pennsylvania on May 1, 1889, to commemorate Agnew's retirement (Photograph courtesy of the University of Pennsylvania School of Medicine)

he denied himself during his whole life the pleasure he would undoubtedly have derived from seeing the masterpieces of the drama, many of which he was fond of quoting, enacted on the stage. In accord with the other, he resigned a valuable hospital position, and, in spite of strong pressure, refused many lucrative consultations."[63]

A moral rejection of the theater might seem to be a contradictory position for a man whose medical lectures were known to "make the boys yell," who performed twice a week, for most of his life, in a space known as an amphitheater, and who is shown, in Eakins's painting *The Agnew Clinic,* in his customary (and quite dramatic) attitude, addressing attentive students, while an assistant finishes surgery (a mastectomy, and therefore at this time a palliative procedure) on the unconscious woman patient.[64] (See figure 13.) It was not that Agnew disliked the performance or even the theater; he found it "fascinating in the extreme." Its very liveliness of representation made it an effective enticement: "Satan could not arrange a more complete programme to seduce the souls of men into actual and mental whoredom."[65] And Agnew's antitheatrical pamphlet deploys the same unstable economy of identification that made the presence of women physicians at the clinical lecture so disturbing. Agnew considered theaters dens of prostitution, hated theatrical dances in which women were "twirled, and handled," but objected most of all to the "distinct personations" of dramatic performance, the fact that vices were there "faithfully imitated." For Agnew, since representations of virtue could never be as exciting as those of vice, the theater must be a display of compelling and exciting images of evil. Those who saw such characters were drawn by their very vividness and variety, no matter how the plot condemned or punished them. For a woman to witness such a performance was to become part of the spectacle: "How dare she meet the vulgar gaze of gaping spectators, the coarse laugh and boisterous plaudits of pit and dome; and mingle with the vilest libertines who disgrace God's footstool."[66] Agnew's objections to women physicians were phrased in quite similar terms. In his inaugural lecture at the School of Medicine of the University of Pennsylvania, given immediately after he had resigned from the Pennsylvania Hospital, Agnew argued that while women were generally mentally and physically unsuited to the demands of medicine, those few who were suited to medical work were monstrous, at once an illicit spectacle and illicit spectators:

> It is within the range of possibility, under modern views, to develop a race of women, who may yet inaugurate a Platonic republic, where men and women may wrestle in the same gymnasium, *nuda cum nudis;* or, like the Greeks, plunge into the same bath; or maidens, like those of Rome, who could witness unmoved the fierce encounters of the Coliseum, and after the slaughter was ended, sit down, in the arena wet with human gore, to enjoy a sumptuous repast.

Agnew chillingly warned that such women would forfeit the protection of men; if a woman sought to "amputate limbs, make perineal section, or cut for stone; let her remember there are laws controlling the social structure of society, the operation of which will disrobe her of all those qualities now the glory of the sex, and will cast her down in the dust of the earth."[67] The woman physician, like the woman at the theater, was both exposed and put at risk by what she saw.

These antitheatrical warnings model the anxieties that attended women's entrance to the clinical amphitheater. That space, that "Holy of Holies,"[68] could easily become a scene of carnival disorder, no better than the vulgar display of the commercial theater, in which the body was excited, betrayed into disorganized identification, and subjected to contagion. A woman who saw, with the eye of science, the spectacle of exposure, disrupted the gender binary that guaranteed scientific detachment. She transformed the men who saw her watching into a disorderly mob. These anxieties became more intense, and also more contained, when the spectacle was staged in yet another privileged space—the dissecting room.

211

THE DISSECTING ROOM

If the clinical lecture was a liminal space where the hospital met the medical college, where patient care met instruction, where students from diverse institutions gathered, the dissecting room was the heart of an individual medical school. Each school maintained its own dissection room and hired a Demonstrator of Anatomy to secure material and supervise students. Although dissection was an optional experience for male medical students, they were expected to perform autopsies, practice surgical procedures on cadavers, and dissect "parts." Those who wanted additional instruction could attend such private institutes as the Philadelphia School of Anatomy, directed by none other than D. Hayes Agnew, which taught 200 to 250 students a year during the 1850s.[69]

In some ways, the practice of the dissecting room was not particularly marked by gender. When Woman's Medical College student Mary Theodora McGavran visited the Hahnemann dissecting room in 1899, she remarked, "A mans dissecting room doesn't differ materially from a womans—Ours is a little larger I think."[70] There is no evidence that women medical students followed dissection procedures different in any way from those of male medical students, although the atmosphere of the room was probably quite different from that of the men's schools. And women students told the same stories of dissection as male medical students: they were frightened or repulsed at first but grew fascinated by what they learned; sometimes they made jokes about the body they were dissecting or imagined it as reanimated. Three accounts of dissection from the 1890s establish the range. Edith Flower Wheeler remarked that the dissecting room "did not smell like a rose garden" and that she had to "beat down the aversion to cutting flesh that had once been living, even as you or I." But, she declared, it could be done, and "in time the interest blotted out the shrinking."[71] Later, practicing surgery on a corpse, Wheeler indulged in gallows humor: "I did a laparotomy on a patient today, a dead one. Had lots of fun. Succeeded in poking holes through everything that I ought not to. If my patient had not been dead to start with, she would have been deader'n a door nail by the time I got through."[72] Anne Walter Fearn, an 1893 graduate of the Woman's Medical College, remembered her dissection experiences forty years later: Just before dawn, as she prepared a corpse for the next day's demonstration, she "tugged at the tendon on the arm outstretched on a board. The arm jerked, clasped itself around my waist, and stayed there."[73] Unlike male students, however, women students do not seem to have been prone to sexual humor in the dissecting room.[74] But they did joke about their fears of dissection and sometimes personified the skeletons they studied. (See figure 14, in which

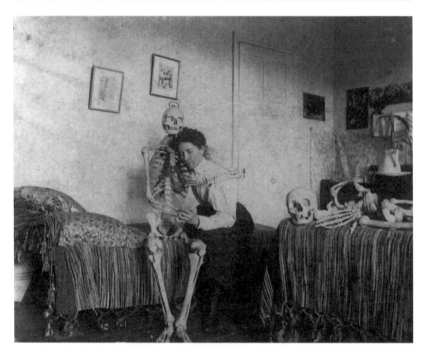

Figure 14. Sylvia Hatton (WMC 1899) with "Chimmie Fadden," her nicknamed skeleton, 1895–96 (Archives and Special Collections on Women in Medicine, MCP Hahnemann University)

Sylvia Hatton [Woman's Medical College graduate, 1899] clowns with "Chimmie Fadden," her skeleton, and figure 15, in which four members of the class of 1896 arrange themselves in a column, embraced by the head and forearms of a skeleton. Both photographs flaunt the medical students' comfort with images of death; both play with the incongruity of the image of death and the maiden transposed into a professional and scientific setting. Sylvia Hatton is studying the articulation of her skeleton's wrist, and the naked, grinning skull in the 1896 photograph is juxtaposed with the new graduates' serious faces, caps, and gowns.)

Early in the history of the Woman's Medical College, the construction of the dissecting room and the appointment of the Demonstrator were sensitive decisions. The first annual announcement assured readers that "**The Anatomical Rooms** will be furnished with every convenience and *kept strictly private*. They will be under the supervision of the Professor of Anatomy, *aided by competent female assistants*."[75] The Demonstrator of Anatomy

213

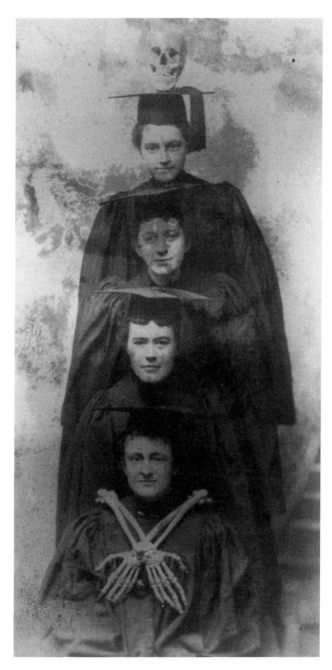

Figure 15. *Top to bottom:* Elizabeth Wray-Howell, M.D., Mary Montgomery Marsh, M.D., Grace Shermerhorn, M.D., and Laura Hills, M.D. (from whose scrapbook this picture was taken), graduates of the Woman's Medical College of Pennsylvania, class of 1896 (Archives and Special Collections on Women in Medicine, MCP Hahnemann University)

was, like the clinic assistant, a highly trusted graduate; she was probably the first woman to work as a professional instructor in an American medical school. When the demonstrator had some difficulty obtaining "material," the faculty passed a resolution that "the Demonstrator in this College has all the rights and privileges of the most favored Demonstrator in this City and she is authorized to purchase and prepare subjects for Demonstration and present or sell them to the class at her own expense."[76] (The minutes often mention the janitor, however, as the person responsible for procuring a corpse.) And the faculty and corporators agreed that the dissecting room should be separate from the school and closed to men; in this space, there would be no untoward mixing of the genders. The act of dissection was to be carried out in privacy, almost in secrecy; the book of the body would open itself only in an enclosed space.

In the mid-nineteenth-century medical economy of the visual, dissection occupied a privileged place. The work was done under an inexorable time constraint; without refrigeration or reliable preservatives, dissection had to be done quickly and only in the winter. (*Frankenstein* is, among other things, a demonstration of the dangers of summer dissection.) The corpse was held and propped, sometimes with the tools that would have restrained the living body for surgery without anesthesia, sometimes with more industrial supports. Such supports are visible in the background of a student group photograph taken in the Woman's Medical College anatomy laboratory in 1897. (See figure 16.) The scene of dissection could become grotesque. Consider, for example, the following directions for dissection of the (male) perineum, from Wilson's *System of Human Anatomy:*

> To dissect the perineum, the subject should be fixed in the position for lithotomy, that is, the hands should be bound to the soles of the feet, and the knees kept apart. An easier plan is the drawing of the feet upwards by means of a cord passed through a hook in the ceiling. Both of these plans of preparation have for their object the full exposure of the perineum. And as this is a dissection which demands some degree of delicacy and nice manipulation, a strong light should be thrown upon the part. Having fixed the subject, and drawn the scrotum upwards by means of string or hook, carry an incision from the base of the scrotum along the ramus of the pubes and ischium and tuberosity of the ischium, to a point parallel with the apex of the coccyx; then describe a curve over the coccyx to the same point on the opposite side, and continue the incision onwards along the opposite tuberosity, and along the ramus of the ischium and of the pubes, to the opposite side of the scrotum, where the two extremities may be connected by a transverse incision. This incision will completely surround the perineum, following very nearly the outline of its boundaries. Now let the student dissect off the integument carefully from the whole of the included space, and he will expose the fatty cellular structure of the common superficial fascia, which exactly resembles the superficial fascia in every other situation. . . .[77]

215

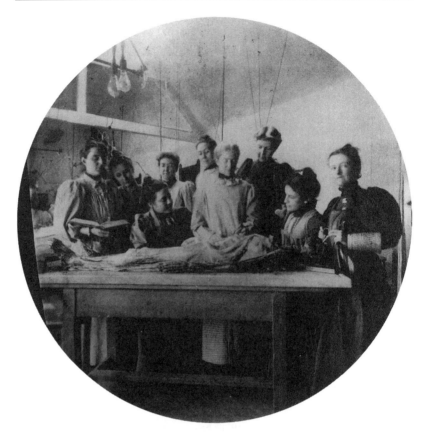

Figure 16. Student group photograph in anatomy laboratory (note supports and apparatus in the background), class of 1897 (Archives and Special Collections on Women in Medicine, MCP Hahnemann University)

The spectacle of the exposed corpse is presented to the presumably male student as a double bind: having secured and exposed his subject and performed what must have seemed to be a castration, the student is to find nothing unusual in the tissues of the genitals, only superficial fascia that resemble those of "every other situation." The work of dissection performed a spectacular exposure of the body in order to assure the student that there was nothing in particular to expose; the student is invited to reframe the corpse and its genitals with the eye of science and then to proceed below the superficial.

The copy of Wilson's *System of Human Anatomy* from which this quote was taken belonged to Ann Preston. Preserved as a relic, it is carefully marked; Preston drew the indexing letters onto the corresponding structures in Wilson's drawings, underlined passages, and kept lists of scientific facts on the flyleaves—complementary colors, distances of the planets from the sun. Presumably, Preston moved from the anatomy's painstaking topographic prose to the engraved illustrations to the material body in front of her. The anatomy text offered her a particular mapping of the body, which she surrounded with other systematic reductions of the natural world. It was her task as a student to transform the corpse before her into an approximation of the anatomical text and figure, to make a "preparation" of an organ or system that "demonstrated" its structures and relations. In dissection, the work of seeing was supported by the work of arranging and constructing; the opening of the body revealed nature, but the labor of the student rendered it intelligible. Preston's copy of *Anatomy* speaks of the struggle of students at the early Woman's Medical College to normalize for themselves the culture of dissection, to find their place in the visual economy of medicine.

Often, their normalization worked; the act of dissection spoke to intense desires of women students for a particular experience of the body and could be articulated with cultural practices, popular in reform circles, of physiological investigation. The Woman's Medical College Alumnae Association memorial notice for Ida Richardson, who graduated from the college in 1879, spoke of her conversion to dissection. Richardson had resisted the whole idea of a medical career because she hated publicity but had finally decided that she was divinely called to be a doctor. Her doubts continued through her first year of medical school, and she decided to test her vocation by beginning to dissect. An older student urged her to "accustom herself to the room."

> At first she resisted, but finally yielded, and consented to sit by while the others worked, and read to them from the anatomy in regard to the tissues uncovered in the dissection. Soon after this she began the work for herself, and instead of its weaning her from her chosen course, she forgot the unpleasantness in the marvelous beauty of the hidden tissues of the human frame. Her enthusiasm over dissection was so great that she aroused all the students around her and carried them with her, and became the life of the room.[78]

This is not the "necessary inhumanity" which historian Ruth Richardson has identified as the dissector's response to "tasks which would, in normal circumstances, be taboo or emotionally repugnant," understandable though that would be.[79] Instead, Ida Richardson seems to have experienced an aesthetic conversion, a slowly staged seduction by the beauty of the interior spaces of the body. Precisely because the dissection room was private, remote from the publicity that she dreaded,[80] Richardson could enter its visual economy by reading aloud, appropriating the voice of the text. Her memorialist uses not the language of scientific conquest but that of bodily care and appropriation; we read of weaning, of arousal, of life.

Many of the early women physicians had been attracted to dissection from girlhood; we might recall Hannah Longshore's dissection of "the bodies of insects, rodents, and domestic animals . . . as at times convenient they fell into my hands," and Mary Putnam Jacobi's designs on the rat's heart in the barn.[81] For others, dissection was, as for Richardson, a trial of their vocation. When Elizabeth Blackwell was preparing for medical study, one of her fellow teachers gave her a dead cockchafer (a large beetle) "as a first subject for dissection":

> I accepted the offer, placed the insect in a shell, held it with a hair-pin, and then tried with my mother-of-pearl handled penknife to cut it open. But the effort to do this was so repugnant that it was some time before I could compel myself to make the necessary incision, which revealed only a little yellowish dust inside.[82]

Striking in this account is Blackwell's attempt to perform a "scientific" dissection with the paraphernalia of feminine charm: a shell, a hairpin, a decorative knife. No wonder she felt queasy. Later, in Philadelphia, Blackwell studied in a private anatomical school. The teacher

> by his thoughtful arrangements enabled me to overcome the natural repulsion to these studies generally felt at the outset. With a tact and delicacy for which I have always felt grateful, he gave me as my first lesson in practical anatomy a demonstration of the human wrist. The beauty of the tendons and exquisite arrangements of this part of the body struck my artistic sense, and appealed to the sentiment of reverence with which this anatomical branch of study was ever afterwards invested in my mind.[83]

Again, Blackwell's dissection is organized as a private study, an inquiry into the subjectivity of the anatomist. She brought the wrist to her room and worked on it there. She demonstrated the tendons and bones of the corpse's wrist, but it was her own hand and wrist that opened them to view. Dissection disclosed the structure of the body, including the body of the dissector.

If dissection was for Galen an opening of the body "in order to see deeper or hidden parts," for nineteenth-century women physicians this act of opening and viewing could become pleasurable.[84] In a culture that did not have x rays or microscopic photographs, not to mention sonograms or MRIs, the pleasures of dissection could be modeled, at least for reform women, on the newly acceptable pleasures of reading fiction. If the clinical lecture aroused the anxieties associated with theatrical performance, dissection, after the first "horrors" were past, could become as interesting, as absorbing, as novel reading. The body, since the Enlightenment, had been seen as a "book of nature": the illustration in Johann Kulmus's 1732 collection of anatomical plates shows a library, unveiled by a female allegorical figure, where a female dissector invites us to inspect a female corpse arranged on the revolving table. (See figure 17.) Both the body and the books are closed, but only for the moment. This trope was still robust in nineteenth-century medical discourse. D. Hayes Agnew, anatomist and opponent of the medical education of women, declared in his 1870 introductory lecture that dissection was "a charming task" and proclaimed: "The lifeless frame is the greatest of all books. Turn over its leaves with untiring diligence. You can never know its contents too well."[85] As we have seen, dissection was itself guided by the directions in an anatomy text; a student not lucky enough to have Ida Richardson reading aloud could keep the anatomy propped before her as a reference, so that there was an unusually intimate correspondence between the written word and the materials of the body that students uncovered. (See figure 18.) That correspondence mediated the labor of dissection; rather than experiencing it as *work,* both Richardson and Blackwell (like Longshore, or Jacobi in "A Martyr for Science")[86] saw dissection as a practice of *seeing,* opening the body to an intent gaze. Paradoxically, dissection at once dissolved the body and revealed it. Familiar limbs and features gave way to fascia, everywhere the same, and revealed the bones, heart, and stomach everyone had experienced in her own body but had never seen before.

The family group, listening to novels about lives like their own, forming themselves as spectators of the newly elaborated institutions of authorship and entertainment, themselves immobile and absorbed, had something in common with these avid women, gathered in a private room, gazing into a (radically) immobile body which they had in a material sense made to disappear, working out the correspondences between its structures and a text arranged before them. Both the dissected body and the literary text required artful arrangement; both displayed the labor of delicate preparation. And, like the readers of domestic fiction, the woman medical student engaged in dissection was also an object of moral instruction, finding religious lessons in the structures she uncovered.[87] If the sensibility developed in the reading of literature was, from the early days of the Republic, an "idiom that specializes in inside-outside transferences," that idiom could structure the work of dissection, the ultimate realignment of bodily borders.[88]

The dissected body could be an intensely particular scene of instruction, both scientific and moral. In 1886, Rachel Bodley, dean of the Woman's Medical College of Pennsylvania, received a "singular request" from a woman with whom she had corresponded on religious matters; the woman wanted her body to be claimed after death as the property of several Woman's Medical College professors and to be dissected as a test of her theory about the continuation of sexual sensation after the ovaries had been removed. The correspondent claimed that a Dr. Mills had published this the-

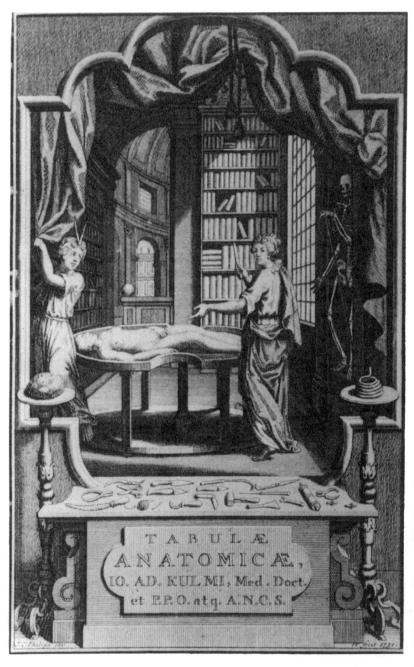

Figure 17. *The Human Body and the Library as Sources of Knowledge*, illustration for Johann Adam Kulmus's *Tabulae anatomicae*, Amsterdam, 1732 (Photograph courtesy of the History of Medicine Division, National Library of Medicine, Washington, D.C.)

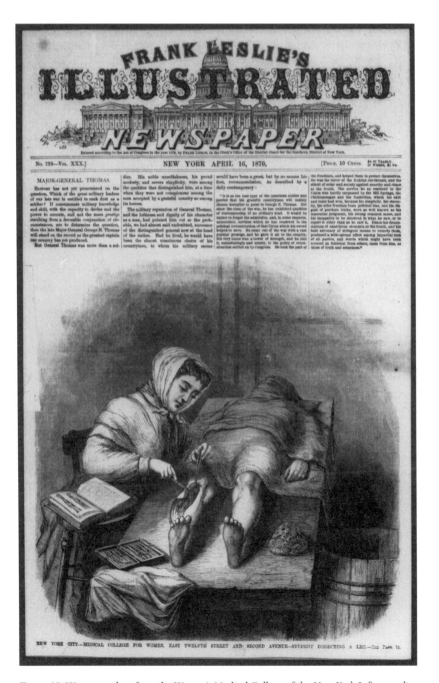

Figure 18. Woman student from the Woman's Medical College of the New York Infirmary dissecting a leg, illustration for *Frank Leslie's Illustrated Newspaper*, April 16, 1870 (Photograph courtesy of the History of Medicine Division, National Library of Medicine, Washington, D.C.)

ory, although she had never seen the publication.[89] She wanted to be dissected so that she could "prove on her body," to use Ann Preston's phrase, "why a consciousness of sensation in the lower sexual organs, remains when there is no motor sensation passing above the space from which the ovaries have been removed." She outlined a theory of a residual nerve connection in the stump; accordingly, she directed that the nerves should be "traced back to their roots so that proof may be had that the cure of nymphomania by oophorectomy is effected by separating some telegraphic connection leading from the sexual organs to the brain." If her theory was proved, the correspondent asked that her case history and the results of the investigation be "read before the students of the Woman's College" and later published "for the benefit of science"; she listed two physicians and two lay people who should be invited to the lecture. But the will was to remain utterly secret until the woman's death. An appended note says that no physician "would have a right to urge this operation upon a patient" and describes her own history as "that of a woman . . . who was willing to lose her life rather than have it stained with shame"; she ends by acknowledging that "the peace God gave her [such as it was] has been dearly bought, but the price is not too much for anyone who wants to do right." Much of this deeply felt document is obscure; it seems that the writer had suffered from something that was diagnosed as nymphomania and that, although she submitted to an oophorectomy, she was surprised to still feel sensations from the "lower sexual organs." Although she had her own ideas about the cause of these sensations, only dissection could settle the case, tracing her sensations to their roots. Through dissection, the intensely private experience that dominated this writer's life would become public. Her case would be known; her body displayed; an appropriately selected audience would witness the physical truth of her condition; and a more anonymous account would enter the scientific record. This dissection would do the work that another writer might have undertaken in an autobiographical novel or memoir: representing to a discerning audience the intractable truth of an embodied life. What the writer could not know about herself would be known because of her; the unresolved contradiction of her final note—at once condemning the operation and enjoining it as not too much for someone who aspired to do right—would be settled by dissection and proclaimed in a systematic scientific discourse. Dissection was so much a practice of reading that, for Bodley's correspondent, it was also a practice of writing.

While it was generally less controversial than attendance at mixed clinical lectures, women's practice of dissection could also be seen as threatening, particularly in mixed settings. At the coeducational National College of Medicine at the Columbian University in Washington, D.C., tensions between men and women students came to a crisis in 1892. Zakrzewska's autobiography reports that some of the male students "so debased themselves by offering insult, not only to the women medical students, but also to the helpless bodies of their fellow beings who had been given to them for scientific study," that official action was required.[90] The faculty and trustees voted not to admit any more women students. In *The Gilded Age*, Ruth Bolton found herself at night in the dissecting room with the corpse of an African American man who is imagined as objecting to the humiliation of ending a life of oppression by being dissected by a woman.[91] Much worse things could be imagined: the *Boston Medical and Surgical Journal* of February 23, 1871, ran a story under the heading "Outrage at a Woman's Medical College," which was reprinted from the *Richmond and Louisville Medical Journal*.[92] It told of students at the Cleveland Medical College who had received the body of a poor woman for postmortem examination and had pledged to give it a decent burial. An Episcopal minister was secured, and rites were performed, but "suspicions were aroused" by the lack of a grave in the cemetery:

> The coffin was then opened and found to contain billets of wood. The body, the "lady students" had retained for their delectable entertainment! Apart from the revolting and repulsive enormities of such a scandalous transaction, and apart, also, from the abhorrent violations of a sacred pledge, how can any one, in terms sufficiently excoriating, denounce those who would thus deliberately have performed over a mass of wood, the most sacred and solemn rites known to man? Such appalling blasphemy is without precedent and beyond description.

The writers seem equally scandalized by the ceremony at the empty grave and the theft of the body; for them, the case demonstrated that a woman who left her sphere was soon "lost to every instinct which brings to her sex its tenderest blessings." Like the staff of Pennsylvania Hospital, zealously regulating the cancellation of indelicate lectures, these writers feared that any change in women's customary place in the visual economy of medicine would lead to unnameable transgressions. The vectors of the moralizing scene of dissection are reversed: the body disappeared, not because it was opened to science, but because it had been stolen. Dissection involved not private instruction but a fraudulent public display. Rather than a confirmation of piety, the dissection led to blasphemy. Only the absorption, the interest, the "delectable entertainment," is the same.

Faced with such intractable discursive energies, women physicians and their supporters drew upon all their rhetorical resources to justify their presence both at clinical lectures and in the dissecting room. Sometimes they argued from consistency, a warhorse of the movement for women's medical education: if women were inherently modest, then respect for their modesty required female doctors. Or consistency could motivate equal treatment: if male students saw female patients in clinical lectures, then women students should see male patients treated: "These ladies had an absolute right there; they were admitted by precisely the same authority that admitted the black-guards; and more than this, it was right that they should accept the privilege offered them if they wished to do so."[93] But the argument from consistency could be complicated by the logic of the separate female sphere. If women's modesty required female physicians, then men's modesty must be protected from the gaze of women. "The women have their own hospital; why not let them attend it?"[94] The Woman's Medical College faculty extended the principle of consistency to the patient exposed in the clinical lecture; this argument was seldom taken up by their supporters:

> Into these clinics, women also—often sensitive and shrinking, albeit poor—are brought as patients to illustrate the lectures, and we maintain that wherever it is proper to introduce women as patients, there also it is but just and in accordance with the instincts of the truest womanhood for women to appear as physicians and students.[95]

But of course, this argument could cut two ways: if male medical students were "coarsened" by viewing women patients, then medical women were tainted by seeing male patients. And of course there was the modesty of the male patient, the male medical students, the male lecturer, all of which found their own advocates.

Against these claims, supporters of women's medical education advanced the proposition we first met in Zakrzewska's autobiography, that "science has no sex." Science was proposed as a neutral ground between the genders. The faculty of the Woman's Medical College argued:

> We maintain, in common with all medical men, that science is impersonal, and that the high aim of relief to suffering humanity sanctifies all duties; and we repel, as derogatory to the profession of medicine, the assertion that the physician who has risen to the level of his high calling need be embarrassed, in treating general diseases, by the presence of earnest women students.[96]

Journalists made the same point more floridly:

> If all medical students could be endowed with a proper conception of the work they have in hand they would quickly part with all restricting observances, would lose their personality in the great search for truth, would be transported to that ideal sphere where mind holds communion with the Infinite, and where no unclean thought is allowed to enter. They would drink in the ultimate aim and scope of scientific revelation, and be so absorbed in their philanthropic mission as to pass beyond the trammels of custom, rank, sex, and occasion.[97]

The sight of the suffering or exposed body of the patient is recuperated through the rhetoric of romantic benevolence, which transforms earnest im-

224

personality into sublime transcendence. The gaze of science, far from being detached and neutral, is both erotically united with its object and released from the social debts of the subject. The visual economy of medicine is re-imagined as a domain where the gaze of the physician can produce both knowledge and pleasure, both science and care.

This book has concentrated on the written texts produced by women physicians and their supporters and has investigated how those texts managed medical care and created medical knowledge. In examining the work of the clinical lecture and the dissecting room, I extend this analysis to include other practices by which medicine created knowledge, knowledge that would eventually find a textual realization, placing these practices in relation to reading and writing. The performances, spectacles, and representations that shape those practices show us how women physicians found pleasure and produced knowledge in the work of medicine.

This book began with the young Marie Zakrzewska calmly spending the night in the dead house, cured of her weak eyes, taking up her two borrowed medical books. It ends with images of women entering the amphitheater, organizing their own dissecting rooms, writing their own books. This is not, of course, the end of the story; after the Flexner report and the admission of women to male medical schools in the late 1880s, the women's schools which had graduated so many physicians and developed so many teachers quickly closed. Only in conservative Philadelphia, where women were excluded from the University of Pennsylvania School of Medicine and the Jefferson Medical College, did the women's medical college remain open. In the early decades of the twentieth century, while women sought higher education in increasing numbers, the absolute number of women physicians declined.[98] Now, as feminists and science educators search for the reasons that women are un-derrepresented in the sciences, Zakrzewska's motto seems quaint, almost sentimental; for contemporary feminists, science has a sex, and that sex is male. This book has been an investigation of what it might mean if we were not to understand science as having a stable sex or if we were to understand the sex of science as evolving under the pressure of women's discursive for-mations. The answer to that question is neither unitary nor universal, since women physicians took up medical writing in a variety of registers, for a variety of aims, in a variety of institutional and scientific rhetorics. Some, like Ann Preston, were virtually anonymous as writers; Preston, however, created the institutional rhetoric for a women's medical school. Others, like Hannah Longshore, wrote very little and withheld any overt statement of the in-forming purposes of their writing. Longshore's work, however deeply idio-syncratic, was also intimately connected with the whole range of political and religious interests known as reform. Some women physicians intended to write, and wrote, a medicine that was indistinguishable from that written by males, but even Mary Putnam Jacobi's writings insisted on the specificity of female physiological experience and developed ways of incorporating the words and experiences of women patients into medical writing. Most of the writing of female physicians, like most contemporary medical writing, was not undertaken for publication; in their academic papers and in their meticulous hospital records, these physicians patiently constructed quotidian rhetorics of scientific care, incorporating the voices of patients, eliding the assumptions that what was male was normal, establishing a certain distance from the institutions of the profession, assuming without argument the specificity of female bodily experience and the neutral benignity of their own impersonal gaze. Nineteenth-century women physicians wrote very different kinds of medicine, with very different understandings of what it meant to write science as a woman. Theirs was a sustained performance of gendered scientific writing, a performance all the more remarkable in that it was often supported by the belief that science is outside gender. What happened to all that labor in the language of medicine? Much of it was lost and forgotten; some of it vanished into the hegemonic registers of medicine; some of it languishes in archives. But the material recovery of that labor suggests a new way of thinking about science, of understanding how women appropriated the pleasures of scientific work, how they made the language of science, if not their mother tongue, a fluent second language or perhaps a creole. These stories suggest that science has had more than one gender and hint that gender (at least in scientific writing) need not eternally be binary. While medicine was emerging as a profession, women shaped and changed its discourses, even as they were being excluded and castigated in other medical registers. For these women, the dead house of medicine was not simply a place of horror but also, as for Zakrzewska, a scene of festive knowledge, "freshly painted . . . with the necessary apparatus . . . while the bodies, clad in white gowns, were ranged on boards along the walls."[99] May it be so again, and for us, and soon.

Notes

Works Cited

Index

Notes

The following abbreviations are used throughout the notes and the works cited:

ASCWM   Archives and Special Collections on Women in Medicine, MCP Hahne-
         mann University, Philadelphia, Pa.
CPP   Library of the College of Physicians of Philadelphia, Philadelphia, Pa.
CSHN   Center for the Study of the History of Nursing, School of Nursing, Uni-
         versity of Pennsylvania, Philadelphia, Pa.
FHL   Friends Historical Library, Swarthmore College, Swarthmore, Pa.
HLPH   Historic Library and Archives Collection, Pennsylvania Hospital, Phila-
         delphia, Pa.
JEFF   Thomas Jefferson University Archives, Philadelphia, Pa.
MCHS   Montgomery County Historical Society, Norristown, Pa.
PA   Rare Book and Manuscript Library, University of Pennsylvania, Phila-
         delphia, Pa.
QC   Quaker Collection, Haverford College Library, Haverford, Pa.
SL   Schlesinger Library, Radcliffe College, Cambridge, Mass.
WMC   Woman's Medical College of Pennsylvania, Philadelphia, Pa.

CHAPTER 1. OUT OF THE DEAD HOUSE

1. Agnes Vietor, M.D., F.A.C.S., *A Woman's Quest: The Life of Marie E. Zakrzew-ska, M.D.* (New York: Appleton, 1924), 16, 17. The account of Zakrzewska's early life was based on a letter she wrote to Mary L. Booth, originally published in 1860 under the title, "A Practical Illustration of 'Woman's Right to Labor': or A Letter from Marie E. Zakrzewska, M.D., late of Berlin, Prussia."

2. Vietor, *Woman's Quest,* 18.

3. Vietor, *Woman's Quest,* 140, 142.

4. Vietor, *Woman's Quest,* 67.

5. Linda Lehmann Goldstein, "'Without Compromising in Any Particular': The Success of Medical Coeducation in Cleveland, 1850–1856," *Caduceus* 10, no. 2 (autumn 1994): 101–15.

6. For a contemporary analysis of women physicians as engaged in masquerade,

see Rosemary Pringle, *Sex and Medicine: Gender, Power, and Authority in the Medical Profession* (Cambridge: Cambridge University Press, 1998).

7. Judith Butler, *Gender Trouble: Feminism and the Subversion of Identity* (New York: Routledge, 1990).

8. For a general introduction to the rich literature of nineteenth-century United States medical history, see Charles E. Rosenberg, *The Care of Strangers: The Rise of America's Hospital System* (New York: Basic, 1987); John Harley Warner, *The Therapeutic Perspective: Medical Practice, Knowledge, and Identity in America, 1820–1885* (Cambridge, Mass.: Harvard University Press, 1986; rpt. Princeton: Princeton University Press, 1997); and Morris Vogel, *The Invention of the Modern Hospital: Boston, 1870–1930* (Chicago: University of Chicago Press, 1980).

9. Kenneth Ludmerer, *Learning to Heal: The Development of American Medical Education* (Baltimore: Johns Hopkins University Press, 1985), 3. For accounts of the ways in which medical students supplemented these experiences, see Rosenberg, *Care of Strangers*, chaps. 7 and 8; and Leo J. O'Hara, *An Emerging Profession: Philadelphia Doctors, 1860–1900* (New York: Garland, 1989).

10. Gloria Moldow, *Women Doctors in Gilded-Age Washington: Race, Gender, and Professionalization* (Urbana: University of Illinois Press, 1987), 37.

11. Regina Markell Morantz-Sanchez, *Sympathy and Science: Women Physicians in American Medicine* (New York: Oxford University Press, 1985), 244–45; Morantz-Sanchez is the indispensable source for the history of women in medicine. Other important works include Ruth Abram, *Send Us a Lady Physician: Women Doctors in America, 1815–1920* (New York: Norton, 1985); Judith Walzer Leavitt, ed., *Women and Health Care in America: Historical Readings* (Madison: University of Wisconsin Press, 1984); Thomas Neville Bonner, *To the Ends of the Earth: Women's Search for Education in Medicine* (Cambridge, Mass.: Harvard University Press, 1992); and Lilian R. Furst, ed., *Women Healers and Physicians: Climbing a Long Hill* (Lexington, Ky.: University Press of Kentucky, 1997).

12. Morantz-Sanchez, *Sympathy and Science*, 92.

13. Morantz-Sanchez, *Sympathy and Science*, 101.

14. Morantz-Sanchez, *Sympathy and Science*, 228.

15. Warner, *Therapeutic Perspective*, 16–36.

16. Abraham Flexner, *Medical Education in the United States and Canada* (New York: Carnegie Foundation for the Advancement of Teaching, 1910).

17. Morantz-Sanchez, *Sympathy and Science*, 245; Bonner, *To the Ends of the Earth*, 149.

18. Ludmerer, *Learning to Heal*, 248.

19. Morantz-Sanchez, *Sympathy and Science*, 234.

20. Londa Schiebinger, *The Mind Has No Sex? Women in the Origins of Modern Science* (Cambridge, Mass.: Harvard University Press, 1989); and Londa Schiebinger, *Nature's Body: Gender in the Making of Early Modern Science* (Boston: Beacon, 1993).

21. For an example of criticism that dismantles tacit gender assumptions, see Emily Martin, "The Egg and the Sperm: How Science Has Constructed a Romance Based on Stereotypical Male-Female Roles," *Signs: Journal of Women in Culture and Society* 16, no. 3 (1991): 485–501. For a comprehensive account of women's

entry into scientific careers, see Margaret Rossiter: *Women Scientists in America: Struggles and Strategies to 1940* (Baltimore: Johns Hopkins University Press, 1982).

22. Carol Gilligan, *In a Different Voice: Psychological Theory and Women's Development* (Cambridge, Mass.: Harvard University Press, 1982); Mary Belenky, B. M. Clinchy, N. R. Goldberger, and J. M. Tarule, *Women's Ways of Knowing: The Development of Self, Voice, and Mind* (New York: Basic Books, 1986).

23. Evelyn Fox Keller, *Reflections on Science and Gender* (New Haven, Conn.: Yale University Press, 1985); and Evelyn Fox Keller, *A Feeling for the Organism: The Life and Work of Barbara McClintock* (San Francisco: Freeman, 1983), 197–207.

24. Bruno Latour and Steve Woolgar, *Laboratory Life: The Construction of Scientific Facts* (Princeton, N.J.: Princeton University Press, 1979); Gillian Beer, *Darwin's Plots: Evolutionary Narrative in Darwin, George Eliot, and Nineteenth-Century Fiction* (London: Routledge, 1983); Steven Shapin and Simon Schaffer, *Leviathan and the Air-Pump: Hobbes, Boyle, and the Experimental Life* (Princeton, N.J.: Princeton University Press, 1985).

25. See Donna Haraway, *Primate Visions: Gender, Race, and Nature in the World of Modern Science* (London: Routledge, 1989); Donna Haraway, *Simians, Cyborgs, and Women* (London: Routledge, 1989); Donna Haraway, "A Game of Cat's Cradle: Science Studies, Feminist Theory, Cultural Studies," *Configurations* 2, no. 1 (1993): 59–72, and the essays based on Haraway's work in Chris Hables Gray, ed., *The Cyborg Handbook* (London: Routledge, 1995).

26. For a brief summary of work in the rhetoric of science, see Susan Wells, *Sweet Reason: Rhetoric and the Discourses of Modernity* (Chicago: University of Chicago Press, 1996), chap. 2; for a useful summary of feminist studies of science, see Evelyn Fox Keller, "Feminism and Science," in *Feminism and Science,* ed. Evelyn Fox Keller and Helen E. Longino (New York: Oxford University Press), 3–65.

27. See Paul Gross and Norman Leavitt, *Higher Superstition: The Academic Left and Its Quarrel with Science* (Baltimore: Johns Hopkins University Press, 1994); and Andrew Ross, ed., *Science Wars* (Durham, N.C.: Duke University Press, 1996).

28. The Biology and Gender Study Group (Athena Beldecos, Sarah Bailey, Scott Gilbert, Karen Hicks, Lori Kenschaft, Nancy Niemczyk, Rebecca Rosenberg, Stephanie Schaertel, and Andrew Wedel), "The Importance of Feminist Critique for Contemporary Cell Biology," in *Feminism and Science,* ed. Nancy Tuana (Bloomington: Indiana University Press, 1989), 172–87.

29. Ann Ruggles Gere, *Intimate Practices: Literacy and Cultural Work in U.S. Women's Clubs, 1880–1920* (Urbana: University of Illinois Press, 1997); Catherine Hobbs, ed., *Nineteenth-Century Women Learn to Write* (Charlottesville: University of Virginia Press, 1994).

30. Bruno Latour, "Socrates' and Callicles' Settlement—or, The Invention of the Impossible Body Politic," *Configurations* 5, no. 2 (spring 1997): 189–240.

31. Charlotte Perkins Gilman, "The Yellow Wall-Paper," in *The Yellow Wall-Paper,* ed. E. Hedges, rev. 2d ed. (Old Westbury, Conn.: Feminist Press, 1996; short story originally published 1892 in *New England Magazine*), 9–36.

CHAPTER 2. MEDICAL CONVERSATIONS AND MEDICAL HISTORIES

1. John Harley Warner, *The Therapeutic Perspective: Medical Practice, Knowledge, and Identity in America, 1820–85* (Princeton, N.J.: Princeton University Press, 1997), 154–55.

2. For a critical account of the patient as "good historian," see William Frank Monroe, Warren Lee Holleman, and Marsha Cline Holleman, "Is There a Person in This Case?" *Literature and Medicine* 11, no. 1 (spring 1992): 45–63.

3. For an overview of sociolinguistic studies of gender differences, see Sally McConnell-Ginet, "Language and Gender," in *Linguistics: The Cambridge Survey*, vol. 4: *Language: The Socio-cultural Context*, ed. Frederick Newmeyer (Cambridge: Cambridge University Press, 1988), 75–99. For an overview of theories of language difference, see Camille Roman, Suzanne Juhasz, and Christanne Miller, eds., *The Women and Language Debate* (New Brunswick, N.J.: Rutgers University Press, 1994).

4. See, for example, the comprehensive summaries of research in Elliot G. Mishler, Lorna Amarsingham, Stuart Hauser, Ramsay Liem, Samuel Osherson, and Nancy Wexler, *Social Contexts of Health, Illness, and Patient Care* (Cambridge: Cambridge University Press, 1981), 104–41. For representative specific studies, see Howard Waitzkin, *The Politics of Medical Encounters: How Patients and Doctors Deal with Social Problems* (New Haven, Conn.: Yale University Press, 1991); Ronald Chenail, ed., *Medical Discourse and Systemic Frames of Comprehension*, vol. 42 in Advances in Discourse Processes (Norwood, N.J.: Ablex, 1991); Alexandra Dundas Todd and Sue Fisher, eds., *The Social Organization of Doctor-Patient Communication*, 2d ed. (Norwood, N.J.: Ablex, 1993; originally published, Washington, D.C.: Center for Applied Linguistics, 1983); Jay Katz, *The Silent World of Doctor and Patient* (New York: Free Press, 1984); Elliot G. Mishler, *The Discourse of Medicine: Dialectics of the Medical Interview* (Norwood, N.J.: Ablex, 1984); Kathy Davis, "Paternalism under the Microscope," in *Gender and Discourse: The Power of Talk*, ed. Alexandra Dundas Todd (Norwood, N.J.: Ablex, 1988), 19–54; Candace West, *Routine Complications: Troubles with Talk between Doctors and Patients* (Bloomington: Indiana University Press, 1984).

5. Talcott Parsons, *The Social System* (Glencoe, Ill.: Free Press, 1951).

6. Charles E. Rosenberg, *The Care of Strangers: The Rise of America's Hospital System* (New York: Basic Books, 1987), 47–68.

7. Pauline Poole Foster, *Anne Preston, M.D. (1813–1872): A Biography: The Struggle to Obtain Training and Acceptance for Women Physicians in Mid-Nineteenth Century America*, Ph.D. dissertation, University of Pennsylvania (Ann Arbor: University Microfilms, 1984).

8. For the structure of the medical interview, see Waitzkin, *Politics of Medical Encounters*, 25–35; and Mishler, *Discourse of Medicine*, chaps. 3–5. For the relationship between spoken medical encounters and their written representations, see Aaron V. Cicourel, "Text and Discourse," *Annual Review of Anthropology* 14 (1985): 159–85.

9. Waitzkin, *Politics of Medical Encounters*, 32.

10. See the special issue of *Literature and Medicine* 11, no. 1 (spring 1992), on

the genre of the case history, especially Julia Epstein, "Historiography, Diagnosis, and Poetics," 23–44; and Rita Charon, "To Build a Case: Medical Histories as Traditions in Conflict," 115–32. The fullest account of the importance of narrative in physicians' accounts is Kathryn Montgomery Hunter's *Doctors' Stories: The Narrative Structure of Medical Knowledge* (Princeton, N.J.: Princeton University Press, 1991). My account of the structure of the medical interview is drawn from Mishler's extensive empirical study; it necessarily flattens the varied contours of individual practices.

11. Worthington Hooker, *Physician and Patient; or, a Practical View of the Mutual Duties, Relations, and Interests of the Medical Profession and the Community* (New York: Arno Press, 1972; original publication, 1849), 443.

12. David Silverman, "Policing the Lying Patient: Surveillance and Self-Regulation in Consultations with Adolescent Diabetics," in *The Social Organization of Doctor-Patient Communication,* ed. Alexandra Dundas Todd and Sue Fisher, 2d ed. (Norwood, N.J.: Ablex, 1993), 213–43.

13. Hooker, *Physician and Patient,* 443.

14. Woman's Medical College, "First Annual Announcement" (Philadelphia: Clarkson and Scattergood, 1850), 4.

15. Edwin Fussell, "Valedictory Address to the Graduating Class of the Female Medical College of Pennsylvania at the Tenth Annual Commencement, March 13, 1861," 7, MCP Collection, ASCWM.

16. Louisa May Alcott, *Hospital Sketches,* in *Alternative Alcott,* ed. E. Showalter (New Brunswick, N.J.: Rutgers University Press, 1988; original publication, 1863), 39.

17. Charles Meigs, *Woman; Her Diseases and Remedies* (Philadelphia: Lea and Blanchard, 1851), 282–83.

18. Pierre Choderlos de Laclos, *Les Liaisons dangereuses* (Paris: Garnier-Flammarion, 1964), 322.

19. Meigs, *Woman,* 155–77.

20. Meigs, *Woman,* 155.

21. Meigs, *Woman,* 155.

22. Meigs, *Woman,* 158.

23. Meigs, *Woman,* 160.

24. Meigs, *Woman,* 162.

25. Meigs, *Woman,* 170.

26. Meigs, *Woman,* 178.

27. Ronald J. Chenail, in *Medical Discourse and Systemic Frames of Comprehension,* discusses how the parents of children whose heart murmurs were being diagnosed understood their doctors' evaluations of their condition. Previous studies had shown that the consequences of parents' understanding their children to be diseased were, in many ways, indistinguishable from the consequences of disease itself (A. B. Bergman and S. J. Stamm, "The Morbidity of Cardiac Nondisease in School Children," *New England Journal of Medicine* 276 [1967]: 1008–13).

28. Dr. W. Fulton, Case and lecture notes by Dr. W. Fulton, 1866, bound handwritten notes on clinical cases of Prof. Ellerslie Wallace and Prof. Jacob Da Costa, Archives MM-207, Thomas Jefferson University Archives. A letter by Joseph Bomeman, of Bradford Book Company, included in the Fulton files, identifies him as a physician "who attended Jefferson Medical College after completing his service in

the Army during the Civil War" (Feb. 27, 1936; letter contained in Fulton's case and lecture notes).

29. Fulton, Case and lecture notes by Dr. W. Fulton, Nov. 1 and 8, 1866.

30. *Medical and Surgical Journal* (Philadelphia), "Women Are Dirty Creatures, Anyhow!" 50, no. 1422 (May 31, 1884): 4.

31. S. E. McCully, "Masturbation in the Female," *American Journal of Obstetrics* 16, no. 8 (Aug. 1883): 844–45.

32. Lister's letter, from the Archives of the Edinburgh Royal Infirmary, is quoted in Shirley Roberts, *Sophia Jex-Blake: A Woman Pioneer in Nineteenth Century Medical Reform* (London: Routledge, 1993), 133. Bell's letter was dated October 30, 1872; no date is given for Lister's.

33. Elizabeth Blackwell, *Pioneer Work in Opening the Medical Profession to Women* (New York: Schocken, 1977; original publication, 1895), 193.

34. Fulton, Case and lecture notes by Dr. W. Fulton, Dec. 21, 1866.

35. Nancy Theriot, "Women's Voices in Nineteenth-Century Medical Discourse: A Step toward Deconstructing Science," in *Gender and Scientific Authority,* ed. Barbara Laslett, Sally Gregory Kohlstedt, Helen Longino, and Evelynn Hammonds (Chicago: University of Chicago Press, 1996), 124–54.

36. Warner, *Therapeutic Perspective,* 20–34.

37. See Charles Rosenberg, "The Therapeutic Revolution: Medicine, Meaning, and Social Change in Nineteenth Century America," in *The Therapeutic Revolution: Essays in the Social History of American Medicine,* ed. Morris J. Vogel and Charles E. Rosenberg (Philadelphia: University of Pennsylvania Press, 1979); and Warner, *Therapeutic Perspective.*

38. Harriot Kezia Hunt, *Glances and Glimpses; or, Fifty Years Social, Including Twenty Years Professional Life* (Boston: Jewett, 1856); Rachel Gleason, *Talks to My Patients: Hints on Getting Well and Keeping Well,* new ed. enlarged with the addition of nineteen "Letters to Ladies" on health, education, society, etc. (New York: Holbrook, 1895). For an account of the association between women physicians and empathic treatment, see Regina Markell Morantz-Sanchez, "The Gendering of Empathic Expertise: How Women Physicians Became More Empathic Than Men," in *The Empathic Practitioner: Empathy, Gender, and Medicine,* ed. Ellen Singer More and Maureen Milligan (New Brunswick, N.J.: Rutgers University Press, 1994), 40–58.

39. Anna Mott was the author of *The Ladies' Medical Oracle; or, Mrs. Mott's Advice to Young Females, Wives, and Mothers,* Being a Non-Medical commentary on the cause, prevention, and cure of the diseases of the female frame, together with an explanation of her system of European vegetable medicine for the cure of diseases, and the patent medicated champoo baths; to which is added, an explanation of the gift, and an exposition of the numerous fabricated reports, "a weak invention of the enemy" (Boston: self-published, 1834). A handwritten note on the flyleaf of the copy owned by the ASCWM directs readers to buy these medicines from the Misses Hunt, Female Doctors.

40. WMC, Faculty Minutes, Jan. 26, 1853, MCP Collection, ASCWM.

41. Hunt, *Glances and Glimpses,* 156; see also 139, 158, 251.

42. Hunt, *Glances and Glimpses,* 151.

43. Hunt, *Glances and Glimpses*, 391.

44. Hunt, *Glances and Glimpses*, 392.

45. See Ann Braude, *Radical Spirits: Spiritualism and Women's Rights in Nineteenth Century America* (Boston: Beacon, 1989).

46. WMC, "Third Annual Announcement, of the Female Medical College of Pennsylvania for the Session of 1852–53, Situated in Philadelphia," 4, MCP Collection, ASCWM.

47. Dr. Elizabeth C. Keller, "A Case of Laparotomy," in WMC, Alumnae Association, *Proceedings of the Twelfth Annual Meeting of the Alumnae Association of the Woman's Medical College of Pennsylvania*, Mar. 18, 1887 (Philadelphia: Rodgers Printing Co., 1887), 61–63, MCP Collection, ASCWM.

48. Keller, "Case of Laparotomy," 61.

49. Keller, "Case of Laparotomy," 62.

50. Keller, "Case of Laparotomy," 62.

51. For a similar enthusiasm for surgery, see the account of Mary Dixon Jones's use of Tait's operation to remove the ovaries and Fallopian tubes, in Regina Morantz-Sanchez, "Making It in a Man's World: The Late-Nineteenth-Century Surgical Career of Mary Amanda Dixon Jones," *Bulletin of the History of Medicine* 69 (1995): 542–68. I am grateful to Prof. Morantz-Sanchez for sharing in draft her biography of Dixon Jones, *Conduct Unbecoming a Woman: Medicine on Trial in Turn-of-the-Century Brooklyn* (New York: Oxford University Press, 1999).

52. Keller, "Case of Laparotomy," 62.

53. Keller, "Case of Laparotomy," 64.

54. But see the use of *orgasm* in S. E. McCully's letter, "Masturbation in the Female": "In some women, so intense is the pleasure of an orgasm proper that it has been described to me as almost painful" (845).

55. Blackwell, *Pioneer Work*, 30.

56. Maria Minnis, "Disquisition on Medical Jurisprudence" Respectfully Submitted to the Faculty of the Female Medical College of Pennsylvania as an Inaugural Thesis for the Degree of the Doctorate in Medicine, by Maria Minnis of Phelps, New York, Period of study, four years, Preceptors, Caleb Bannister, M.D., and G. F. Horton. Philadelphia, January 10th, 1853, ASCWM. Minnis writes about means of identifying criminal abortions but also laments that the lack of physician's privilege violates the sacred confidence between physician and patient. See also Sarah Hall, "A Thesis on the Physical and Moral Effects of Abortion," Presented to the Faculty of Woman's Medical College of Pennsylvania by Sarah C. Hall, Philadelphia Session of 1869–70, ASCWM. Hall states that the only safe course for the physician was "to be deaf to *all* entreaties of this nature, from whatever source, since no finite being can foretell what modifying influences may be brought to bear upon the most inauspicious birth, it is the very acme of impious assumption to thus deliberately try to thwart Laws that are unchangeable" (15–16).

(Note: In nineteenth-century thesis titles throughout the volume, I have reproduced the orthography of the title page as closely as possible, adding quotation marks to designate the main title.)

57. Gleason, *Talks to My Patients*, 160.

58. Gleason, *Talks to My Patients*, 159.

59. Gleason, *Talks to My Patients,* 161.

60. Todd and Fisher, *Social Organization of Doctor-Patient Communication;* Mishler, *Discourse of Medicine;* and Waitzkin, *Politics of Medical Encounters.*

61. Candace West, "'Ask Me No Questions . . .': An Analysis of Queries and Replies in Physician-Patient Dialogues," in *The Social Organization of Doctor-Patient Communication,* ed. Alexandra Dundas Todd and Sue Fisher, 2d ed. (Norwood: Ablex, 1993), 127–60.

62. Mishler, *Discourse of Medicine,* 85.

63. M. Balint, *The Doctor, His Patient and the Illness* (New York: International University Press, 1957).

64. For a striking instance of a plausible fantasy, see G. Raimbault, O. Cachin, J. Limal, C. Eliacheff, and R. Rapaport, "Aspects of Communication between Patients and Doctors: An Analysis of the Discourse in Medical Interviews," *Pediatrics* 55 (1975): 401–5, in which a patient diagnosed with Taylor's syndrome interprets the physician's explanation of a missing chromosome as meaning that she is only her father's daughter and has no genetic inheritance from her mother.

65. Michel Foucault, *Discipline and Punish: The Birth of the Prison,* trans. Alan Sheridan (New York: Vintage, 1979).

66. Zakrzewska writes:

> From the very beginning, I had instituted record books in which the name, age, residence, occupation, diagnosis and treatment of every individual case were written—of those who were in the hospital, those who came to the dispensary clinics, and those who were attended at their homes.
>
> These books revealed to the visitors our activity, and they were admired also by our professional brethren. No such records then existed in their dispensaries but were introduced after our example, primitive as it was in those years.

Agnes C. Vietor, ed., *A Woman's Quest: The Life of Marie Zakrzewska, M.D.* (New York: Appleton, 1924), 234.

67. John W. H. Reber, Surgical Clinic Notebook, 1866, Jefferson Medical College, Philadelphia, Oct. 14, 1865, MM-25, Thomas Jefferson University Archives. Here and in other transcriptions, empty square brackets indicate illegible words. All patient names, when given in the original, have been disguised.

68. Jefferson Medical College, Notebook of Clinical Cases, anonymous medical student, Oct.–Dec. 1853, quotation from entry for October 6, MM-289, Thomas Jefferson University Archives.

69. Jefferson Medical College, Notebook of Clinical Cases, anonymous medical student, Oct. 1853.

70. See Waitzkin, *Politics of Medical Encounters,* chap. 8, for material on the regulation of drugs and alcohol in the doctor-patient conversation; it is also significant that many of the interactions that Waitzkin found "nonproblematic" were trauma cases (240–48).

71. Jefferson Medical College, Clinical Notes (probably of the general dispensary), 1866–69, UA-JMC 014, Thomas Jefferson University Archives.

72. Waitzkin, *Politics of Medical Encounters,* 30.

73. Reber, Surgical Clinic Notebook, Oct. 14, 1865.

74. Kersey Thomas, Notebook, "Female Medical College of Pennsylvania, N 229 Arch Street, Philadelphia," 1854–55, ASCWM. Thomas was a professor at the Woman's Medical College of Pennsylvania. The book includes accounts of 176 cases treated in 1854 and 1855, including 23 men, 135 women, 15 children, and 3 who could not be determined.

75. Thomas, Notebook, patient #2.

76. Thomas, Notebook, patient #42.

77. Thomas, Notebook, patient #60.

78. See, for example, Jefferson Medical College, Notebook of Clinical Cases, Oct.–Dec. 1853; Eli Carithers, Notebook of Clinical Cases, Jefferson Medical College, 1849–50, MM-014; J. Francis Dunlap, Notebook of Clinical Cases, Jefferson Medical College, 1873–77, MM-029; Reber, Surgical Clinic Notebook; Fulton, Case and lecture notes by Dr. W. Fulton, 1866; and Jefferson Medical College, Clinical Notes, probably of the general dispensary; all from JEFF. The closest approximation to a criticism of medical practice in any of these notebooks occurs in the Jefferson Medical College, Notebook of Clinical Cases, 1853; the student records, in his notes for the November 12, 1854, clinic, Dr. Norris's story of an unnamed doctor who diagnosed a fracture as a luxation and crippled a patient; the student remarks, "May the God of Mercies ever direct me and keep me from taking a fracture for a luxation."

79. Students were instructed to follow such a form in taking histories. See Charles Meigs's demonstration history in *Woman,* where he directs students to "gather up the whole history of the case" in a series of fourteen questions, after which the doctor concludes:

> "You must let me examine the case; I can't tell what it is except you allow that."
> "Well, I suppose if I must I must. But don't hurt me."
> "Not in the least, not at all." (p. 243)

80. See Epstein, "Historiography, Diagnosis, and Poetics"; Charon, "To Build a Case"; and Ellen Barton, "Literacy in (Inter)Action," *College English* 59, no. 4 (Apr. 1997): 408–37.

81. Warner, *Therapeutic Perspective.*

82. For a collaborative analysis and critique of problem-oriented notes, see Suzanne Poirier, Lorie Rosenblum, Lioness Ayre, Daniel Brauner, Barbara Sharf, and Ann Folwell Stanford, "Charting the Chart—an Exercise in Interpretation(s)," *Literature and Medicine* 11, no. 1 (spring 1992): 1–22.

83. These cases and the longer histories that follow are included in a small collection of 1868 patient records (Woman's Hospital of Pennsylvania, Patient Records, 1868–76, Center for the Study of the History of Nursing, School of Nursing, University of Pennsylvania); the handwriting in these short cases is very similar to Emeline Horton Cleveland's.

84. These records therefore demonstrate simultaneously specific and prolonged attention to the patient's description of her illness and a willingness to deploy the full range of available numerical measurements of bodily functions, a combination that John Harley Warner's survey of hospital histories suggests was rare (*Therapeutic Perspective*, 90–92, 107).

85. Woman's Hospital of Pennsylvania, Patient Records, Case 2071, Sept. 22, 1875.

86. Warner, *Therapeutic Perspectives*, 159.

87. Woman's Hospital of Pennsylvania, Patient Records, Case 2213, Apr. 20, 1876.

88. David H. Flood and Rhonda Soricelli, "Development of the Physician's Narrative Voice in the Medical Case History," *Literature and Medicine* 11, no. 1 (spring 1992): 64–83, 70.

89. Woman's Hospital of Pennsylvania, Patient Records, Case 2315, July 29, 1876.

90. Regina Markell Morantz and Sue Zschoche, "Professionalism, Feminism, and Gender Roles: A Comparative Study of Nineteenth-Century Medical Therapeutics," *Journal of American History* 67 (Dec. 1980): 568–88.

91. Rebecca Cole, "First Meeting of the Women's Missionary Society of Philadelphia," *Woman's Era* 3, no. 4 (Oct./Nov. 1896): 4–5.

92. Gloria Moldow, *Women Doctors in Gilded-Age Washington: Race, Gender, and Professionalization* (Urbana: University of Illinois Press, 1987), 130.

93. Blackwell, *Pioneer Work,* 227–28.

94. Margaret Jerrido, "Rebecca Cole," typed manuscript, undated, Black Women Physicians Project, Rebecca Cole file, ASCWM.

95. M. J. Scarlett, "Valedictory Address of Prof. M. J. Scarlett, before the Graduating Class of the Female Medical College of Pennsylvania, March 16, 1867," 6–7, Additional Holdings, Publications, MCP Collection, ASCWM.

96. Black Women Physicians Project, Rebecca Lee [Crumpler] file, transcription of Faculty Notes for Feb. 25, 1864, ASCWM.

97. Charles Epps, M.D., Davis Johnson, Ph.D., Audrey Vaughan, M.S., "Black Medical Pioneers: African-American 'Firsts' in Academic and Organized Medicine," *Journal of the National Medical Association* 85, nos. 8, 9, 10 (Aug. and Sept. 1993): 629–44, 703–20. See also the local historical research by Ann Rollins, described in the Boston University *University News* 2 (summer 1995), 60 (located in Black Women Physician's Project, Rebecca Lee [Crumpler] file, [clipping], ASCWM).

98. Rebecca Crumpler, M.D., *A Book of Medical Discourses in Two Parts* (Boston: Cashman, Keating & Co., Printers, 1883).

99. Crumpler, *Medical Discourses,* 3–4.

100. Crumpler's *Medical Discourses* references are as follows: doctors' attendance for poor women (14), customs of old-fashioned people (28), children caring for younger siblings (29, 38, 89), hungry children (39), children who failed to thrive (62), treating cholera (68), and the seamstress (131).

101. Crumpler, *Medical Discourses,* 119, 16.

102. Crumpler, *Medical Discourses,* 26.

103. Crumpler, *Medical Discourses,* 8.

104. Crumpler, *Medical Discourses,* 14.

105. Crumpler, *Medical Discourses,* 114.

106. For patient fantasies, see the images of women doctors in novels by nineteenth-century women, including Elizabeth Stuart Phelps, *Doctor Zay* (New York: Feminist Press, 1987; original publication, 1882); Sarah Orne Jewett, *A Country Doctor* (Boston: Houghton Mifflin, 1884; reprinted, New York: Penguin, 1986); and Annie Nathan Meyer, *Helen Brent, M.D.: A Social Study* (New York: Cassell

Publishing, 1892); as well as the discussion of these novels and others in Lilian Furst, "Halfway up the Hill: Doctresses in Late Nineteenth-Century American Fiction," in Lilian Furst, ed., *Women Healers and Physicians: Climbing a Long Hill* (Lexington: University Press of Kentucky, 1997), 221–38. There is reason to read these texts as representations of the patient's desire; in a letter to S. Weir Mitchell, Elizabeth Stuart Phelps wrote that she had written *Doctor Zay* as a "professional invalid . . . in good and regular standing" and that she "tried to draw a Doctor by reflection, or by reflex action, the result is, at least, I hope, a patient" (Elizabeth Stuart Phelps, correspondence with S. Weir Mitchell, Jan. 25, 1884, Mitchell files, Library of the College of Physicians of Philadelphia).

CHAPTER 3. INVISIBLE WRITING I: ANN PRESTON
INVENTS AN INSTITUTION

1. Ann Preston, letter to Hannah Monaghan Darlington, May 26, 1833, MCP Deans Files, Preston Papers, ASCWM.
2. For details of Ann Preston's early life, see the exhaustive and invaluable Pauline Poole Foster, *Ann Preston, M.D. (1813–1872): A Biography: The Struggle to Obtain Training and Acceptance for Women Physicians in Mid-Nineteenth Century America*, Ph.D. dissertation, University of Pennsylvania (Ann Arbor: University Microfilms, 1984).
3. Ann Preston, *Cousin Ann's Stories for Children* (Philadelphia: McKim, 1849).
4. Foster, *Ann Preston*, 89, 92, 98.
5. Ann Preston, letter to Lavinia Passmore, Oct. 8, 1843, Letter Collection, Chester County Historical Society, West Chester, Pa.
6. Eliza Judson, "Address in Memory of Ann Preston, M.D., Delivered by Request of the Corporators and Faculty of the Woman's Medical College of Pennsylvania," Mar. 11, 1873, 14, MCP Deans Files, ASCWM.
7. Ann Preston, letter to Hannah Monaghan Darlington, Jan. 4, 1851, WMC, Deceased Alumnae Files, Preston Papers, ASCWM.
8. Sarah Mapps Douglass, letters to Hannah White Richardson (a member of the Board of Lady Corporators), 1850–82, RG5/187: Richardson Family Papers, ser. 4, Friends Historical Library of Swarthmore College.
9. Anna L. Wharton, letter to her husband, Joseph Wharton, Mar. 12, 1856, RG5/162: Joseph Wharton Papers, ser. 4.2, Friends Historical Library of Swarthmore College.
10. See Harold J. Abrahams, *Extinct Medical Schools of Nineteenth-Century Philadelphia* (Philadelphia: University of Pennsylvania Press, 1966), 213.
11. Ann Preston, "Women as Physicians," [1875], 7, CSHN. This document was originally published (with the same title) as a letter to the *Medical and Surgical Reporter* (Philadelphia) 16, no. 18 (May 4, 1867): 391–94. The document now held at the CSHN was reprinted by the Woman's Medical College of Pennsylvania; no date or printer's address are given, but a postscript refers to an upcoming series of lectures in the spring of 1875, which is the year to which Foster dates the document. Quotations in this chapter are from the WMC reprint.

12. Judith Butler, *Bodies That Matter: On the Discursive Limits of "Sex"* (New York: Routledge, 1993), 127.

13. Ann Preston, T. Morris Perot, Joseph Jeanes, and Emeline Cleveland, letter to Pennsylvania State Medical Society, June 8, 1866, reprinted in Clara Marshall, *The Woman's Medical College, an Historical Outline* (Philadelphia: Lea and Blanchard, 1898), 40–41; Ann Preston and Emeline Cleveland, "Statement of the Woman's Medical College of Pennsylvania," in Marshall, *Woman's Medical College,* 24–27. The jeering incident will be discussed further in the final chapter of this book.

14. WMC, Faculty Minutes, 1850–64, MCP Collection, ASCWM. Regarding the memorial resolutions, see minutes for Dec. 29, 1854; on revising the bylaws, see minutes for Jan. 2, 1855, and also for Feb. 7, 1863; on writing the college history, see Jan. 5, 1855.

15. The announcements we can be certain Preston helped to write, on the basis of the evidence in the faculty minutes, are: WMC, "Fourth Annual Announcement of the Female Medical College of Pennsylvania . . . for the Session 1853–54," MCP Collection, ASCWM (see Faculty Minutes I, May 12, 1853); WMC, "Sixth Annual Announcement of the Female Medical College of Pennsylvania . . . for the Session of 1855–56," MCP Collection, ASCWM (see Faculty Minutes I, Feb. 12, Mar. 1, and Mar. 2, 1855); WMC, "Tenth Annual Announcement of the Female Medical College of Pennsylvania . . . for the Session of 1859–60," MCP Collection, ASCWM (see Faculty Minutes I, Dec. 27, 1858); WMC, "Fourteenth Annual Announcement of the Female Medical College of Pennsylvania . . . for the Session of 1863–64" (bound with "Valedictory Address to the Graduating Class of the Female Medical College of Pennsylvania at the Eleventh Annual Commencement, March 14, 1863, by Emeline H. Cleveland, M.D."), MCP Collection, ASCWM (the announcement is very short; see Faculty Minutes I, Feb. 7, 1863).

There is a gap in the faculty minutes from 1864 until after Preston's death; Foster assigns the seventeenth to the twenty-third annual announcement to her, since they were published during her deanship and are mentioned in Judson's memorial address: WMC, "Seventeenth Annual Announcement of the Female Medical College . . . for the Session of 1866–67," MCP Collection, ASCWM; WMC, "Eighteenth Annual Announcement of the Woman's Medical College of Pennsylvania . . . for the Session of 1867–68," MCP Collection, ASCWM; WMC, "Nineteenth Annual Announcement of the Woman's Medical College of Pennsylvania . . . for the Session of 1868–69," MCP Collection, ASCWM; WMC, "Twentieth Annual Announcement of the Woman's Medical College of Pennsylvania . . . for the Session of 1869–70," MCP Collection, ASCWM; WMC, "Twenty-first Annual Announcement of the Woman's Medical College of Pennsylvania . . . for the Session of 1870–71," MCP Collection, ASCWM; Woman's Medical College of Pennsylvania, "Twenty-second Annual Announcement of the Woman's Medical College of Pennsylvania . . . for the Session of 1871–72," MCP Collection, ASCWM; WMC, "Twenty-third Annual Announcement of the Woman's Medical College of Pennsylvania . . . for the Session of 1872–73," MCP Collection, ASCWM.

16. Ann Preston gave a number of introductory and valedictory lectures; according to the custom of all medical schools, after the lecture, students (or some other group within the college) requested that she supply a copy for publication,

240

and the lecture was printed. All these lectures show Ann Preston as their author: "Introductory Lecture to the Course of Instruction in the Female Medical College of Pennsylvania for the Session 1855–56," by Ann Preston, M.D., Professor of Physiology, MCP Deans Files, Preston Papers, ASCWM; "Valedictory Address to the Graduating Class of the Female Medical College of Pennsylvania for the Session of 1857–58," by Ann Preston, M.D., Professor of Physiology and Hygiene, MCP Deans Files, Preston Papers, ASCWM; "Introductory Lecture to the Class of the Female Medical College of Pennsylvania, Delivered at the Opening of the Tenth Annual Session, Oct. 19, 1859," by Ann Preston, M.D., Professor of Physiology and Hygiene, CSHN; "Valedictory Address to the Graduating Class of the Female Medical College of Pennsylvania at the Twelfth Annual Commencement, March 16, 1864," by Ann Preston, M.D., Professor of Physiology and Hygiene, with Announcement of the Fifteenth Annual Session, MCP Deans Files, Preston Papers, ASCWM; "Valedictory Address to the Graduating Class of the Woman's Medical College of Pennsylvania at the Eighteenth Annual Commencement, March 12th, 1870," by Ann Preston, M.D., Professor of Physiology and Hygiene, CSHN.

17. Ann Preston, "Nursing the Sick and the Training of Nurses," an Address Delivered at the Request of the Board of Managers of the Woman's Hospital, at Philadelphia, by Ann Preston, M.D., 1863, CSHN; Ann Preston, "Women as Physicians."

18. Eliza Judson, in her "Address in Memory of Ann Preston, M.D.," Delivered by Request of the Corporators and Faculty of the Woman's Medical College of Pennsylvania, Mar. 11, 1873 (MCP Deans Files, ASCWM), speaks of Preston's journal and quotes from it. Gulielma Fell Alsop, in her *History of the Woman's Medical College, Philadelphia, Pennsylvania (1850–1950)* (Philadelphia: Lippincott, 1950), refers to the journal as something she has in hand. However, Pauline Poole Foster, in researching her dissertation on Preston, was not able to locate the journal; nor have successive archivists at the ASCWM.

19. Mary Mumford, "Remarks at the Woman's Medical College Golden Jubilee," 1900, MCP Collection, ASCWM.

20. Mary P. Ryan, *Women in Public: Between Banners and Ballots* (Baltimore: Johns Hopkins University Press, 1990).

21. Preston, "Introductory Lecture . . . 1855–56," 2.

22. Preston, "Introductory Lecture . . . 1855–56," 8.

23. Preston, "Valedictory Address . . . 1857–58," 8.

24. Preston, "Valedictory Address . . . 1864," 4.

25. Margaret Hope Bacon, *Mothers of Feminism: The Story of Quaker Women in America* (New York: Harper and Row, 1986).

26. Lucretia Coffin Mott, *Discourse on Woman,* Delivered at the Assembly Buildings, December 17, 1849 (Philadelphia: T. B. Peterson, 1850); reprinted in Karlyn Kohrs Campbell, *Man Cannot Speak for Her,* vol. 2: *Key Texts of the Early Feminists* (New York: Praeger, 1989). See also Campbell's analysis of the speech in *Man Cannot Speak for Her,* vol. 1: *A Critical Study of Early Feminist Rhetoric* (New York: Praeger, 1989), 37–48.

27. Preston, "Introductory Lecture . . . 1855–56," 7.

28. Charles Meigs, *Woman; Her Diseases and Remedies* (Philadelphia: Lea and Blanchard, 1851), 27.

29. Meigs, *Woman*, 28.

30. Cambell, *Man Cannot Speak for Her*, vol. 1, 105–21.

31. Preston, "Introductory Lecture . . . 1855–56," 8.

32. Preston, "Introductory Lecture . . . 1855–56," 9–10.

33. Preston, "Introductory Lecture . . . 1855–56," 10.

34. John Harley Warner, *The Therapeutic Perspective: Medical Practice, Knowledge, and Identity in America, 1820–1885* (Princeton, N.J.: Princeton University Press, 1997), 75–77.

35. Preston, "Introductory Lecture . . . 1855–56," 11.

36. Preston, "Valedictory Address . . . 1857–58," 11.

37. Preston, "Introductory Lecture . . . 1855–56," 13.

38. Preston, letter to Lavinia Passmore, Oct. 8, 1843.

39. The 1870 valedictory address, which would have been written almost immediately after the jeering incident, is somewhat different in organization and tone. It is realistically sober in its opening promises: "We can none of us map out the exact road before you, nor foresee the changes and trials which await you; but there are unchanging principles of action which can guide safely through all vicissitudes, and these we trust you will make your own" (Preston, "Valedictory Address . . . 1870," 1). The speech is organized as a plea for truth, for the progress of medicine, for a moral therapy.

40. WMC, Faculty Minutes, Nov. 15, 1859.

41. Campbell, *Man Cannot Speak for Her*, vol. 1, 11.

42. Marjorie Garber, *Vested Interests: Cross-Dressing and Cultural Anxiety* (New York: Harper, 1992), 234.

43. See WMC, "Fourth Annual Announcement of the Female Medical College of Pennsylvania."

44. WMC, Faculty Minutes, Mar. 1 and Mar. 2, 1855.

45. WMC, "Sixth Annual Announcement," 2.

46. WMC, "Sixth Annual Announcement," 6.

47. John S. Haller, Jr., *Medical Protestants: The Eclectics in American Medicine, 1825–1939* (Carbondale: Southern Illinois University Press, 1994), 158.

48. See, for example, Woman's Medical College of Pennsylvania, "First Annual Announcement of the Female Medical College of Pennsylvania for the session of 1850–51 . . . ," MCP Collection, ASCWM:

> **The Anatomical Rooms** will be furnished with every convenience and *kept strictly private.*
>
> They will be under the supervision of the Professor of Anatomy, *aided by competent female assistants.* (12)

49. Quoted in Charles E. Rosenberg, *The Care of Strangers: The Rise of America's Hospital System* (New York: Basic Books, 1987), 156; Pennsylvania Hospital, Minute Book of the Board of Managers, minutes for Nov. 28, 1855, R11D12, HLPH.

50. T. L. Savitt, "'A Journal of Our Own': The *Medical and Surgical Observer* at the Beginnings of an African-American Medical Profession in Late Nineteenth Century America," part 2, *Journal of the National Medical Association* 88, no. 2 (Feb. 1996): 115–22.

51. Rebecca Crumpler, *A Book of Medical Discourses in Two Parts* (Boston: Cashman, Keating & Co., 1883), 114–16, Historical Collection, National Library of Medicine, Washington, D.C.

52. Rosi Braidotti, *Nomadic Subjects: Embodiment and Sexual Difference in Contemporary Feminist Theory* (New York: Columbia University Press, 1994), 199.

53. WMC, "Sixth Annual Announcement," 8, 1.

54. WMC, "Tenth Annual Announcement," 5.

55. WMC, "Twenty-first Annual Announcement," 4.

56. Judson, "Address in the Memory of Ann Preston," 41–42.

57. Judson, "Address in the Memory of Ann Preston," 16.

58. Foster, *Ann Preston,* 262.

59. In an anonymous pamphlet titled *Men and Women Medical Students and the Woman Movement* (Apr. 1870), we read, "Filling the public office of Dean to a college and bellwether to the flock, suggests to our mind, either that the cure by Dr. Kirkebride [*sic*] was incomplete, or that the disease has revived *in pantaloons,*" an eerie invocation of the cross-dressing theme. The pamphlet is bound with the Minute Book of the Board of Managers of the Pennsylvania Hospital, R11D12, HLPH.

60. Preston, "Nursing the Sick," 2.

61. Judson, "Address in the Memory of Ann Preston," 20.

62. Garber, *Vested Interests,* 16.

63. Alsop, *History of the Woman's Medical College,* 61.

64. Foster, *Ann Preston,* 302.

65. Woman's Hospital of Pennsylvania, Board of Managers Minutes, Sept. 1 and Sept. 22, 1864, Hospitals, MCP-G3a, ASCWM.

66. Philadelphia County Medical Society, "Proceedings," in the Philadelphia *Medical and Surgical Reporter,* "Report of Committee on Status of Female Physicians, Philadelphia County Medical Society," 16, no. 13 (Mar. 30, 1867): 256–62.

67. Philadelphia County Medical Society, "Proceedings," in the Philadelphia *Medical and Surgical Reporter,* "Report of Committee on Status of Female Physicians," 260, 258.

68. Preston, "Women as Physicians," 1.

69. Preston, "Women as Physicians," 2–4.

70. Preston, "Women as Physicians," 5.

71. Mary P. Ryan, *Womanhood in America: From Colonial Times to the Present,* 3d ed. (New York: Franklin Watts, 1983), 113–67.

72. Preston, "Women as Physicians," 6.

73. Preston, "Women as Physicians," 7.

CHAPTER 4. LEARNING TO WRITE MEDICINE

1. For a general history of nineteenth-century medical education, see Kenneth Ludmerer, *Learning to Heal: The Development of American Medical Education* (Baltimore: Johns Hopkins University Press, 1985). For a specific account of the curriculum at the University of Pennsylvania, see Thomas Huddle, "Competition and Re-

form at the University of Pennsylvania, 1847–77," *Journal of the History of Medicine and Allied Sciences* 51, no. 3 (July 1996): 251–92.

2. Joseph Longshore, letter to Thomas Longshore, Jan. 24, 1834, Longshore Papers, ASCWM.

3. For struggles to define the thesis requirements in the University of Pennsylvania School of Medicine at the end of the eighteenth century, see Lisa Rosner, "Student Culture at the Turn of the Nineteenth-Century: Edinburgh and Philadelphia," *Caduceus* 10, no. 2 (autumn 1994): 65–86.

4. University of Pennsylvania Medical Faculty, "Report on the Medical Department of the University of Pennsylvania," for the Session of 1851–52, to the Alumni of the School, by the Medical Faculty (Philadelphia: Lippincott, Grambo and Company, 1852), unpaginated, bound with University of Pennsylvania School of Medicine pamphlets (M378.748 PZME.8), Rare Book and Manuscript Library, University of Pennsylvania, Philadelphia.

5. Leo J. O'Hara, *An Emerging Profession: Philadelphia Doctors, 1860–1900* (New York: Garland, 1989), 27–28.

6. Daniel Drake, *Practical Essays on Medical Education and the Medical Profession in the United States* (Cincinnati: Roff and Young, 1832), reprinted in Gert Brieger, ed., *Medical America in the Nineteenth Century: Readings from the Literature* (Baltimore: Johns Hopkins University Press, 1972), 13.

7. *Boston Herald*, Sept. 10, 1847, quoted in Thomas Neville Bonner, *To the Ends of the Earth: Women's Search for Education in Medicine* (Cambridge, Mass.: Harvard University Press), 17.

8. See, for example, F. Campbell Stewart, "The Actual Condition of the Medical Profession in This Country; with a Brief Account of Some of the Causes Which Tend to Impede Its Progress, and Interfere with Its Honors and Interests," *New York Journal of Medicine* 6 (1846): 151–71, reprinted in Brieger, *Medical America*, 62–74.

9. *Medical and Surgical Reporter* (Philadelphia), "Minutes of the Medical Society of the State of Penn'a.," (June 18, 1870): 529.

10. Letter from D. L. Rogers, quoted in Andrew Boardman, "An Essay on the Means of Improving Medical Education and Elevating Medical Character," reprinted in Brieger, *Medical America*, 27–28.

11. John Dickson Bruns, *Life, Its Relations, Animal and Mental: An Inaugural Dissertation* (Charleston, S.C.: Steam Power Press of Walker, Evans, and Co., 1857), CPP.

12. Elisha K. Kane, M.D., *Experiments on Kiesteine, with Remarks on Its Application to the Diagnosis of Pregnancy* (Philadelphia: Medical Faculty of the University of Pennsylvania, 1842), reprinted from the *American Journal of the Medical Sciences* 4 (1842): 13–38, CPP.

13. Oliver Wendell Holmes, "Report of the Committee on Medical Literature," *Transactions of the American Medical Association* 1 (1848): 249–88.

14. WMC, "Third Annual Announcement, of the Female Medical College of Pennsylvania for the Session of 1852–53," MCP Collection, ASCWM.

15. WMC, Faculty Minutes, Feb. 17–19, 1859, MCP Collection, ASCWM. For the enormous range of nineteenth-century approaches to literacy instruction for

women, see Catherine Hobbs, ed., *Nineteenth-Century Women Learn to Write* (Charlottesville: University Press of Virginia), 1995.

16. For a list of publications of the early graduates of the Woman's Medical College of Pennsylvania, see Clara Marshall, *The Woman's Medical College of Pennsylvania: An Historical Outline* (Philadelphia: P. Blakiston, 1897).

17. See the list of theses in University of Pennsylvania Medical Faculty, "Report on the Medical Department of the University of Pennsylvania," for the Session of 1851–52.

18. The full titles of the theses I have studied in the register of health from the University of Pennsylvania, all of which are in the Rare Book and Manuscript Library of the University of Pennsylvania, are as follows:

Joshua Allen. "An Essay on Organic Life Force" for the Degree of Doctor of Medicine, by Joshua G. Allen, County of Delaware, State of Pennsylvania. Preceptor Dr. Charles J. Morton of Pa. Duration of studies three years. Presented 2nd mo. 15th, 1850.

Thomas Corson, "An Essay on Health versus Fashion" for the Degree of Doctor of Medicine, in the University of Pennsylvania. By Thomas J. Corson, of New Hope, Bucks county, State of Pennsylvania. Residence in city, 293 Race Stre., Preceptor, Chas. Foulke, M.D., Duration of studies, three and a half years. Presented, Jany 18th, 1851.

Abram Smith. "An Essay on the Moral and Physical Education of Females" For the Degree of Doctor of Medicine in the University of Pennsylvania by Abram Smith, of Easton, Northampton County, State of Pennsylvania, Residence No. 91 South Eighth Street, Philada. Preceptor S. Morton Zulich, M.D. Duration of Studies 3 years. Presented Feby 1850.

As in the discussion of medical forensics (chap. 2), I have reproduced the orthography of thesis title pages as closely as possible, adding quotation marks to designate the main title.

I would also categorize in the register of health such theses as James Brown (1851), "Physical Effects of Heat and Cold"; John Cummings (1851), "Medical Reform"; B. Fancuil Craig (1851), "Phenomena of Human Vision"; Frisby Newcomer (1851), "Origin of Medicine, &c."; James Wilson (1851), "Effects of Habit."

19. *Transactions of the Medical Society of New Jersey,* Thomas Corson obituary (Newark, N.J.: Hardham, 1879), 209; Thomas Corson, *Physician and Patient: Address Delivered before the State Medical Society of New Jersey (1869),* by Thos. J. Corson, M.D., President of the Society, pamphlet, 1869, CPP.

20. See, for example, Michael Halloran, "Rhetoric in the American College Curriculum: The Decline of Public Discourse," *Pre/Text* 3 (1982): 245–69; James Berlin, *Writing Instruction in Nineteenth-Century American Colleges* (Carbondale: Southern Illinois University Press, 1984); Albert Kitzhaber, *Rhetoric in American Colleges, 1850–1900* (Dallas: Southern Methodist University Press, 1990); Susan Miller, *Textual Carnivals: The Politics of Composition* (Carbondale: Southern Illinois University Press, 1991); Nan Johnson, *Nineteenth Century Rhetoric in North America* (Carbondale: Southern Illinois University Press, 1991); and the documents collected in John C. Brereton, ed., *The Origins of Composition Studies in the American College, 1875–*

1925, a Documentary History (Pittsburgh: University of Pittsburgh Press, 1995). Anne Ruggles Gere's *Intimate Practices: Literacy and Cultural Work in U.S. Women's Clubs, 1880–1920* (Urbana: University of Illinois Press, 1997) investigates the alternate practices of women's clubs.

21. Ann La Berge and Mordechai Feingold, eds., *French Medical Culture in the Nineteenth Century* (Amsterdam and Atlanta, Ga.: Rodopi, 1994); therein, see especially Jacalyn Duffin, "Private Practice and Public Research: The Patients of R. T. H. Laennec" (118–49); and Ann La Berge, "Medical Microscopy in Paris, 1830–65" (296–326).

22. Charles E. Rosenberg, *The Care of Strangers: The Rise of America's Hospital System* (New York: Basic Books, 1987).

23. M. A. K. Halliday and J. R. Martin, *Writing Science: Literacy and Discursive Power* (Pittsburgh: University of Pittsburgh Press, 1993).

24. Halliday and Martin, *Writing Science*, 61.

25. Rosenberg, *Care of Strangers*, see esp. chap. 3. For a more focused account, oriented to changes in therapy, see John Harley Warner, *The Therapeutic Perspective: Medical Practice, Knowledge, and Identity in America, 1820–1885*, reprint ed. (Princeton, N.J.: Princeton University Press; original publication, Cambridge, Mass.: Harvard University Press, 1986). For early responses to these theories, see Morris Vogel and Charles Rosenberg, eds., *The Therapeutic Revolution: Essays in the Social History of American Medicine* (Philadelphia: University of Pennsylvania Press, 1979); and Charles Rosenberg and Janet Golden, eds., *Framing Disease: Studies in Cultural History* (New Brunswick, N.J.: Rutgers University Press, 1992).

26. Rosenberg, *Care of Strangers*, chap. 3.

27. For the discourses of scientific medicine, see Michel Foucault, *The Birth of the Clinic: An Archaeology of Medical Perception* (New York: Random House, 1973). For a historical treatment of scientific medicine in the United States, see the works cited above and Rosenberg, *Care of Strangers,* chap. 6.

28. Halliday and Martin, *Writing Science*, 65.

29. Corson, "Health versus Fashion," 12–14.

30. Corson, "Physician and Patient," 7.

31. For a discussion of transactional writing by students for teachers, see James Britton, *The Development of Writing Abilities (11–18)* (London: Macmillan Education, 1975).

32. Corson, "Health versus Fashion," 20. A whole chapter might be written about such spellings as Corson's *develope*, common enough in all these theses, both from Penn and the WMC texts, to seem standard. Nonstandard spellings of both technical and nontechnical terms are common in many theses, as they are in many handwritten contemporary documents.

33. See Sheila M. Rothman, *Living in the Shadow of Death: Tuberculosis and the Social Experience of Illness in American History* (New York: Basic Books, 1994). Since the term *phthisis* could include both tuberculosis and many less serious diseases, including pneumonia and bronchitis, the disease was of course confusing and unpredictable. It could lead to sudden death, linger, go into remission, or be cured. Both Rothman and Barbara Bates (*Bargaining for Life: A Social History of Tuberculosis, 1876–1938* [Philadelphia: University of Pennsylvania Press, 1992]) recount

many instances of tubercular patients negotiating the management of their disease with physicians.

34. *The Eclectic Medical Journal of Philadelphia,* ed. William Paine, M.D., and Marshall Calkins, M.D., Professor of the Institutes and Practice of Surgery in the Eclectic Medical College of Pennsylvania, Philadelphia, CPP. See, for example, vol. 3, no. 6 (June 1860), which includes a brief notice in "Miscellany" lamenting how few people can cook potatoes well. The New York *Medical Gazette,* on the other hand, satirically reprinted such notices from irregular publications as evidence of quackery.

35. Samuel Gross, "The Factors of Disease and Death after Injuries, Parturition, and Surgical Operations," *Reports and Papers, A.P.H.A.* 2 (1874–75): 400–14, reprinted in Brieger, ed., *Medical America,* 190–200, quotation on 194.

36. For another University of Pennsylvania thesis in the discourse of health, see Abram Smith's "Essay on the Moral and Physical Education of Females." Smith follows Corson's organization, nearly topic for topic. The thesis raises interesting questions about varying cultural norms for plagiarism and originality, an issue recently researched by Candace Spigelman, "Dialectics of Ownership in Peer Writing Groups," Ph.D. dissertation, Temple University, Philadelphia, 1996.

37. The following theses are all from the Woman's Medical College in the register of health and are housed in the ASCWM, WMCP Theses, 1851–56. Their title pages read:

Angenette Hunt. "A Disquisition on the True Physician." Respectfully submitted to the Faculty of the Medical College of Pennsylvania, as inaugural Thesis for the degree of M.D. by Angenette Hunt of Hamilton, N.Y. Term of study 3 years. Preceptor Dr. H. N. Hunt. Philadelphia, Nov. 26th, 1851.

Ann Preston. "A Disquicition on General Diagnosis," Respectfully submitted to the Faculty of the Female Medical College of Pennsylvania as an Inaugural Thesis for the Degree of M.D. by Ann Preston of West Grove, Penna, term of study 3 years, preceptor, N. R. Moseley, M.D., Phila, Nov. 26th, 1851.

Anna M. Longshore [Anna Longshore-Potts]. "A Disquisition on Electricity." Respectfully submitted to the Faculty of the Female Medical College of Pennsylvania As an Inaugural Thesis For the Degree of M.D. By Anna M. Longshore of Bucks County Pa. Period of Study three years. Preceptor J. S. Longshore, M.D. November 1851.

Augusta R. Montgomery. "A Disquisition on the Medical Education of Woman" Respectfully Submitted to the Faculty of the Female Medical College of Pennsylvania as an Inaugural Thesis for the Degree of Doctor of Medicine. By Augusta R. Montgomery. Residence: Attica, New York. Term of Study. Three years. Preceptors: Drs. Hayes and Hadley. Philadelphia, January 1st, 1853.

Maria Minnis. "A Disquisition on Medical Jurisprudence." Respectfully submitted to the Faculty of the Female Medial College of Pennsylvania as an Inaugural Thesis for the Doctorate in Medicine by Maria Minnis of Phelps, New York. Period of Study, four years. Preceptors, Caleb Bannister M.D. and G. F. Horton. Philadelphia, January 10th 1853.

38. WMC, Deceased Alumnae Files, Angenette A. Hunt, ASCWM. This information is from a newspaper obituary, no author or newspaper name given, dated Dec. 29, 1901.

39. A. Hunt, "True Physician," 3. Hunt's punctuation, relying heavily on dashes joined to commas, is more colloquial than that of most of the theses produced at the University of Pennsylvania School of Medicine but not unusual for theses produced at the Woman's Medical College of Pennsylvania.

40. See Warner, *Therapeutic Perspective,* 163.

41. See, for example, the founding statement of the Organization of the American Eclectic Medical Association of Philadelphia, "for the purpose of informing the public of the true resources of all the one idea systems of medicine, and of the great advantage obtained by combining the important and valuable features of each, into one general American system of medicine." This call by Prof. William Paine is quoted in the *Eclectic Medical Journal of Philadelphia,* "Organization of the American Eclectic Medical Association of Philadelphia," 1, no. 4 (April 1858): 166. For a general account of Eclectic medicine, see John S. Haller, *Medical Protestants: The Eclectics in American Medicine, 1825–1939* (Carbondale: Southern Illinois University Press, 1994).

42. A. Hunt, "True Physician," 10.

43. A. Hunt, "True Physician," 10–11.

44. A. Hunt, "True Physician," 7–8.

45. Harriot Kezia Hunt, *Glances and Glimpses: Or Fifty Years Social, Including Twenty Years Professional Life* (Boston: Jewett, 1856), 87.

46. Ann Preston, "Valedictory Address to the Graduating Class of the Female Medical College of Pennsylvania for the Session of 1857–58," by Ann Preston, M.D., Professor of Physiology and Hygiene, 1–2, MCP Deans Files, Preston Papers, ASCWM.

47. Rachel Gleason, *Talks to My Patients: Hints on Getting Well and Keeping Well,* new ed., enlarged with the addition of nineteen "Letters to Ladies" on health, education, society, etc. (New York: Holbrook, 1895), 61.

48. A. Hunt, "True Physician," 11–12.

49. A. M. Longshore, "Electricity," 8, 12.

50. Anna Longshore-Potts, *Love, Courtship, and Marriage* (Paradise Valley Sanitarium, National City, San Diego Co., Calif.: self-published, 1891), ASCWM.

51. WMC, Faculty Minutes I, Dec. 1851. Each faculty member voted whether to pass or fail each student; the votes were recorded with black and white balls. Anna Longshore and Angenette Hunt passed with seven white balls apiece.

52. Jacques Lacan, *Feminine Sexuality: Jacques Lacan and the école freudienne,* ed. Juliet Mitchell and Jacqueline Rose (New York: Norton, 1985).

53. For accounts of standpoint theory, see Evelyn Fox Keller, "Feminism and Science," in *Feminism and Science,* ed. Evelyn Fox Keller and Helen Longino (New York: Oxford University Press, 1996); Sandra Harding, "Rethinking Standpoint Epistemology: What Is 'Strong Objectivity'?" in *Feminist Epistemologies,* ed. Linda Alcott and Elizabeth Potter (New York: Routledge, 1993); and Sandra Harding, *Whose Science? Whose Knowledge? Thinking from Women's Lives* (Ithaca, N.Y.: Cornell University Press, 1991).

54. Evelyn Fox Keller, *Reflections on Gender and Science* (New Haven, Conn.: Yale University Press, 1985); for the gender of the medical gaze see Ludmilla Jordanova, *Sexual Visions: Images of Gender in Science and Medicine between the Eigh-*

teenth and Twentieth Centuries (New York: Harvester, 1989). None of this argument should be taken to mean that there was an earlier state of medical writing in which gender was not reified; see Laurinda Dixon, *Perilous Chastity: Women and Illness in Pre-Enlightenment Art and Medicine* (Ithaca: Cornell University Press, 1995).

55. For wax models, see Ludmilla Jordanova, *Sexual Visions,* 87–111. For flap anatomies and the reluctance of anatomical atlases to illustrate the female body, see K. B. Roberts, "The Contexts of Anatomical Illustrations," in *The Ingenious Machine of Nature: Four Centuries of Art and Anatomy,* by Mimi Cazort, Monique Kornell, and K. B. Roberts (Ottawa: National Gallery of Canada, 1996), 78–92.

56. Mary Ryan, *Women in Public: Between Banners and Ballots* (Baltimore: Johns Hopkins University Press, 1990).

57. Jordanova, *Sexual Visions,* 87.

58. Harding, "Rethinking Standpoint Epistemology: What Is 'Strong Objectivity'?" 51.

59. Keller, "Feminism and Science," 31.

60. Rosenberg, *The Care of Strangers,* 138–40; and W. F. Bynum, *Science and the Practice of Medicine in the Nineteenth Century* (Cambridge: Cambridge University Press, 1994), 130.

61. All theses in the register of medicine at the Woman's Medical College of Pennsylvania are from the ASCWM. The full title pages for the 1851 theses (class of 1852) read:

Susanna H. Ellis. "A Disquisition on the Influence of the Nervous System on the Functions of Respiration and Digestion." Respectfully submitted to the Faculty of the Female M. College of Pennsylvania as an inaugural thesis; for the Degree of M.D. By Susanna H. Ellis of Philadelphia. Preceptor J. W. Comfort, M.D. Period of study 3 years, 1851.

Frances Mitchell. "A Disquisition on Chlorosis." Respectfully submitted to the Faculty of the Female Medical College of Pennsylvania as an Inaugural Thesis for the degree of the Doctorate in the Female Medical College of Pennsylvania. By Frances G. Mitchell of England. Period of Study three years. Preceptor J. F. X. Mc-Closkey, M.D., Philadelphia, Dec 1st 1851.

Phebe Way. "A Disquisition on Wounds." Respectfully submitted to the Faculty of the Female Medical College of Pennsylvania. As an Inaugural Thesis for the Degree of M.D. by Phebe M. Way of Chester County, Pennsylvania. Preceptor, J. W. Comfort.

Hannah Longshore. "A Disquisition on Neuralgia, its Treatments," respectfully Submitted to the Faculty of the Female Medical College of Pennsylvania as an Inaugural Thesis for the Degree of M.D. by Hannah E. Longshore of Philadelphia. Period of Study, Three Years. Preceptor, Dr. Joseph S. Longshore. November 1851.

Martha Sawin. "A Disquisition on Anaemia." Respectfully Submitted to the Faculty of the Female Medical College of Pennsylvania as an Inaugural Thesis for the Degree of M.D. by Martha A. Sawin of Boston, Mass. Period of Study 3 years. Preceptors, E. C. Rolfe, M.D., W. M. Cornell, M.D.

The full title pages of the 1852 theses (class of 1853) in the register of medicine read as follows:

Charlotte Adams. "Disquisitio De Physiologus Effectis Nutricum A Lactatione

Nimia." Verecundie Submittitur ad Professores Feminae Medicinalis Collegii Pennsylvaniae, Quasi Inauguratum Propositum Pro Grado Doctoris Medicinae. Per Charlotte G. Adams, Bostonae. Praeceptores Guilielmus M. Cornell M.D., Enochus C.
Rolfe, MD., Tempus Studii—Tres Annos. Philadelphia, Januaris Primo Die. Annodomini MDCCCLII.

Annah N. S. Anderson. "A Disquisition on General Physiology," Respectfully Submitted to the Faculty of the Female Medical College of Pennsylvania as an Inaugural
thesis, for the Degree of Doctorate of Medicine. By Annah N. S. Anderson of Bristol,
Bucks County Pennsylvania. Period of study 3 years. Preceptor Dr. Benjamin Malone, Philadelphia, January 1853 [underlining on original title page].

Julia A. Beverly. "A disquistion on Iron," respectfully Submitted to the Faculty of
the Female Medical College of Pennsylvania As an Inaugural Thesis for the Degree
of Doctor in Medicine, January 7th, 1853 by Julia A. Beverly of Prov. Rhode Island.
Preceptors, W. M. Cornell, M.D. and E. C. Rolfe, M.D. Period of study three years.

Hannah W. Ellis. "A Disquisition on Labor." Respectfully submitted to the Faculty
of the Female Medical College of Pennsylvania as an Inaugural Thesis for the Degree
of Doctorate of Medicine by Hannah W. Ellis of Pennsylvania. Period of study 3
years. Preceptor   Philadelphia, 1853.

Henrietta W. Johnson. "A disquisition on the Skin and its Functions": Respectfully
Submitted to the Faculty of the Female Medical College of Pennsylvania as an Inaugural thesis For the degree of M.D. by Henrietta W. Johnson of New Jersey. Preceptor I. W. Redfield M.D., Term of Study Three Years.

Margaret Richardson. "A Disquisition on Phthisis Pulmonalis," respectfully Submitted to the Faculty of the Female Medical College of Pennsylvania as an Inaugural
Theses for the Degree of the Doctorate in Medicine. By Margaret Richardson of
Pennsylvania. Period of Study, three years, Preceptor, J. S. Longshore, M.D., Philadelphia, December 30th, 1852.

The theses from the University of Pennsylvania in the register of medicine that will
be discussed in this chapter are all found in the Rare Book and Manuscript Library,
University of Pennsylvania (PA). They are:

S. Wylie Crawford. "An Essay on Hypertrophy and Atrophy" for the Degree of
Doctor of Medicine in the University of Pennsylvania. by S. Wylie Crawford of Philad., State of Pennsylvania. Residence—Philadelphia, Arch St. above. Preceptor,
Wm. E. Horner, M.D., Duration of Studies, three years; Presented, February 4th,
1850.

Jesse A. Rivins. "An Essay on Auscultation in the Diagnosis of Pulmonary Disease."
For the Degree of Doctor of Medicine in the University of Pennsylvania by Jesse A.
Rivins of Rutherford County, Tennessee. Preceptors. Watson and Wendel. Duration
of studies 3 years and 4 months. Presented Jan 22nd, 1850 [note on front of thesis
reads "ad eundum Louisville," the usual nomenclature for a student who had begun
medical training elsewhere].

John W. Sale. "An Essay on Haemoptysis" For the Degree of Doctor of Medicine
in the University of Pennsylvania, by John W. Sale, of Bedford County, State of Virginia. Residence in the City No 13th Filbert St. Preceptor R. A. Sale, M.D. Duration
of Studies 3 years. Presented on the 15th of Jany, 1850.

62. WMC, Alumnae Association, *Transactions of the Thirty-fourth Annual Meet-*

ing of the Alumnae Association of the Woman's Medical College of Pennsylvania, May 27–28, 1909, Obituaries (Philadelphia: Published by the association, 1909), MCP Collection, ASCWM. The fullest biography of Richardson is in Theodore W. Bean, *A History of Montgomery County, Pennsylvania*, vol. 1 (Philadelphia: Everts and Peck, 1884), 667–68, MCHS. The same source shows Margaret Richardson as a practicing physician but not as a member of the Montgomery County Medical Society (677); members of the county medical society, however, served as her pallbearers in 1909 (*Norristown Daily Herald*, May 18, 1909, MCHS). Bean's history is the source for Richardson's obituary in the *Norristown Daily Herald*.

63. Bynum (*Science and the Practice of Medicine*) offers valuable caution against dichotomizing traditional and scientific understandings of disease. For an influential article on the specificity of disease, see Owei Temkin, "The Scientific Approach to Disease: Specific Entity and Individual Sickness," in *The Double Face of Janus and Other Essays in the History of Medicine* (Baltimore: Johns Hopkins University Press, 1977), 441–55.

64. John Harley Warner, *Against the Spirit of System: The French Impulse in Nineteenth-Century American Medicine* (Princeton, N.J.: Princeton University Press, 1998), 185–206.

65. Bynum, *Science and the Practice of Medicine*, 17.

66. Rothman, *Living in the Shadow of Death*.

67. Richardson, "Phthisis Pulmonalis," 8.

68. Richardson, "Phthisis Pulmonalis," 9.

69. For physiognomy, see Barbara Stafford, *Body Criticism: Imaging the Unseen in Enlightenment Art and Medicine* (Cambridge, Mass.: MIT Press, 1991); and Christopher Rivers, *Face Value: Physiognomical Thought and the Legible Body in Marivaux, Lavater, Balzac, Gautier, and Zola* (Madison: University of Wisconsin Press, 1994).

70. William Carpenter, *Principles of Human Physiology with the Chief Applications to Psychology, Pathology, Therapeutics, Hygiéne, and Forensic Medicine*, by William B. Carpenter, M.D., F.R.S., F.G.S., ed. with additions by Francis Gurney Smith, M.D., new American from the last London ed. (Philadelphia: Blanchard and Lea, 1856), 190.

71. Richardson, "Phthisis Pulmonalis," 10–11.

72. Bynum, *Science and the Practice of Medicine*, 36.

73. Richardson, "Phthisis Pulmonalis," 16.

74. Bynum, *Science and the Practice of Medicine*, 40.

75. Richardson, "Phthisis Pulmonalis," 13.

76. Richardson, "Phthisis Pulmonalis," 13.

77. Richardson, "Phthisis Pulmonalis," 7–8.

78. Kane, *Experiments on Kiesteine*, 14.

79. Richardson, "Phthisis Pulmonalis," 14–15.

80. Bonner, *To the Ends of the Earth*, 15–16.

81. A cognate "disguised" thesis from the Department of Medicine at the University of Pennsylvania, written in the register of health, has as its official title "An Essay on Organic Life Force." On the first inside page, the author, Joshua G. Allen, has painstakingly inscribed, "An essay on Organic Life force: an Independent Vital Prin-

ciple contended for and explained upon a New Theory." See Allen, "An Essay on Organic Life Force."

82. Way discussed the general effects of various kinds of wounds on the body, recommended specific materials for and placements of sutures, and offered advice on the course of treatment for wound patients. But Robert Liston's *Elements of Surgery*, ed. Samuel D. Gross (Philadelphia: Ed. Barrington and Geo. Haswell, 1846), one of the recommended surgery texts, discussed wounds in detail (167 and passim), describing the effects of laceration on various levels of vascular tissue, the process of coagulation, and possible complications of treatment. Another recommended text, Alf. A. L. M. Velpeau's *New Elements of Operative Surgery*, first American from the last Paris ed. (New York: Langley, 1845), offered, besides an inimitable chapter on the "sang-froid of the surgeon," a discussion of the differences between lacerations of veins and those of arteries.

83. Sawin, "Anaemia," 6, quoting Carpenter, *Principles of Human Physiology*.

84. This passage is found in the 1856 edition of Carpenter, *Principles of Human Physiology*, which would not, of course, have been available to students graduating in 1853; I have not been able to locate the earlier edition of this text, but the coherence between Sawin's quotation and Carpenter's treatment of blood constituents leads me to believe that this section did not change substantially.

85. For the classic critique of "male as norm," see Helen Longino and Ruth Doell, "Body, Bias, and Behavior: A Comparative Analysis of Reasoning in Two Areas of Biological Science," *Signs: Journal of Women in Culture and Society* 9, no. 2 (winter 1983): 206–27.

86. Carpenter, *Principles of Human Physiology*, 189.

87. Gulielma Fell Alsop, *History of the Woman's Medical College, Philadelphia, Pennsylvania (1850–1950)* (Philadelphia: Lippincott, 1950), 35.

88. H. K. Hunt, *Glances and Glimpses*, 370.

89. WMC, Faculty Minutes, Nov. 18, 1850.

90. Alsop, *History of the Woman's Medical College*, 307; *Medical and Surgical Reporter* (Philadelphia), obituary, Francis McCloskey, n.s. 2 (1859): 189. Steven Peitzman drew my attention to this notice.

91. See Joseph Longshore, "The Ovular Theory of Menstruation, and Its History," *Eclectic Medical Journal of Philadelphia* 8, no. 6 (June 1865): 241–45.

92. H. W. Ellis, "Labor," 9.

93. WMC, Faculty Minutes, Jan. 19, 1853.

94. H. W. Johnson, "Skin and its Functions," 5.

95. Sale, "Haemoptysis," 9–10.

96. Sale, "Haemoptysis," 6.

97. Warner, *Therapeutic Perspective*, 208–20.

98. O'Hara, *An Emerging Profession*, 38.

99. John P. Richardson, "Enteric or Typhoid Fever," Department of Medicine, University of Pennsylvania, Preceptor H. D. W. Pawling, Department of Medicine. Feb 17, 1863, PA.

100. Edgar E. Hume, *Orthinologists of the US Army Medical Corps: Thirty-Six Biographies* (Baltimore: Johns Hopkins University Press, 1942), 90–104.

101. Hume, *Ornithologists*, 101.

102. Crawford, "Hypertrophy and Atrophy," 1–2.

103. John S. Cook, "An Essay on Diabetes" for the Degree of Doctor of Medicine, by John S. Cook, Easton, Northampton County, Penna., Preceptor Lewis C. Cook, M.D., 1850, 22, Rare Book and Manuscript Library, University of Pennsylvania.

104. Rivens, "Diagnosis of Pulmonary Disease," 21.

105. Black Women Physicians Project, 1864–1995, Carolyn Still Wiley Anderson file, ASCWM.

106. Caroline V. Wiley, "A Thesis on Fibromata," Presented to the Faculty of the Woman's Medical College of Pennsylvania for Degree of Doctor of Medicine by Caroline Wiley, Philadelphia, Session of 1877–78.

107. Matthew Anderson, *Presbyterianism. Its Relation to the Negro*, Illustrated by The Berean Presbyterian Church, Philadelphia, with Sketch of the Church and Autobiography of the Author (Philadelphia: John McGill, White, and Co., 1897), 251.

108. See *The Berean Manual Training and Industrial School* (Philadelphia: n.d., probably 1914); and *The Berean Manual Training and Industrial School* (Philadelphia, 1907–8); both in the Black Women Physicians Project, Anderson file, ASCWM.

109. Caroline V. Wiley-Anderson, "Popliteal Aneurism," in WMC, Alumnae Association, *Report of the Proceedings of the Thirteenth Annual Meeting of the Alumnae Association of the Woman's Medical College of Pennsylvania*, Mar. 16, 1888 (Philadelphia: Rodgers Printing, 1888), 33–35, MCP Collection, ASCWM.

110. Black Women Physicians Project, 1864–1995, Eliza Grier file, "Coal Black Woman Doctor," *North American Medical Review*, MCP clipping file, Acc. #133, ASCWM.

111. Ruth Lathrop, letter, Jan. 6, 1898, Black Women Physicians Project, Grier file.

112. The "emancipated slave" quotation is from Grier's letter to the president and proprietor of the Woman's Medical College, dated Dec. 6, 1890, Black Women Physicians Project, Grier file. An account of Grier's earlier education can be found in Darlene Clark Hine, *Black Women in America: An Historical Encyclopedia* (Bloomington: Indiana University Press, 1994). The story of Grier supporting her medical education by picking cotton is from Dorothy Salem, ed., *African American Women: A Biographical Dictionary* (New York: Garland, 1993). All documents from Black Women Physicians Project, Grier file.

113. Eliza Grier, letter to Susan B. Anthony, Mar. 7, 1901, Black Women Physicians Project, Grier file.

114. Georgia Fraser-Goins, "Miss Doc," 110, 111, Georgia Fraser-Goins Collection, Moorland-Spingarn Research Center, Manuscript Division, Howard University Library, quoted in Gloria Moldow, *Women Doctors in Gilded-Age Washington: Race, Gender, and Professionalization* (Urbana: University of Illinois Press, 1987), 130.

115. Wiley, "Fibromata," 44.

116. Wiley, "Fibromata," 1–2.

117. Wiley, "Fibromata," 8.

118. Wiley, "Fibromata," 15.

119. Wiley, "Fibromata," 36–37.

120. Wiley, "Fibromata," 20, 42.

121. Wiley, "Fibromata," 22.

122. WMC, Alumnae Association, *Report of the Proceedings of the Nineteenth An-*

nual Meeting of the Alumnae Association of the Woman's Medical College of Pennsylvania, May 9–10, 1894 (Philadelphia: Buchanan, 1894), 104.

123. WMC, Alumnae Association, *Report of the Proceedings of the Nineteenth Annual Meeting*, 104.

124. Georgiana Young, "A Thesis on Opium," Presented to the Faculty of the Woman's Medical College of Pennsylvania, for degree of Doctor of Medicine by Georgie E. Young, Philadelphia, Session of 1877–78. ASCWM.

125. Dr. C. Bruce Lee, letter to the dean of the Woman's Medical College of Pennsylvania, Apr. 20, 1964, Black Women Physicians Project, Georgiana Young file, ASCWM.

126. Young, "Opium," 40.

127. Young, "Opium," 19–20.

128. Young, "Opium," 27.

129. Juan F. Bennett, "Sanitary Chemistry," Submitted to the Faculty and Corporators of the Woman's Medical College for the Degree of Doctor of Medicine, Juan F. Bennett, 1888. ASCWM.

130. Elizabeth Blackwell, *Pioneer Work in Opening the Medical Profession to Women* (New York: Schocken, 1977; original publication, 1895), 288.

131. Bennett, "Sanitary Chemistry," 8, 9.

132. Bennett, "Sanitary Chemistry," 15.

133. Bennett, "Sanitary Chemistry," 34.

134. Bennett, "Sanitary Chemistry," 36.

135. Regina Morantz-Sanchez, *Sympathy and Science: Women Physicians in American Medicine* (New York: Oxford University Press, 1985).

CHAPTER 5. INVISIBLE WRITING II: HANNAH LONGSHORE AND THE BORDERS OF REGULARITY

1. Resources on the lives of the Longshore family are collected in the Longshore Papers, ASCWM. They include Hannah Longshore's autobiographical speech, catalogued as "Autobiography," and several of her letters. Works in the Longshore Papers at ASCWM by her husband, Thomas Longshore, include his "Sketch of Her Early Years," an undated manuscript; the unsigned "Biography of Hannah E. Longshore," an undated manuscript in two versions; and the unsigned "Biography of Joseph Skelton Longshore," an undated manuscript in two versions; both of the unsigned manuscripts are in Thomas Longshore's handwriting. Thomas E. Longshore's "History of the College," an undated manuscript notebook catalogued as his "Autobiography" (file 11), and miscellaneous clippings, articles, and correspondence are also included in the Longshore Papers. The New York Academy of Medicine holds Jane Campbell's "Sketch of the Life of Dr. Hannah Longshore, a Pioneer Woman Physician of Philadelphia," manuscript dated Oct. 29, 1901 (date crossed out).

Additional Longshore family letters and publications by Thomas Longshore are at the Friends Historical Library of Swarthmore College. The Friends Historical Library includes Thomas Longshore's published works, the pamphlets *"The Christ" Interpreted*, signed T. E. L. (Philadelphia, July 1884), 3 pages; *Father, Son, and Holy*

Ghost, by T. E. Longshore (n.d., n.p.), 22 pages; *The Spiritual Religion of Jesus and Salvation by Christ. Not Judaism nor Paganism; neither Greek nor Roman Mythology; Nor the Religion of Christianity as Taught by the Church in Ancient or Modern Times*, signed T. E. L. (Philadelphia: John Hiestand, Printer, July 1884), 15 pages; and *Our Lord and Savior Jesus Christ*, by T. E. Longshore (Philadelphia, Mar. 1888). Finally, the Friends Historical Library includes both Thomas Longshore's *George Fox Interpreted: The Religion, Revelations, Motives and Mission of George Fox Interpreted in the Light of the Nineteenth Century and Applied to the Present Condition of the Church* (Philadelphia: self-published, 1881); and his major work, *The Higher Criticism in Theology and Religion Contrasted with Ancient Myths and Miracles as Factors of Human Evolution and Other Essays on Reform* (New York: Somesby, 1892).

Joseph Longshore, brother of Thomas Longshore and brother-in-law of Hannah Longshore, is the author of the following: *The Principles and Practice of Nursing, or a Guide to the Inexperienced* (Philadelphia: Merrihew and Thompson, 1842); *The Philadelphia System of Obstetrics* (Philadelphia: University Publication Society, 1868); *Woman and Her Maladies: The Little Book of Forbidden Knowledge* (Philadelphia: Grant, Faires, and Rodgers, 1878); and *The Centennial Liberty Bell* (Philadelphia: Claxton, Remsen and Haffelfinger, 1876); all can be found in the general collection of the University of Pennsylvania Library but are also widely held. His "Introductory Lecture, delivered before the class, at the opening of the Female Medical College of Pennsylvania, Oct. 12, 1850" was published (Philadelphia: Young, 1850), as was his "Valedictory Address delivered before the graduating class, at the first annual commencement of the Female Medical College of Pennsylvania, held at the Musical Fund Hall, Dec. 30, 1851" (Philadelphia: Published by the graduates, 1852); both are in the collections of the ASCWM and CPP. The Longshore Papers at the ASCWM include several of his early letters.

Anna Longshore-Potts, sister of Joseph and Thomas and sister-in-law of Hannah Longshore, is the author of *Love, Courtship, and Marriage* (Paradise Valley Sanitarium, National City, San Diego County, Calif.: self-published, 1891), ASCWM; and *Discourses to Women on Medical Subjects* (London: self-published, 1897), ASCWM.

2. For short biographies of the three Myers sisters, see Fredrick C. Waite, "The Three Myers Sisters—Pioneer Women Physicians," *Medical Review of Reviews* (Mar. 1933): 1–7. For Mary Frame Myers Thomas's connections to suffrage journals, see Margaret Hope Bacon, *Mothers of Feminism: The Story of Quaker Women in America* (New York: Harper and Row), 90–91, 141.

3. A note on Anna Longshore-Potts is added, on a small piece of paper, to Thomas Longshore's undated manuscript notebook, catalogued as his "Autobiography."

4. WMC, Alumnae Association, *Transactions of the Thirty-eighth Annual Meeting of the Alumnae Association of the Woman's Medical College of Pennsylvania*, June 5–6, 1913 (Philadelphia: Published by the association, 1913), 38, MCP Collection, ASCWM.

5. Included among the Longshore Papers in the ASCWM are Lucretia Blankenburg, "Notes on an Interview with Mrs. Blankenburg" (no date or interviewer given). Here, Lucretia Blankenburg characterizes her mother as "a very conscientious woman of great hypnotic power. [She] hypnotized a child once unconsciously and

had to get another doctor to awaken the child." Mrs. Blankenburg speaks of Hannah Longshore's dedication, of her homeopathic tendencies, and ascribes to her a rivalry with Ann Preston: "Ann Preston, a school teacher friend of Dr. Longshore and a diligently trained Quaker, graduated the same time she did from the WMC. Dr. Preston was very frail. Went to a sanitarium. Mentally off. Was cured and became connected with the College. . . . Very jealous of Dr. Longshore. Dr. Longshore won out." She speculates that Hannah Longshore developed strength in her arms while driving her own horse that helped her to use forceps in a delivery, even though Ann Preston said it was not "ladylike" for Dr. Longshore to drive her own horse. Blankenburg concludes, "All the women that persecuted Dr. Longshore so are dead."

6. WMC, Alumnae Association, *Report of the Proceedings of the Seventeenth Annual Meeting of the Alumnae Association of the Woman's Medical College of Pennsylvania,* May 6–7, 1892 (Philadelphia: Smith and Salmon, 1892), 125, MCP Collection, ASCWM.

7. The Woman's Medical College toasts were not usually published, but an account of the toasts and replies for the first alumnae supper can be found in the WMC, Alumnae Association, *Report of Proceedings of the Seventeenth Annual Alumnae Meeting,* and the names of the toast-givers and their topics were often published by the alumnae (see 172–90).

8. WMC, Alumnae Association, *Report of the Proceedings of the Seventeenth Annual Alumnae Meeting,* 127.

9. WMC, Alumnae Association, *Report of the Proceedings of the Seventeenth Annual Alumnae Meeting,* 178, 179.

10. *Philadelphia Inquirer,* "Reunion, University of Pennsylvania," clipping dated Dec. 20, 1875, in the William Pepper Papers, PA.

11. Bacon, *Mothers of Feminism;* Karlyn Kohrs Campbell, *Man Cannot Speak for Her,* vol. 1: *A Critical Study of Early Feminist Rhetoric,* vol. 2: *Key Texts of the Early Feminists* (New York: Praeger, 1989).

12. See Ann Braude, *Radical Spirits: Spiritualism and Women's Rights in Nineteenth Century America* (Boston: Beacon, 1989); and A. Owen, *The Darkened Room: Women, Power, and Spiritualism in Late Victorian England* (Philadelphia: University of Pennsylvania Press, 1990).

13. Campbell, *Man Cannot Speak for Her,* vols. 1 and 2.

14. This speech exists as an untitled, undated holograph, in four versions: one final draft and three preliminary drafts, collected in the Longshore Papers as Hannah Longshore, "Autobiography," ASCWM. The final manuscript begins "Madam toast Mistress and co workers," and internal references date it at about 1895. In her unpublished "Sketch of the Life of Dr. Hannah Longshore," held at the New York Academy of Medicine, Jane Campbell tells the story of Longshore, "nearly fifty years after she had graduated from the infant Woman's Medical College," arising "at the Banquet now given annually by the Alumnae of the College, to answer the Toast 'Memories of Early Years.'" Campbell asserts that Longshore's reminiscences of the "days of Auld Lang Syne" made "one of the special features of the occasion." In date, form, and topic, the manuscript seems coherent with Campbell's account; the manuscript is surely a toast, and there is no other likely context in which a woman physician would have given such a speech. It is therefore very likely

that Longshore's manuscript was a reply to a toast given at the alumnae banquet.

15. In quoting Hannah Longshore throughout the chapter, I've presented the punctuation and spelling exactly as they appeared in the original sources.

16. In fact, although the charter of the Woman's Medical College was often invoked in its early history, successive archivists and institutional historians have never located that document.

17. Harold J. Abrahams, *Extinct Medical Schools of Nineteenth-Century Philadelphia* (Philadelphia: University of Pennsylvania Press, 1966).

18. Joseph Longshore, "Woman," *Eclectic Medical Journal of Philadelphia* 8, no. 1 (Jan. 1865): 14–19; and his "History of Obstetrics," *Eclectic Medical Journal of Philadelphia* 8, no. 3 (Mar. 1865): 117–20; 8, no. 4 (Apr. 1865): 160–63; 8, no. 5 (May 1865): 1–97.

19. T. Longshore, "History of the College," 28–29.

20. Rev. H. B. Elliot, "Woman as Physician," in *Eminent Women of the Age: Being Narratives of the Lives and Deeds of the Most Prominent Women of the Present Generation,* by James Parton and others (Hartford, Conn.: S. M. Betts and Company, 1868), 544.

21. Thomas and Hannah Longshore, letter to "you all," May 10, 1850, Longshore Papers, Family Correspondence file, ASCWM.

22. T. Longshore, "Autobiography," 95–100.

23. The story was dramatized in a radio play suggested by Lucretia Blankenburg, described in the Philadelphia Club of Advertising Women, "Notes of Philadelphia Friendship Dinner," typescript, May 2, 1936, Longshore Papers, ASCWM.

24. Ella Upham, "Women in Medicine," *North American Journal of Homeopathy* reprint, no date, 3.

25. Upham, "Women in Medicine," 5–6.

26. Warner, *Therapeutic Perspective,* 151.

27. T. Longshore, "Autobiography," 106.

28. J. Longshore, "A Valedictory Address," 4.

29. J. Longshore, "A Valedictory Address," 7.

30. J. Longshore, "A Valedictory Address," 11.

31. For the literature on women and autobiography, see Virginia Brereton, *From Sin to Salvation: Stories of Women's Conversions, 1800 to the Present* (Bloomington: Indiana University Press, 1991); Mary Jean Corbett, *Representing Femininity: Middle-Class Subjectivity in Victorian and Edwardian Women's Autobiographies* (New York: Oxford University Press, 1992); Susan Stanford Friedman, "Women's Autobiographical Selves," in *The Private Self: Theory and Practice of Women's Autobiographical Writings,* ed. Shari Benstock (Chapel Hill: University of North Carolina Press, 1988), 34–62; Estelle Jelinek, *The Tradition of Women's Autobiography: From Antiquity to the Present* (Boston: Twayne, 1986); and her *Women's Autobiography: Essays in Criticism* (Bloomington: Indiana University Press, 1980); Linda Peterson, *Victorian Autobiography: The Tradition of Self-Interpretation* (New Haven, Conn.: Yale University Press, 1986); Sidonie Smith, *A Poetics of Women's Autobiography: Marginality and the Fictions of Self-Representation* (Bloomington: Indiana University Press, 1987); Liz Stanley, *The Auto/Biographical I: The Theory and Practice*

of Feminist Auto/Biography (Manchester, England: Manchester University Press, 1992).

For a concise statement of the episodic nature of women's autobiographies, see Jelinek, *Tradition of Women's Autobiography,* 17. For women's autobiography as defined by relationship and connection, see, for example, Friedman, "Women's Autobiographical Selves," 41.

32. Ellen Fussell Cope, in her manuscript "Bits of Background," quotes from a letter of Graceanna Lewis on the Indiana antislavery campaign:

> Upon the platform with other women of Pendleton sat Rebecca Fussell, with her infant son in her arms. Frederick Douglass was speaking when the attack of the mob was made. A large man, wild with excitement, who had forced his way to the platform, with raised club was rushing toward the speaker to strike him down. On the impulse of the moment, she held up her child between the two. The man hesitated, looked ashamed, and with a muttered oath said, "We are not here to fight women and babies," and turned aside.

Graceanna Lewis letter, no recipient or date noted, quoted in Ellen Fussell Cope, "Bits of Background," 6–7, Friends Historical Library of Swarthmore College, SC 045: Alice Fussell, Fussell-Lewis Family Papers, folder 3.

33. Howard Brinton, *Quaker Journals: Varieties of Religious Experience among Friends* (Wallingford, Pa.: Pendle Hill, 1972), 1. The journal in question is that of John Woolman, 1720–70.

34. William Osler, *An Alabama Student and Other Biographical Essays,* 2d impression (New York: Oxford University Press, 1909). The biography of William Pepper (210–31) was delivered at the opening of the 1898 session of the Johns Hopkins Medical School.

35. Osler once remarked that "human kind might be divided into three groups— men, women, and women physicians." See Lillian Welsh, *Reminiscences of Thirty Years in Baltimore* (Baltimore: Norman, Remington, 1925), 44–45, quoted in Regina Markell Morantz-Sanchez, *Sympathy and Science: Women Physicians in American Medicine* (New York: Oxford University Press, 1985), 142.

36. See, for example, *The Journal,* "Gershom M. Fitch: A Biographical Sketch," 9, no. 9 (May 4, 1881): 67, FHL; or *Friends' Intelligencer,* "Life of James Parnel and Francis Howgill," 37 (1880): 21–22, 320–24, 337–41, FHL.

37. Peterson, *Victorian Autobiography,* 124–28.

38. T. Longshore, "Autobiography," 73.

39. T. Longshore, *George Fox Interpreted,* 124, 123.

40. T. Longshore, *George Fox Interpreted,* 24–25.

41. T. Longshore, *George Fox Interpreted,* 124.

42. T. Longshore, "Autobiography," 42–43.

43. T. Longshore, "Autobiography," 70; H. Longshore, "Autobiography," draft 2.

44. Bruno Latour and Steve Woolgar, *Laboratory Life: The Construction of Scientific Facts* (Princeton, N.J.: Princeton University Press, 1979).

45. Steven Shapin and Simon Schaffer, *Leviathan and the Air Pump: Hobbes, Boyle, and the Experimental Life* (Princeton: Princeton University Press, 1985).

46. Hannah Longshore, "A Case of Conception without Intromission," *Medical and Surgical Reporter* (Philadelphia) 50, no. 22 (May 31, 1884): 700–701.

47. J. Longshore, "A Valedictory Address," 14.

48. Anne Fausto-Sterling, *Myths of Gender: Biological Theories about Women and Men* (New York: Basic Books, 1992; originally published, 1985); Emily Martin, *The Woman in the Body: A Cultural Analysis of Reproduction* (Boston: Beacon, 1987); Max Charlesworth, "Whose Body? Feminist Views on Reproductive Technology," in *Troubled Bodies: Critical Perspectives on Postmodernism, Medical Ethics, and the Body,* ed. Paul A. Komesaroff (Durham, N.C.: Duke University Press, 1995), 125–41.

49. Edward Cass, "Letter from Ohio," *Medical and Surgical Reporter* (Philadelphia) 50, no. 22 (May 31, 1884): 685.

50. For connections between nineteenth-century scientific writing and literary and imaginative forms, see Jonathan Smith, *Between Fact and Feeling: Baconian Science and the Nineteenth-Century Literary Imagination* (Madison: University of Wisconsin Press, 1994).

51. Evelyn Fox Keller, *Reflections on Gender and Science* (New Haven, Conn.: Yale University Press, 1985), 86.

52. Sandra Harding, *Whose Science? Whose Knowledge? Thinking from Women's Lives* (Ithaca, N.Y.: Cornell University Press, 1991).

53. Sheila M. Rothman, *Living in the Shadow of Death: Tuberculosis and the Social Experience of Illness in American History* (New York: Basic Books, 1994).

54. G. Kass-Simon and Patricia Farnes, *Women of Science: Righting the Record* (Bloomington: University of Indiana Press, 1990), xii.

55. T. Longshore, "Autobiography," 45.

CHAPTER 6. MARY PUTNAM JACOBI: MEDICINE AS WILL AND IDEA

1. The case history is reprinted in Mary Putnam Jacobi, *Mary Putnam Jacobi, M.D.: A Pathfinder in Medicine,* ed. Women's Medical Association of New York City (New York: Putnam's Sons, 1925), 501–4, an important and generally reliable source for Mary Putnam Jacobi's medical writing (hereafter cited as Jacobi, *Pathfinder*). A typescript with Putnam Jacobi's handwritten corrections is held in the Mary Putnam Jacobi Collection, Jacobi Papers, folder 35, Schlesinger Library, Radcliffe College. Putnam Jacobi seems to have sent the case history to a number of physicians, asking their advice. The corrected typescript differs from the published document in several details: It is entitled "Case. Description of the Early Symptoms of the Meningeal Tumor Compressing the Cerebellum. From Which the Writer Dies. Written by Herself," with an epigraph from George Eliot: "The mention of ourselves is always affecting." The editors of *Pathfinder* make many small changes in punctuation and arrangement from the typescript, omitting place names and modifying dates; they do not include the handwritten additions. In the quoted section, the manuscript adds "to making a *plan*" after "exertion," and "*his* own" before "personal weakness."

The other easily available published source for Mary Putnam Jacobi's writing is Mary Putnam Jacobi, *Life and Letters of Mary Putnam Jacobi,* ed. Ruth Putnam (New York: Putnam's Sons, 1925).

(Note that even though I refer to Putnam Jacobi most often with the combined last names, her sources are all found under "Jacobi" in Works Cited, for that is how they are routinely catalogued in libraries and archives.)

2. For discussions of "so-called anti-sepsis," see Mary Putnam Jacobi, "Some Details on the Pathogeny of Pyaemia and Septicaemia," originally published in the *Medical Record* 7 (1872): 73–101 (see the reprint in Jacobi, *Pathfinder*, 171–200; quotation above on p. 197); for her discussion of Bright's disease, see the undated last letter to the editor (*Medical Record* 4 [1869–70]: 548–67) in Mary Putnam Jacobi, "Letters to the *Medical Record*, 1867–70—Medical Matters in Paris," signed P. C. M. (*Pathfinder*, 159–70).

3. Ann Preston, letter to Hannah Monaghan Darlington, May 26, 1833, MCP Deans Files, Preston Papers, ASCWM. For Putnam Jacobi's positivism, see her *The Value of Life: A Reply to Mr. Mallock's Essay "Is Life Worth Living?"* (New York: Putnam's Sons, 1879).

4. Mary Putnam Jacobi, *The Question of Rest for Women during Menstruation*, The Boylston Prize Essay of Harvard University, 1876 (New York: Putnam's Sons, 1877).

5. For marked and unmarked cross-dressing, see Marjorie Garber, *Vested Interests: Cross-Dressing and Cultural Anxiety* (New York: Routledge, 1992), 353–74.

6. Ann Douglas, *The Feminization of American Culture* (New York: Knopf, 1977).

7. Mary Putnam Jacobi, "Found and Lost," in Mary Putnam Jacobi, *Stories and Sketches* (New York: Putnam's Sons: 1907), 1–49 (first published in *Atlantic Monthly*, Apr. 1860).

8. Mary Putnam Jacobi, autobiographical manuscript, typescript, 1902, Mary Putnam Jacobi Collection, Jacobi Papers, a-26, folder 3, Schlesinger Library, Radcliffe College.

9. Jacobi, autobiographical manuscript, 4.

10. Jacobi, autobiographical manuscript, 5.

11. See her letters in Mary Putnam Jacobi, Correspondence, Mary Putnam Jacobi Collection, Jacobi Papers, Schlesinger Library, Radcliffe College: from her grandmother, Oct. 1, 1854, on her sense of sin, and her reply Oct. 1854 (folder 5); to her brother, in 1857, urging conversion (folder 6); to her grandmother, Sept. 15, 1861, agreeing to continue church attendance (folder 7); the 1854 letters are reprinted in Jacobi, *Life and Letters*. In 1863, she wrote that she was "a total disbeliever in the distinctive tenets of the technically called orthodox system of divinity" but swore not to attend any stage performance for ten years, lest anyone believe that she had left the church in search of amusement (Jacobi, *Life and Letters*, 58).

12. Mary Putnam Jacobi, "Fragment at the thought of her twelfth birthday," filed with Correspondence, Mary Putnam Jacobi Collection, Jacobi Papers, folder 5, Schlesinger Library, Radcliffe College.

13. Mary Putnam Jacobi, "Foreword to the Family," Mary Putnam Jacobi Collection, Jacobi Papers, a-26, folder 3, SL.

14. See her father's letter about the "repulsive pursuit" of medical science (Jacobi, *Life and Letters*, 70) and also his letters urging her to delay her medical studies and to return home from Paris (Jacobi, Correspondence, 1871, folder 8). George Putnam did become reconciled to his daughter's medical career.

15. See Jacobi, *Life and Letters*, 110, Feb. 1, 1867. As a mother, Mary Putnam

Jacobi wrote to her daughter in terms that recalled those she had used toward her father. During a serious illness, Putnam Jacobi wrote a letter to be read by her daughter after Mary's death; she urged her daughter "always to seek to know the most that can be known, so as to be able to live the largest life" (Jacobi, Correspondence, letter to Marjorie Jacobi, July 3, 1889, Mary Putnam Jacobi Collection, Jacobi Papers, folder 14, Schlesinger Library, Radcliffe College).

16. Jacobi's letter to Dr. J. V. Ingham, 1900, autograph case, CPP, details her professional memberships.

17. Mary Putnam Jacobi, "Woman in Medicine," in *Woman's Work in America*, ed. Annie Nathan Meyer (New York: Holt, 1891), 139–205. Full bibliographies of Mary Putnam Jacobi's work can be found in *Life and Letters* and in *Pathfinder*.

18. Mary Putnam Jacobi, M.D., and Victoria White, M.D., *On the Use of the Cold Pack Followed by Massage in the Treatment of Anaemia* (New York: Putnam's Sons, 1880); and Mary Putnam Jacobi, *Essays on Hysteria, Brain Tumor and Some Other Causes of Nervous Disease* (New York: Putnam's Sons, 1888).

19. See, for example, Elizabeth Blackwell's collection *Essays in Medical Sociology* (New York: Arno Press, 1972; original publication, 1902); and her *Laws of Life: With Special Reference to the Physical Education of Girls* (New York: Garland, 1986; original publication, 1852).

20. See the list of publications by members of the Woman's Medical College of Pennsylvania Alumnae Association in Clara Marshall, *The Woman's Medical College of Pennsylvania: An Historical Outline* (Philadelphia: P. Blakiston, 1897), 89–142.

21. Mary Putnam Jacobi, "Urethral Irritation," *Proceedings of the Philadelphia County Medical Society* 13 (1892): 450–62; quotation from Henry, 457; quotation from Tyson, 458; quotation from Roberts, 460.

22. Jacobi, Correspondence, 1861, folder 7.

23. Jacobi, *Life and Letters*, 266.

24. Mary Putnam, "Theorae ad Lienis officium," Thesis Medicinae Collegii Foeminis Pennsylvaniae Facultati submissa ad gradem obtinendum Medicinae Doctoris, Maria C. Putname scripta, New York, 1864.

25. WMC, Faculty Minutes, Feb. 26, 1864, MCP Collection, ASCWM.

26. For a full account of the controversy concerning Mary Putnam's status at the Woman's Medical College, see Carol Gartner, "Fussell's Folly: Academic Standards and the Case of Mary Putnam Jacobi," *Academic Medicine* 71, no. 5 (May 1996): 470–77.

27. Jacobi, "Woman in Medicine," 161–62.

28. Jacobi, "Woman in Medicine," 163.

29. Jacobi, letter to her mother, June 1864, in Jacobi, *Life and Letters*, 275.

30. Jacobi, *Life and Letters*, 76.

31. Some of the *New Orleans Sunday Times* columns are collected in the Mary Putnam Jacobi Collection, Jacobi Papers, folder 28, SL; they are signed "Mary Israel" and begin as sketches written while Putnam was tutoring in New Orleans. The sketches began to be published in October 1866 (Jacobi, *Life and Letters*, 106); they were "cut back" early in 1867 and came to an end sometime before May 1867 (Jacobi, *Life and Letters*, 110, 133). The essays in the *Medical Record*, signed "P. C. M.," were written from 1867 to 1870 and are reprinted in Jacobi, *Pathfinder*, 1–171. The letters

to the New York *Evening Post* began as compilations from French newspapers, for which she was paid ten dollars a week, and they developed into notes on "gossip." Putnam began writing them in December 1866; they were cut back in the summer of 1867 and resumed as weekly columns in September 1867, although the editor became dissatisfied with them in November, and they seem to have been discontinued soon after (Jacobi, *Life and Letters,* 107, 112, 147, 153). In October 1867, the *Philadelphia Reporter* also began to carry her letters (Jacobi, *Life and Letters,* 150). I have not made a complete search for this journalism.

32. For the *Medical Record* correspondence, see Joy Harvey, "La Visite: Mary Putnam Jacobi and the Paris Medical Clinics," in *French Medical Culture in the Nineteenth Century,* ed. Ann La Berge and Mordechai Feingold, Wellcome Institute Series in the History of Medicine (Amsterdam and Atlanta, Ga.: Clio Medica 25, 1994), 350–71. The correspondence is also discussed in John Harley Warner, *Against the Spirit of System: The French Impulse in Nineteenth-Century American Medicine* (Princeton, N.J.: Princeton University Press, 1998), 322–29. Warner concludes that "it is quite possible that Putnam, during her time abroad, wrote more on Paris than any other nineteenth-century American physician—in private letters, in professional journals, in popular periodicals, and in newspapers," but that Putnam, coming to Paris after French empiricism had been disseminated to the United States, did not experience Parisian medicine as deeply at odds with American scientific medicine (328).

33. Jacobi, *Life and Letters,* 134–37.

34. Jacobi, *Life and Letters,* 146–47.

35. Jacobi, *Life and Letters,* 217.

36. "Imagination and Language," originally published in *Putnam's Monthly,* Mar. 1868; "A Study of Still-Life, Paris," from *Putnam's Monthly,* Dec. 1868; "A Sermon at Notre-Dame," from *Putnam's Monthly,* Dec. 1868 and Feb. 1869; "A Martyr to Science," from *Putnam's Monthly,* Aug. 1869; *Concerning Charlotte,* from *Putnam's Monthly,* Jan., Feb., and Mar. 1870; and "Some of the French Leaders," from *Scribner's Monthly,* Aug. 1871, are reprinted with the early stories "Found and Lost" and "Hair Chains" in Mary Putnam Jacobi, *Stories and Sketches* (New York: Putnam's Sons, 1907). All citations to these stories pertain to *Stories and Sketches.* Her letter to her family of Sept. 4, 1871, was reprinted in *Putnam's Monthly,* Nov. 1870; it is included in Jacobi, *Life and Letters,* 255–69. She also wrote "The Clubs of Paris," *Scribner's Monthly* 3 (Nov. 1871): 105–8, which is not included in *Stories and Sketches.*

37. Jacobi, *Life and Letters,* 188.

38. Jacobi, *Life and Letters,* 98.

39. Jacobi, *Life and Letters,* 132–33.

40. Jacobi, *Life and Letters,* 174.

41. For an account of Mary Putnam Jacobi's political activity and relationship to the Réclus family, see Joy Harvey, "Medicine and Politics: Dr. Mary Putnam Jacobi and the Paris Commune," *Dialectical Anthropology* 15 (1990): 107–17.

42. Jacobi, *Life and Letters,* 147.

43. Jacobi, *Life and Letters,* 190.

44. Nancy Cervetti, "S. Weir Mitchell: Literature and Medicine," unpublished talk, Wood Institute for the History of Medicine, Mar. 1997, CPP.

45. See the use of woorara in Mary Putnam Jacobi, "Pathogeny of Infantile Paralysis," a paper originally read before the New York County Medical Society, Dec. 22, 1873, first published in the *American Journal of Obstetrics* 8 (1874): 1–24, and included in Jacobi, *Pathfinder*, 240–83; and Mary Putnam Jacobi, "The Indication for Quinine in Pneumonia," first published in the *New York Medical Journal*, 1887, and included in Jacobi, *Pathfinder*, 419–45.

46. Jacobi, *Life and Letters*, 200.

47. Jacobi, *Stories and Sketches*, 223.

48. Jacobi, *Stories and Sketches*, 246.

49. Jacobi, *Stories and Sketches*, 354.

50. Jacobi, *Stories and Sketches*, 368.

51. Mary Putnam Jacobi, "Inaugural Address at the Opening of the Woman's Medical College of the New York Infirmary, October 1, 1880," in Jacobi, *Pathfinder*, 347.

52. Mary Putnam Jacobi, "Modern Female Invalidism," in Jacobi, *Pathfinder*, 482.

53. Charles Reade, *The Woman-Hater* (Paris and Boston: Grolier Society, n.d.). *The Woman-Hater* was originally published in *Blackwood's Magazine* from June 1876 to June 1877 and then issued in three volumes in June 1877. See the interesting discussion of the relation between this novel and British physician Sophia Jex-Blake in Frederick Wegener, "'A Line of Her Own': Henry James's 'Sturdy Little Doctress' and the Medical Woman as Literary Type in Gilded-Age America," *Texas Studies in Language and Literature* 39, no. 2 (summer 1997): 139–80.

54. Harvey, "La Visite."

55. Jacobi, *Pathfinder*, 34.

56. Jacobi, *Pathfinder*, 46, 57.

57. Jacobi, *Pathfinder*, 62–67, 96–97, 114.

58. Jacobi, *Pathfinder*, 38.

59. Margaret Richardson, "A Disquisition on Phthisis Pulmonalis," respectfully Submitted to the Faculty of the Female Medical College of Pennsylvania as an Inaugural Thesis for the Degree of the Doctorate in Medicine, By Margaret Richardson of Pennsylvania, Period of Study, three years, Preceptor, J. S. Longshore, M.D., Philadelphia, December 30th, 1852, 16–17, ASCWM. See the discussion of Richardson's thesis in chapter 4 of this book.

60. John W. Sale, "An Essay on Haemoptysis" For the Degree of Doctor of Medicine in the University of Pennsylvania, by John W. Sale, of Bedford County, State of Virginia, Residence in the City No. 13th Filbert St. Preceptor R. A. Sale, M.D., Duration of Studies 3 years, Presented on the 15th of Jany, 1850, 5–7, PA.

61. Steven Peitzman, *A New and Untried Course: Woman's Medical College and Medical College of Pennsylvania* (New Brunswick, N.J.: Rutgers University Press, 2000), chap. 4.

62. Jacobi, *Pathfinder*, 39.

63. Barbara Stafford, *Body Criticism: Imaging the Unseen in Enlightenment Art and Medicine* (Cambridge, Mass.: MIT Press, 1991).

64. Sir Walter Scott, *Waverly* (New York: Penguin, 1972; original publication, 1814), 175.

65. Ralph Waldo Emerson, "Nature," in *Emerson: Essays, First and Second Series*, ed. Douglas Crane (New York: Vintage, 1990), 313.

66. Jacobi, *Pathfinder,* 39.

67. Jacobi, *Pathfinder,* 8.

68. Jacobi, *Pathfinder,* 114–33, 28–31, 73–75, 137–43.

69. M. A. K. Halliday and J. R. Martin, *Writing Science: Literacy and Discursive Power* (Pittsburgh: University of Pittsburgh Press), 13–15.

70. Jacobi, *Pathfinder,* 134.

71. Jacobi, *Pathfinder,* 136.

72. Jacobi, *Pathfinder,* 22–24, 41–44, 65–72, 143–70.

73. Ludmilla Jordanova, *Sexual Visions: Images of Gender in Science and Medicine between the Eighteenth and Twentieth Centuries* (New York: Harvester, 1989), 87–110.

74. Jacobi, *Pathfinder,* 48.

75. Jacobi, Correspondence, 1871.

76. Putnam to her mother, in Jacobi, *Life and Letters,* 271.

77. Jacobi, *Life and Letters,* 276.

78. Jacobi, "The Clubs of Paris," 105–8.

79. See Jacobi, *Stories and Sketches,* 390–443.

80. Jacobi, *Stories and Sketches,* 390.

81. Gilder's remarks were made at a memorial meeting, Jan. 4, 1907. Addresses were also given by William Osler, Dr. Elizabeth Cushier, Prof. Felix Adler, Mrs. Florence Kelley, Dr. Charles Dana, Mr. Richard Watson Gilder, and Dr. Annie S. Daniel. An invitation to the meeting is included in Jacobi, Correspondence, folder 20. The address itself was published as Richard Watson Gilder, "Address," in *In Memory of Mary Putnam Jacobi* (New York: Academy of Medicine, 1907), 43–56, quotation on 53. The comments in *The Nation* are reported in Jacobi, *Life and Letters,* 294.

82. Jacobi, "Clubs of Paris," 107.

83. Jacobi, "Clubs of Paris," 107.

84. Jacobi, *Life and Letters,* 298.

85. For summaries of Putnam Jacobi's early presentations to the Pathological Society, see Mary Putnam Jacobi: "Anomalous Malformation of the Heart," 111; "Intestinal Obstruction," 208; "Thrombosis of Ovarian Veins," 215; "Scarlatinous Nephritis," 354 (all in *Medical Record* 7 [1872]); and "Phenomena Attending Section of the Right Restiform Body," 17; "A Case of Malignant Icterus," 65; and "Ovarian Tumor," 342 (all in *Medical Record* 8 [1873]).

For Mary Putnam's entrance into professional societies, I have drawn on the account in "Member of Medical Societies," in Jacobi, *Pathfinder* (xxviii–xxx), and the list included in her letter to Dr. J. V. Ingham, 1900, autograph case, CPP. The *Pathfinder* account gives two dates for Mary Putnam's admission to the New York County Medical Society, locating it on November 27, 1871, and in 1873. The first date is correct.

86. Jacobi, "Some Details," *Pathfinder,* 177–78.

87. I am deeply indebted to Russell Viner for his paper "Radical Medicine in Ante-Bellum New York City: Abraham Jacobi and German Social Medicine in America," Fall 1996 Workshop Series of the Department of History and Sociology of Science at the University of Pennsylvania, Oct. 7, 1996. The standard published contemporary source on Mary Putnam Jacobi's relation with Abraham Jacobi is Joy Harvey, "Clanging Eagles: The Marriage and Collaboration between Two Nineteenth-

Century Physicians, Mary Putnam Jacobi and Abraham Jacobi," in *Creative Couples in the Sciences*, ed. Helena Pycior, Nancy Slack, and Pnina Abir-am (New Brunswick, N.J.: Rutgers University Press, 1995), 185–95.

88. Rhoda Truax, *The Doctors Jacobi* (Boston: Little, Brown, 1952).

89. See the undated letter from Abraham Jacobi, asking Mary Putnam Jacobi, apparently living elsewhere after a quarrel, to return home (Jacobi, Correspondence, folder 21). Harvey dates this letter in spring 1883.

90. Letter from Mary Putnam to her mother, Jan. 25, 1868, in Jacobi, *Life and Letters*, 168.

91. Gilder, "Address," 53.

92. "Croup and Diphtheria," *Medical Record* 12 (1876): 397, was signed "M. P. Jacobi"; "Note on the Cause of Sudden Death during the Operation of Thoracentesis," letter to the editor, *Medical Record* 16 (1879): 139, was signed "M. Putnam-Jacobi"; "Case of Facial and Palatine Paralysis and Loss of Equilibrium Produced by a Fall on the Head," *Independent Practitioner* 2 (1881): 69, was signed "M. Putnam Jacobi, M.D." Her most common signature was "Mary Putnam Jacobi, M.D."; this was her signature for both *The Question of Rest for Women during Menstruation* and the *Essays on Hysteria*. Many of these signatures conceal Jacobi's gender; they also alternate between hyphenating her paternal name with her husband's or keeping it as a middle name.

Some of Mary Putnam Jacobi's many drafts of her name survived; the memorial tablet in her honor at the Woman's Medical College of Pennsylvania is inscribed to "Mary Putnam Jacobi," but the account of unveiling the tablet records her name as "Mary Putnam-Jacobi" (WMC, Alumnae Association, "Addresses at the Unveiling of a Memorial Tablet in Honor of Mary Putnam-Jacobi," in WMC, *Transactions of the Thirty-second Annual Meeting of the Alumnae Association of the Woman's Medical College of Pennsylvania*, May 23–24, 1907 [Philadelphia: Published by the association, 1907], 56–71, MCP Collection, ASCWM). The *Life and Letters* and *Pathfinder* volumes both speak of her as Mary Putnam Jacobi. In this book, I have used the most common forms of her name, referring to her as Mary Putnam before her marriage and as Mary Putnam Jacobi after her marriage, using "Putnam Jacobi" as the surname.

93. The first edition of this work is a fifty-page pamphlet: Abraham Jacobi, *Infant Diet, a Paper Read before the Public Health Association of New York*, by A. Jacobi, M.D. (New York: Putnam's Sons, 1873). It was reissued in 1874 as A. Jacobi, *Infant Diet, Revised, Enlarged, and Adapted to Popular Use* by Mary Putnam Jacobi, M.D. (New York: Putnam's Sons), 119 pp.; it was part of the Putnam's Handy Book Series of popular educational materials.

94. A. Jacobi, *Infant Diet*, rev. ed., iii.

95. A. Jacobi, *Infant Diet*, rev. ed., v.

96. A. Jacobi, *Infant Diet*, rev. ed., iv.

97. A. Jacobi, *Infant Diet*, rev. ed., iv.

98. Mary Putnam Jacobi, "Reply to Prof. Munsterberg on American Women's Education," typescript, Mary Putman Jacobi Collection, Jacobi Papers, Writings, 1873, folder 30, 3, Schlesinger Library, Radcliffe College.

99. Jacobi, "Reply to Prof. Munsterberg," 14.

100. Jacobi, "Reply to Prof. Munsterberg," 14.

101. Edward H. Clarke, *Sex in Ediucation: Or, A Fair Chance for Girls* (Boston: Osgood, 1873).

102. Vern Bullough and Martha Voght, "Women, Menstruation, and Nineteenth-Century Medicine," *Bulletin of the History of Medicine* 47 (1973): 66–82. See also Thomas Laqueur, *Making Sex: Body and Gender from the Greeks to Freud* (Cambridge, Mass.: Harvard University Press, 1990), 220–24. Laqueur locates Putnam Jacobi's innovation in the assimilation of reproduction to nutrition but does not understand that Putnam Jacobi saw nutrition as the broad process, involving both nerves and blood, both food and stimulation. Although Laqueur's critique places Putnam Jacobi's essay within the millennial controversy between one-sex and two-sex theories, it does not place the essay within specific nineteenth-century understandings of nutrition, and it ignores the performative aspects of the essay, including its use of survey information.

103. Jacobi, *Pathfinder,* xxvii.

104. C. Alice Baker reported this to Mary Putnam Jacobi in a letter to her, Nov. 7, 1874, Mary Putnam Jacobi Collection, Jacobi Papers, Baker correspondence, Schlesinger Library, Radcliffe College.

105. Baker, letter to Putnam Jacobi, Nov. 7, 1874. Baker refers to an essay of Jacobi's in "Miss Brockett's book," which does not appear in any of the Putnam Jacobi bibliographies.

106. Agnes C. Vietor, ed., *A Woman's Quest: The Life of Marie Zakrzewska, M.D.* (New York: Appleton, 1924), 67.

107. This event was reported in the London *Echo* (Monday, Aug. 29, 1870, 4); the prizewinner's name is given as "Margaret Webster." In a cognate account in the *New Republic* (June 25, 1870; WMC, College Scrapbooks, #3, Jan. 1870–Aug. 1871, 10, ASCWM), the name of the sponsoring journal is given as the *Medical Gazette.* No journal by that name was published in Philadelphia; the New York *Medical Gazette* ran a contest for the largest number of publishable clinical accounts but did not publish during this period. I am grateful to Sally Mitchell for the original *Echo* account.

108. Jacobi, *The Question of Rest,* 78.

109. Laqueur, *Making Sex,* 221–23.

110. Laqueur, *Making Sex,* 223–24.

111. Jacobi, *The Question of Rest,* 27.

112. Jacobi, *The Question of Rest,* 27.

113. D. Armstrong, *Political Anatomy of the Body: Medical Knowledge in Britain in the Twentieth Century* (Cambridge: Cambridge University Press, 1983), 51.

114. Jacobi, *The Question of Rest,* 62.

115. Jacobi, *The Question of Rest,* 46.

116. Catherine Beecher, *Letters to the People on Health and Happiness* (New York: Harper and Row, 1855); see also the useful discussion of Beecher, Weir Mitchell, and Elizabeth Blackwell in Ann Douglas Wood's "'The Fashionable Diseases': Women's Complaints and Their Treatment in Nineteenth-Century America," *Journal of Interdisciplinary History* 4 (1973): 25–52.

117. Beecher, *Letters to the People,* 124.

118. Elizabeth Blackwell, "The Influence of Women in the Profession of Medi-

NOTES TO PAGES 177–179

cine," in *Essays in Medical Sociology,* vol. 2 (New York: Arno Press, 1972; original publication, 1902), 20.

119. For an extended comparison of Putnam Jacobi and Elizabeth Blackwell, see Regina Markell Morantz-Sanchez, *Sympathy and Science: Women Physicians in American Medicine* (New York: Oxford University Press), 184–202.

120. Jacobi, *Pathfinder,* 355.

121. See Mary Putnam Jacobi, "Nitrite of Amyl and Belladonna in Dysmenor-rhoea," *Medical Record* 10 (1875): 11; and Mary Putnam Jacobi, "Remarks upon the Action of Nitrate of Silver on Epithelial and Gland Cells," *Transactions of the New York State Medical Society* (1875): 251, reprinted in Jacobi, *Pathfinder,* 284–94; Mary Putnam Jacobi, "Provisional Report on the Effect of Quinine upon the Cerebral Circula-tion," *Archives of Medicine* 1 (1879): 33. The bibliography printed in *Pathfinder* also lists "The Treatment of Hydrophobia by Woorara," in the *Transactions of the New York State Medical Society* (1877): 23, an essay I have not been able to locate or confirm.

For other essays written during the 1870s, see, for example, Mary Putnam Jacobi, "Curious Congenital Deformities of Upper and Lower Extremities," *Medical Record* 12 (1878): 115; and Mary Putnam Jacobi, "Acute Fatty Degeneration of the New-born," *American Journal of Obstetrics* 2 (1878): 499, reprinted in Jacobi, *Pathfinder,* 311–25. For presentations at the Pathological Society, see Mary Putnam Jacobi, "Pu-erperal Fever, Infection from Ovary through Retroperitoneal Glands," *Medical Rec-ord* 11 (1876): 307 (not 387, as in Jacobi, *Pathfinder* bibliography); or Mary Putnam Jacobi, "Malignant Icterus with Great Enlargement of the Liver," *Transactions of the New York State Pathological Society* 3 (1879): 50.

122. For sphygmographic investigations see Mary Putnam Jacobi, "Sphygmo-graphic Experiments upon a Human Brain Exposed by an Opening in the Cranium," *American Journal of the Medical Sciences* 76 (1878): 10–21, reprinted in Jacobi, *Path-finder,* 299–310; and Mary Putnam Jacobi, "Contribution to Sphygmography: The Influence of Pain on the Pulse Trace," *Archives of Medicine* 1 (1879): 33–35, re-printed in Jacobi, *Pathfinder,* 326–28.

123. "Studies in Endometritis" was published in successive numbers of the *Ameri-can Journal of Obstetrics* 18 (1885): 36–50, 113–28, 262–83, 519–37, 596–606. A series of related articles continues in that same issue of the journal as "Morbid Varia-tions in the Greater or Parturient Cycle, Subinvolution and Chronic Metritis (Studies in Endometritis)," 802–30; and "Menstrual Subinvolution or Metritis of the Non-parturient Uterus (Studies in Endometritis)," 915–25. And in a subsequent issue of the journal, the series continues with "The Ovarian Complication of Endometritis (Studies in Endometritis)," *American Journal of Obstetrics* 19 (1886): 352–67; "Theo-ries of Menstruation: New Theory (Studies in Menstruation)," *American Journal of Obstetrics* 18 (1885): 376.

Essays on Hysteria, Brain-Tumor and Some Other Cases of Nervous Disease con-tains a number of essays not reprinted elsewhere, although "A Case of Probable Tu-mor of the Pons" is reprinted in Jacobi, *Pathfinder,* 446–57. For Putnam Jacobi's earliest work in nervous diseases, see her publication with Victoria White, *On the Use of the Cold Pack Followed by Massage in the Treatment of Anaemia.*

124. Silas Weir Mitchell, *Fat and Blood: And How to Make Them,* 2d ed. (Phila-delphia: Lippincott, 1878; original publication, 1877); the library of the College of

Physicians of Philadelphia shows eight editions. Charlotte Perkins Gilman, "The Yellow Wall-Paper," in *The Yellow Wall-Paper,* ed. E. Hedges, rev. 2d ed. (Old Westbury, Conn.: Feminist Press, 1996; short story originally published 1892 in *New England Magazine*), 9–36.

125. Jacobi and White, *On the Use of the Cold Pack,* 4.

126. Jacobi and White, *On the Use of the Cold Pack,* 46.

127. Mary Putnam Jacobi, "Some Considerations on Hysteria," in Jacobi, *Essays on Hysteria,* 1.

128. See, for example, Mitchell's advice that the physician "seize the proper occasions to direct the thoughts of his patients to the lapse from duties to others, and to the selfishness which a life of invalidism is apt to bring about. Such moral medication belongs to the higher sphere of the doctor's duties, and if he means to cure his patient permanently, he cannot afford to neglect them" (*Fat and Blood,* 46). Putnam Jacobi sent Weir Mitchell a copy of her hysteria book; he wrote a letter praising what he had read, confessing that he envied Putnam Jacobi her "strong logical use of facts in theory. . . . I reason with difficulty on these complex questions with which your mind seems to play" (Mitchell, undated letter in Jacobi, Correspondence, 1901–2, folder 17).

129. Jacobi, "Some Considerations on Hysteria," 12.

130. Jacobi, "Some Considerations on Hysteria," 13.

131. Jacobi, "Some Considerations on Hysteria," 16.

132. Jacobi, "Some Considerations on Hysteria," 64–65.

133. WMC, Alumnae Association, "Addresses at the Unveiling of a Memorial Tablet in Honor of Mary Putnam-Jacobi," 56–71, 66.

134. Charlotte Perkins Gilman, *The Diaries of Charlotte Perkins Gilman,* vol. 2: *1890–1935,* ed. Denise D. Knight (Charlottesville: University Press of Virginia, 1994), 819–23. See also Gilman's account in *The Living of Charlotte Perkins Gilman: An Autobiography* (New York: Appleton-Century, 1935), where she writes that "the distinctive feature of her method was to set that inert brain to work under her direct suggestion and supervision, on small, irrelevant tasks; this to re-establish the capacity for action, without demanding any effort from me. We began with kindergarten blocks, just building things, for slowly increasing periods of application, but before she was through with me I was reading, still at her desk and under her direction, Wilson on *The Cell*" (291).

135. Jacobi, "Some Considerations on Hysteria," 20.

136. Jacobi, "Some Considerations on Hysteria," 64.

137. Jacobi, "Some Considerations on Hysteria," 66.

138. Truax, *The Doctors Jacobi,* 202–9; Jacobi, *Pathfinder,* 349.

139. See, besides "Studies in Endometritis," previously noted, Mary Putnam Jacobi: "The Nature and Dangers of Intra-uterine Medication," *Medical Record* 33 (1888): 23; "Intra-Uterine Therapeutics," *American Journal of Obstetrics* 22 (1889): 449; "Limitations and Dangers of Intra-Uterine Medication," *American Journal of Obstetrics* 22 (1889): 598, 697; "The Use of Electricity in Gynaecology," WMC, *Report of the Proceedings of the Fourteenth Annual Meeting of the Alumnae Association of the Woman's Medical College of Pennsylvania,* Mar. 15, 1889 (Philadelphia: Rodgers Printing Co, 1889), 60, MCP Collection, ASCWM.

140. Mary Putnam Jacobi: "A Case of Trephining of Sternum for Osteomyelitis,"

American Journal of Obstetrics 14 (1881): 981; "Salpingo-oophorectomy," *New York Medical Journal* 29 (1884): 673; "Cystic Ovaries; Battey's Operation," *Medical Record* 25 (1884): 705. For further examples of surgical cases see Mary Putnam Jacobi: "Aspiration of Dermoid Cysts Followed by Inflammation," *American Journal of Obstetrics* 16 (1883): 1160–70; and Mary Putnam Jacobi, "Case of Uterine Fibroid Treated by Apostoli's Method: Enucleation of the Tumor," *American Journal of Obstetrics* 21 (1888): 806.

141. Jacobi, *Essays on Hysteria*, 178.
142. Jacobi, "Studies in Endometritis," 283.
143. Jacobi, *Essays on Hysteria*, 178.
144. Jacobi, "Studies on Endometritis," 37.
145. Illustrations appear in Jacobi, "Studies in Endometritis" on 126, 262–63, 266–67, 269, 811–16, and 923. Other significant illustrations occur in Mary Putnam Jacobi: "Case of Absent Uterus: With Considerations of the Significance of the Hermaphrodism," *American Journal of Obstetrics* 32, no. 4 (Oct. 1895): 512; and "Remarks upon Empyema," *Medical News* 56 (1890): 120–21, 172–73.
146. Jacobi, "Studies in Endometritis," 814.
147. Jacobi, "Studies in Endometritis," 813.
148. Jacobi, *Pathfinder*, 461.
149. Jacobi, *Pathfinder*, 462.
150. Jacobi, *Pathfinder*, 462.
151. Judith Butler, *Gender Trouble: Feminism and the Subversion of Identity* (New York: Routledge, 1990), 24–25.
152. But see Regina Morantz-Sanchez, "Making It in a Man's World: The Late-Nineteenth-Century Surgical Career of Mary Amanda Dixon Jones," *Bulletin of the History of Medicine* 69 (1995): 542–68.
153. Jacobi, *Life and Letters*, 221.
154. Jacobi, *Life and Letters*, 286.
155. Jacobi, *Pathfinder*, 291.
156. Jacobi, "Woman in Medicine," 156.
157. Jacobi, "Woman in Medicine," 177.
158. Jacobi, "Woman in Medicine," 199.
159. Jacobi, *Pathfinder*, 352.
160. Jacobi, *Pathfinder*, 480. The specific essay is "Modern Female Invalidism," unpublished before its inclusion in *Pathfinder*, 478–82.
161. Jacobi, *Pathfinder*, 393.
162. Jacobi, *Pathfinder*, 394, 397.
163. Jacobi, *Pathfinder*, 401.
164. Jacobi, "Woman in Medicine," 196.

CHAPTER 7. FORBIDDEN SIGHTS: WOMEN AND THE VISUAL ECONOMY OF MEDICINE

1. This account is drawn from Pennsylvania Hospital, Minute Book of the Board of Managers, Oct.–Dec. 1869, R11D12, HLPH; and from WMC, College Scrap-

books, MCP-C7, Acc. #133, ASCWM, which is a collection of many (often unidentified) press clippings on the event. I have also consulted the accounts given, usually
many years later, by students who were present at the jeering incident: Anna
Broomall and Eliza Wood-Armitage, all included in the WMC Deceased Alumnae
Files, ASCWM; Sarah Hibbard, manuscript draft of lectures and sermons, Manuscripts, MS 54, Acc. #189, ASCWM; and the recollections by Evelyn Keller, in her
reply to a toast at the 1906 alumnae banquet, "Report of the Entertainment Committee," in WMC, Alumnae Association, *Transactions of the Thirty-first Annual Meeting
of the Alumnae Association of the Woman's Medical College of Pennsylvania,* May
24–25, 1906 (Philadelphia: Published by the association, 1906), 36, MCP Collection,
ASCWM. The medical press covered these incidents; there were regular articles in
the Philadelphia *Medical and Surgical Reporter,* the New York *Medical Gazette,* and
the *Boston Medical and Surgical Journal,* and accounts were included in the standard
histories of the Pennsylvania Hospital: J. Forsyth Meigs, M.D., *A History of the First
Quarter of the Second Century of the Pennsylvania Hospital, read before the board
of managers at their stated meeting held 9th mo 25th, 1876* (Philadelphia: Board
of Managers, 1877), CPP; Thomas Morton, M.D., *The History of the Pennsylvania
Hospital, 1751–1895* (Philadelphia: Times Printing House, 1897); and Francis R.
Packard, M.D., "The Pennsylvania Hospital," in *Founders' Week Memorial Volume,*
ed. Frederick P. Penry, A.M., M.D., Published by the City of Philadelphia in Commemoration of the Two Hundred and Twenty-fifth Anniversary of Its Founding (Philadelphia, 1909), 595–612. I am grateful to Steven Peitzman for showing me the account of this incident in his *A New and Untried Course: Woman's Medical College
and Medical College of Pennsylvania* ((New Brunswick, N.J.: Rutgers University Press,
2000). And Michael Sappol's *A Traffic in Dead Bodies: Anatomy and Embodied Social
Identity in Nineteenth-Century America* (Princeton, N.J.: Princeton University Press,
2001), invaluable throughout this project, has been especially useful in this chapter.

    2. Packard, "The Pennsylvania Hospital," 602.

    3. Charles E. Rosenberg, *The Care of Strangers: The Rise of America's Hospital
System* (New York: Basic Books, 1987), 50–51.

    4. Leo J. O'Hara, *An Emerging Profession: Philadelphia Doctors, 1860–1890*
(New York: Garland, 1989), 85.

    5. Meigs, *A History of the First Quarter,* 23; Morton, *History of the Pennsylvania
Hospital,* 360.

    6. Meigs, *A History of the First Quarter,* 25.

    7. Meigs, *A History of the First Quarter,* 27.

    8. Numbers vary in different accounts. Anna Broomall's recollection, retold at her
seventy-ninth birthday in 1926, was that "there were twenty of us" (Anna Broomall,
Deceased Alumnae Files, newspaper clipping). At the memorial held for her in 1932
by the Delaware County Historical Society, Dr. Mary Griscom spoke of the "valiant
nine" women medical students who were mobbed at the clinical lectures at Pennsylvania Hospital (Mary Griscom, M.D., "Memorial Meeting for Dr. Anna E. Broomall,"
Apr. 4, 1932, in Anna E. Broomall, Deceased Alumnae Files). A clipping in the Eliza
Wood-Armitage scrapbook puts the number at thirty-five ("Our Philadelphia Correspondence," Nov. 7, 1869, in Eliza Wood-Armitage, Scrapbook, 1, Deceased Alumnae Files, ASCWM). Evelyn Keller, replying to a toast at the 1906 alumnae banquet,

said that "thirty-five of us" attended the lecture (WMC, Alumnae Association, *Transactions of the Thirty-first Annual Meeting*, 36). A resolution by the Pennsylvania Hospital Board of Managers, Nov. 13, 1869, speaks of thirty students (Pennsylvania Hospital, Minute Book of the Board of Managers, R11D12, HLPH). The *New York Citizen and Round Table*, quoted in a *Philadelphia Press* article in the Wood-Armitage scrapbook, speaks anxiously of "twenty-five Wild Women, determined to witness the carving and cutting of the masculine form divine" (Wood-Armitage, Scrapbook, 7). The New York *World*, surprised to see such goings on in "Philadelphia, the dullest village in America," gives the number as thirty-four, attended by a "senior female physician" (Wood-Armitage, Scrapbook, 8). The New York *Medical Gazette*, "The Pennsylvania Hospital Scandal," 3 (Nov. 20, 1869): 294, spoke of twenty-seven women students.

9. Again, accounts vary. Corson's note is recounted in Anna Broomall's birthday recollection (how the fortunes of that family were linked to those of women physicians!), which speaks of "pandemonium" at the women's entrance, with students standing on their seats, hooting, and throwing spitballs (Broomall, Deceased Alumnae Files). Evelyn Keller, writing in 1906, describes an entry "amidst jeers and groanings, whistling and stamping of feet" (WMC, Alumnae Association, *Transactions of the Thirty-first Annual Meeting*, 36). The Wood-Armitage clipping, "Our Philadelphia Correspondence," speaks of "a tumultuous uproar" (Wood-Armitage, Scrapbook, 1). The board of managers' resolution refers to "hissing" and "other conduct unbecoming in any well-regulated institution" (Morton, *History of the Pennsylvania Hospital*, 365). Some male medical students claimed that their stamping, laughter, applause, and hissing were normal occurrences at the lectures; a letter signed "Jefferson" in the *Evening Star* claims that the women students "were treated the same as the male students, who often stamp and hoot at each other, and we propose that the ladies shall enjoy the same rights that we ourselves enjoy." Another letter to the *Evening Star*, signed "Aggrieved Male Student," suggested that it was the Eclectics and irregular students, rather than those from the University of Pennsylvania or Jefferson, who had been abusive (both letters in Wood-Armitage, Scrapbook, 9–10).

10. Anna Broomall, in a newspaper account of a celebration of her seventy-ninth birthday, gives the names of the managers as Dilwyn Parrish, a Hicksite, and William Biddle (Anna Broomall, Deceased Alumnae Files). All contemporaneous accounts agree on Biddle's impressive presence; the second manager, however, is usually identified as A. J. Derbyshire (see "Our Philadelphia Correspondence," Wood-Armitage, Scrapbook, 1). Other newspaper accounts quoting from this article identify the source of "Our Philadelphia Correspondence" as the *Anti-Slavery Standard*.

11. Anna Broomall, in the newspaper account of a celebration of her seventy-ninth birthday, gave the names of the lecturers as Dr. Hutchinson (medicine) and Dr. Levis (surgery). But all other contemporaneous accounts agreed that Hunt and Da Costa were the lecturers (see, for example, "Our Philadelphia Correspondence," Nov. 7, 1869, in the Wood-Armitage Scrapbook, 1); no Levis was on medical or surgical staff of the Pennsylvania Hospital in 1869 (Meigs, *A History of the First Quarter*, 95). A Dr. Levis did lecture on surgery at the Blockley (WMC, College Scrapbooks, A, 1816–48, 27).

12. Quoted in Robert M. Kaiser, Sandra L. Chaff, and Steven J. Peitzman, "A

Philadelphia Medical Student of the 1890's: The Diary of Mary Theodora McGavran," *Pennsylvania Magazine of History and Biography* 108, no. 2 (Apr. 1984): 217–36, quotation on 227.

13. WMC, College Scrapbooks, A, 1816–48, 11.

14. "Women Medical Students," *New York Tribune,* Nov. 13, 1869, clipping pasted in a bound volume (1866–79) of the Woman's Medical College Annual Announcements, MCP Collection, ASCWM.

15. R. C., letter to the *New Republic,* in WMC, College Scrapbooks, A, 1816–48, 31.

16. In A. Broomall's birthday recollection, she says, "We were hustled and jostled into the hall. Dilwyn Parrish had sent men to close the gates against the boys. They burst the barriers open and knocked him over in the fracas. He raised his trembling hands in protest, crying: 'The Pennsylvania Hospital will not have this!' Borne along as on the crest of a wave, we found ourselves in 8th street and went twenty different ways, still pursued by taunts and jeers" (A. Broomall, Deceased Alumnae Files). (It is very unlikely that Parrish was there; see n. 10 above.) Griscom's memorial speech has the managers "hustled and pushed" by students, locking the women in a safe room, and sending them home a few at a time (Griscom, "Memorial Meeting"). The writer of "Our Philadelphia Correspondence" says that the male students blocked the walk leading through the yard, so that women students were forced into the carriage way. When they reached the street, they were followed, "greatly to their annoyance," by male students "uttering various uncouth noises and indecent comments, and making other manifestations peculiar to this class of 'gentlemen.'" Another article in the Wood-Armitage scrapbook describes the male students forming "a line on each side of the walk, intending the ladies to run the gauntlet of their stares, and intending a salutation also." When the women left by the road rather than the footpath, "a mock procession was formed, and the insults kept up for some distance" (Wood-Armitage, Scrapbook, 3). A similar account appears in the *Ledger* for November 8 (WMC, College Scrapbooks, A, 1816–48, 17a), which describes the twenty-seven students passing "between the double lines of the male students, whilst the later saluted them with taunts and jeers, mock applause, and real hisses." The New York *Medical Gazette,* in "The Pennsylvania Hospital Scandal," does not mention any harassment inside the hall but describes "the sidewalk lined on either side by the male students who had been in attendance, and who undertook to express their disapprobation of the course adopted by the hospital authorities, by forcing a handful of defenseless women to run the gauntlet of their jeers. To escape this peril, the terrified victims took to the roadway, whereupon their persecutors formed a mock procession and followed them for some distance with hisses and jibes" (294).

17. Elizabeth Keller, in reply to a toast to the "Pathfinders," quoted in H. Frances Bartlett, "Report of the Entertainment Committee," in WMC, Alumnae Association, *Transactions of the Thirty-first Annual Meeting,* 1906, 36.

18. The clipping scrapbook of Eliza Wood-Armitage includes "Our Philadelphia Correspondence," from the Nov. 7, 1869, *Anti-Slavery Standard* (Wood-Armitage, Scrapbook). The article observes that during the Civil War, medical students, "especially those who were born in the baleful shadow of slavery," were known for their "ribaldry and jest, their violence, indecency and scurrility on manifold occasions" (1). Another clipping in her file, from the Philadelphia *Sunday Transcript* (Nov. 14,

1869), speaks of "a time when 'the students' used to exercise their loaded canes and their knives and even pistols, at the expense of public order" and worries that the jeering incident had returned such "respectable outlawry" to the city (9).

Similar responses can be found in the College Scrapbook A (1816–48), which includes clippings dated November 1869 referring to a time "prior to the rebellion" when a typical southern medical student carried "a large size club and a bowie knife" and recalling that "Anti-slavery Fairs were held for years under the shadow of violence and threats, and the doors closed upon them by the Sheriff, in the name of the Commonwealth, because it hurt the students' feelings. . . . colored children, and men and women too, held their lives cheap, when they met a party of students" (WMC, College Scrapbooks, A, 4). Both writers felt that the jeering incident was a return to those bad old days. A long article from the *Philadelphia Press* in the College Scrapbook A (1816–48) recalls regular fights "every Saturday night for months together" in the Walnut Street Theater (23). The writer notes, however, that the three students he interviewed were "neither long-haired, nor slouch-hatted, nor nicotine-stained, nor bowied and pistolled, nor in any way alarming to look upon or to contemplate" (24).

19. In the regular medical press, support for the male medical students was not universal, although the terms of criticism were muted. In "Medical Lectures to Mixed Classes," the first statement on the jeering incident to appear in the Philadelphia *Medical and Surgical Reporter*, the editors mention "demonstrations, not be approved in every respect" (21 [Nov. 20, 1869]: 325).

20. See the New York *Medical Gazette*, generally sympathetic to the women students, which, in "The Pennsylvania Hospital Scandal," advised them that "those who needlessly seek martyrdom in opposition to established usages, seldom attract the sympathy of the community, and rather weaken than strengthen the cause they advocate" (294).

21. *Medical and Surgical Reporter*, "The Medical Profession and the Management of Hospitals," 21 (Dec. 11, 1869): 386. For the doctors' petition, which was signed by the entire medical establishment of Philadelphia, see WMC, College Scrapbooks, A, 1816–48, 43, a newspaper clipping; or *Medical and Surgical Reporter*, "Remonstrance against Mixed Clinics," 21 (Nov. 27, 1869): 345–46.

22. *Medical and Surgical Reporter*, "The Pennsylvania Hospital Clinics," 25 (Aug. 26, 1871), noted that the annual report of the Pennsylvania Hospital records complaints from the medical staff that the separate clinics given to women students "have much increased their labors, diminishing the time appropriated to patients" and that the number of students attending the hospital clinics has declined from 500, including 42 women, to 206, including 32 women. The report asked contributors for instructions and stated that if no instructions were received, "they [the managers] will conceive that the whole matter of lectures to females is left to their judgment and discretion" (200–201).

23. The statement by Ann Preston is collected in WMC, College Scrapbooks, A, 1816–48, 27–29, and was first printed as "Women as Physicians," in the Philadelphia *Medical and Surgical Reporter* 16, no. 18 (May 4, 1867): 391–94. Other newspaper stories speak of a "card" circulated by Dean Ann Preston stating that the women medical students only desired to attend clinics once a week and to see cases not requiring exposure. I have not located that card, which may have been an alternate

publication of this statement. The most accessible copy of the letter is in Clara Marshall, *The Woman's Medical College of Pennsylvania: An Historical Outline* (Philadelphia: P. Blakiston, 1897), 45–53.

24. J. William White, M.D., "Memoir of D. Hayes Agnew, M.D., LL.D.," *Transactions of the College of Physicians*, 3d ser., 15 (Jan. 4, 1893): xxix–lxv.

25. *Medical and Surgical Reporter* (Philadelphia), "The Pennsylvania Hospital and Female Students," 22 (May 14, 1870): 420–21.

26. "The Medical Students Again," *Evening Bulletin* (Apr. 28, 1870), clipping in WMC, College Scrapbooks, #3, 1868, 1869, Jan. 1870–Aug. 1871, 85, ASCWM. For additional responses to these pamphlets, see also pp. 86–89. The pamphlets are collected in *Men and Women Medical Students*, No. 2 (Philadelphia, Apr. 1870), bound with the Minute Book of the Pennsylvania Hospital Board of Managers, HLPH; see also George Wood, M.D., et al., *To the Contributors of the Pennsylvania Hospital* (Philadelphia, spring 1870), HLPH.

27. *Medical and Surgical Reporter*, "Philadelphia Hospital and Female Students," 421.

28. See *Medical and Surgical Reporter* (Philadelphia), "The Female Students Again," 23 (Jan. 28, 1871): 85; and *Medical and Surgical Reporter* (Philadelphia), "The Woman's Medical College of Pennsylvania," 23 (Feb. 11, 1871): 130.

29. Peitzman, "A New and Untried Course."

30. O'Hara, *Emerging Profession*, 194–96.

31. For early feminist studies of science, see Evelyn Fox Keller, *A Feeling for the Organism: The Life and Work of Barbara McClintock* (San Francisco: Freeman, 1983); Evelyn Fox Keller, *Reflections on Gender and Science* (New Haven, Conn.: Yale University Press, 1985); and Sandra Harding, *The Science Question in Feminism* (Ithaca, N.Y.: Cornell University Press, 1986). Early studies have been collected in Nancy Tuana, ed., *Feminism and Science* (Bloomington: Indiana University Press, 1989). More recent work is included in Barbara Laslett, Sally Gregory Kohlstedt, Helen Longino, and Evelynn Hammonds, eds., *Gender and Scientific Authority* (Chicago: University of Chicago Press, 1996). A convenient account of this line of study can be found in Evelyn Fox Keller and Helen Longino, eds., *Feminism and Science* (New York: Oxford University Press, 1996).

32. Harriot Kezia Hunt, *Glances and Glimpses: Or Fifty Years Social, Including Twenty Years Professional Life* (Boston: Jewett, 1856), 270.

33. Ruth Abram, "Will There Be a Monument?" in her *"Send Us a Lady Physician": Women Doctors in America, 1835–1920* (New York: Norton, 1985), 89.

34. See the Wood-Armitage scrapbook for a letter in the *Philadelphia Press* from "A Woman" (Wood-Armitage, Scrapbook, no page number shown); and WMC, College Scrapbooks, #3, 1868, 1869, Jan. 1870–Aug 1871, 87, for a letter signed "A Mother" (not to be confused with the letter titled "A Mother" recounting the story of the exposed maiden). The letters describe similar incidents at a mixed clinic held either in 1863, according to "A Woman," or in 1864–65, according to "A Mother." At a clinic on the use of forceps, the entire lecture was a discussion of the propriety of mixed clinical lectures. The next Saturday, a prisoner was subjected to amputation of his lower lip without anesthesia, "for the purpose of trying the nerves of the ladies present, in the hope that the groans of the patient might drive them from the clinic"

("A Mother"). The patient was held down, his lip was removed, and the points of his mouth were drawn together so that his upper lip protruded "like a ruffle," to the "laughter and cruel jeers" of the male medical students ("A Mother"). The next patient, an Irishman whose dislocated hip had healed, was brought into the clinic and told to strip, "Pat, never mind the ladies; take off your pants" ("A Woman") or perhaps, "Down with them, Sir; that is what the ladies come for" ("A Mother"). When the patient complied, "the professor laughed and looked around upon the male students, who, with but a few exceptions, hooted, laughed, clapped their hands and stamped their feet." After the lectures "we were compelled to march through a double file of men, subject to their jeers and gazes."

In response to the Philadelphia jeering incident, male students at Bellevue met to consider the question of the continued presence of women students to the clinical lectures; the 150 students who met were generally opposed to mixed lectures (*Medical and Surgical Reporter* [Philadelphia], "The Woman Question in New York," 21 [Dec. 4, 1869]: 362–63) but refused to vote in support of a resolution against women's attendance at clinics (*Medical Gazette*, "Professional Items," 3 [Nov. 27, 1869]: 307).

35. Thomas Neville Bonner, *To the Ends of the Earth: Women's Search for Education in Medicine* (Cambridge, Mass.: Harvard University Press, 1992), 140–42.

36. Bonner, *To the Ends of the Earth*, 145–46.

37. Bonner, *To the Ends of the Earth*, 127–28.

38. Mary Putnam Jacobi, "The Practical Study of Biology," *Boston Medical and Surgical Reporter* 120 (1889): 631–36, reprinted in Jacobi, *Pathfinder*, 458–62. "Practical Study" was given as a talk at the 1889 annual dinner of the Massachusetts Medical Society.

39. Anna L. Wharton, letter to her husband, Joseph Wharton, Mar. 12, 1856, RG5/162: Joseph Wharton Papers, ser. 4.2, FHL.

40. Audrey B. Davis, "Louis Thomas Jerôme Auzoux and the Papier Mâché Anatomical Model," *Estratto da atti del I congresso internazionale sulla ceroplastica nella scienza e nell'arte*, vol. 20 of series (Firenze: Biblioteca della "Rivista di storia della scienze mediche e naturali," 1977), 257–79. Thanks to Gretchen Worden of the Mütter Museum for this citation.

41. Ladies' Physiological Institute of Boston and Vicinity, Secretary's Reports and Board Meetings, vol. 1, Dec. 1850, Apr. 1851, Ladies' Physiological Society Papers, MC-236, Schlesinger Library, Radcliffe College. Tickets for the microscopic soirées can be found in WMC, Deans Files, MCP-C4, Rachel Bodley, folder 11, 1886, Acc. #291, ASCWM.

42. Sarah Mapps Douglass, letters to Rebecca White, Philadelphia, Feb. 9, 1862, and two undated letters, Quaker Collection, Haverford College Library.

43. Barbara Stafford, *Body Criticism: Imaging the Unseen in Enlightenment Art and Medicine* (Cambridge, Mass.: MIT Press, 1991). Emily Jane Cohen has extended and qualified this analysis in her meditation on the medical hand as source of knowledge, "Enlightenment and the Dirty Philosopher," *Configurations* 5, no. 3 (fall 1997): 369–424. For a useful history of medical illustration, see Mimi Cazort, Monique Kornell, and K. B. Roberts, *The Ingenious Machine of Nature: Four Centuries of Art and Anatomy* (Ottawa: National Gallery of Canada, 1996).

44. For the edifying power of dissection, see Sappol, *A Traffic of Dead Bodies*.

45. For an account of mail-order physiology texts, see Michael Sappol, "Sammy Tubbs and Dr. Hubbs: Anatomical Dissection, Minstrelsy, and the Technology of Self-Making in Postbellum America," *Configurations* 4, no. 2 (1996): 131–83.

46. "A Mother," letter to the *Herald Tribune,* Mar. 5, 1870, WMC, College Scrapbooks, #3, 1868, 1869, Jan. 1870–Aug.1871, 86.

47. The *Herald Tribune*'s letter could not have been the first publication of this story. The *Tribune* letter was published on March 5, 1870, but the editor of the New York *Medical Gazette* had already read a version of it in the *Church Union* by March 4. As the *Medical Gazette* quotes it, the *Church Union* account reads:

> We know of a recent case in an eminent medical school, in which a young woman suffering from rheumatic fever was brought before the class without any matronly attendance. With closed eyes she lay while the professor called attention to her case, point by point. The final statement made was, that in such a case, at such a stage of development, a minute rash might be expected upon the stomach and bowels—and the professor, without a thought of its indelicacy, before the whole class, made an open examination! The girl lay as one dead. But with the act of denuding the color rose along her face to the roots of her hair. (*Medical Gazette,* "Cliniques for Women," 4 [Mar. 4, 1870]: 164)

The editors of the *Medical Gazette* did not approve of this examination: "To uncover an unfortunate woman in a college amphitheatre . . . is a proceeding, the agony of which to the patient is not compensated for by any adequate advantage to the class." It seemed unlikely to them that a rheumatic fever patient would have an abdominal rash; they were skeptical of the eminence of the medical school. But, unlike the editors of the *Church Union,* they did not therefore conclude that women should attend clinical lectures: exposure before "a promiscuous assemblage of both sexes" would be even more shocking than before an audience of men; instead, clinical instruction should take place on the ward, in small groups.

48. Emily A. Varney-Brownell, M.D., "A Case of Hemoptysis," in WMC, Alumnae Association, *Report of the Proceedings of the Fourteenth Annual Meeting of the Alumnae Association of the Woman's Medical College of Pennsylvania* (Philadelphia: Rodgers Printing Co., 1889), 89–90, MCP Collection, ASCWM.

49. Clipping of Mary Pratt, M.D., "Clinics—the Other Side," letter to the New York *Herald Tribune* (Mar. 1870), in WMC, College Scrapbooks, #3, 1868, 1869, Jan. 1870–Aug. 1871, 86.

50. Charles Reade, *The Woman-Hater* (Paris and Boston: Grolier Society, n.d.; original publication 1877), vol. 1, 218.

51. For praise of the women medical students at the Blockley, see WMC, College Scrapbooks, A, 1816–48, 22. For similar comments on Zurich, see p. 12 in the same scrapbook.

52. Stephen Smith, M.D., "The Medical Co-education of Women," appendix to Elizabeth Blackwell, *Pioneer Work in Opening the Medical Profession to Women* (New York: Schocken, 1977; original publication, 1895), 255–59, quotation on 258. Among the many interesting issues in this story is the question of Blackwell's awareness of the situation: her note argued that the professor of anatomy must necessarily be a "reverent" man, and in the text of her autobiography, she does not even raise

the question of his propriety. But the essay by Smith, written in New York City in 1892, must have been based on information given by Blackwell. Reversing Preston's kidnaping of Meigs, Blackwell gave her most transgressive account of her own education as a hostage to a male writer.

53. WMC, College Scrapbooks, A, 1816–48, 25, clipping from the *Philadelphia Press*, Nov. 12, 1869.

54. WMC, College Scrapbooks, A, 1816–48, "Hospital Clinics," letter to the *Evening Bulletin* (no page number shown).

55. *Medical and Surgical Reporter*, "Remonstrance against Mixed Clinics," 345–46. The "Remonstrance" was widely reprinted and commented upon in the general press, often unfavorably.

56. WMC, College Scrapbooks, A, 1816–48, "Hospital Clinics"; for the threat posed to male spectators by female immodesty, see Mary Ryan, *Women in Public: Between Banners and Ballots* (Baltimore: Johns Hopkins University Press, 1990), 72.

57. WMC, bound volume of annual announcements for 1866 through 1879, clipping pasted in at the end of the announcement for 1870–71, MCP Collection, ASCWM.

58. Sarah Hibbard, manuscript draft of lectures and sermons.

59. Ryan, *Women in Public*, 79–80.

60. The quotation is from p. 22 of Abram Smith, "An Essay on the Moral and Physical Education of Females" For the Degree of Doctor of Medicine in the University of Pennsylvania by Abram Smith of Easton, Northampton County, State of Pennsylvania, Residence No. 91 South Eighth Street, Philada., Preceptor S. Morton Zulich M.D., Duration of Studies 3 years, Presented Feby 1850, 22, PA.

61. Smith, "Moral and Physcial Education of Females," 24.

62. Smith, "Moral and Physical Education of Females," 23.

63. White, "Memoir of D. Hayes Agnew," lvi.

64. Diana Long Hall, "Eakins's Agnew Clinic: The Medical World in Transition," *Transactions and Studies of the College of Physicians of Philadelphia: Medicine and History*, ser. 5, 7, no. 1 (Mar. 1985): 26–31, brief quotation on 26.

65. D. Hayes Agnew, M.D., *Theatrical Amusements; with Some Remarks on the Rev. Henry W. Bellows' Address before the Dramatic Fund Society*, N.Y. (Philadelphia: Wm. S. Young, 1857), 10, 12.

66. Agnew, *Theatrical Amusements*, 7, 8.

67. D. Hayes Agnew, M.D., *Lecture Introductory to the One Hundred and Fifth Course of Instruction in the Medical Department of the University of Pennsylvania, delivered Monday, October 10, 1870* (Philadelphia: Published by the class, 1870), 18.

68. WMC, College Scrapbooks, A, 1816–48, 41.

69. O'Hara, *Emerging Profession*, 88.

70. Kaiser, Chaff, and Peitzman, "A Philadelphia Medical Student of the 1890's," 233.

71. Edith Flower Wheeler, M.D., "She Saunters Off into Her Past," autobiography, typescript, 1946, 83, Wheeler Papers, Deceased Alumnae Files, MCP Collection, ASCWM. I am grateful to Steven Peitzman for this reference.

72. Wheeler, "She Saunters Off into Her Past," 108.

73. Anne Walter Fearn, *My Days of Strength: An American Woman Doctor's Forty Years in China* (New York: Harper and Brothers, 1939), 14. I am grateful to Steven Peitzman for this reference.

74. Michael Sappol, in his *Traffic in Dead Bodies,* discusses dissection as a constituting practice of the masculine medical profession and argues that dissection practices by women physicians, or at women's schools, were distinct from those at men's schools and much less intense (chap. 3).

75. WMC, "First Annual Announcement of the Female Medical College of Pennsylvania for the session of 1850–51 . . . ," 12, MCP Collection, ASCWM.

76. WMC, Faculty Minutes, 1850–74, Oct. 28, 1850, MCP Collection, ASCWM.

77. Erasmus Wilson, M.D., *A System of Human Anatomy, General and Special,* ed. Paul Goddard, fourth American from the last London ed. (Philadelphia: Lea and Blanchard, 1850), 219. Preston's copy is held in the ASCWM.

78. WMC, Alumnae Association, *Transactions of the Twenty-seventh Annual Meeting,* 1902, "Ida E. Richardson," 25–26.

79. Ruth Richardson, *Death, Dissection, and the Destitute* (Harmondsworth: Penguin, 1989), 31.

80. WMC, Alumnae Association, *Transactions of the Twenty-seventh Annual Meeting,* "Ida E. Richardson," 25.

81. Hannah Longshore, "Autobiography," second draft, undated, Longshore Papers, ASCWM; Mary Putnam Jacobi, autobiographical manuscript, typescript, 1902, Mary Putnam Jacobi Collection, Jacobi Papers, a-26, folder 2, SL.

82. Elizabeth Blackwell, *Pioneer Work in Opening the Medical Profession to Women* (New York: Schocken, 1977; original publication, 1895), 85.

83. Blackwell, *Pioneer Work,* 59.

84. Galen, *On the Natural Faculties,* trans. Arthur John Brock, Loeb Classical Library (Cambridge, Mass.: Harvard University Press, 1952), 2.3.

85. Agnew, *Lecture Introductory,* 24–25.

86. Mary Putnam Jacobi, "A Martyr for Science," reprinted in her *Stories and Sketches* (New York: Putnam's Sons, 1907).

87. For nineteenth-century reading practices, see Jane Tompkins, *Sensational Designs: The Cultural Work of American Fiction, 1790–1860* (New York: Oxford University Press, 1985); and Richard Brodhead, *Cultures of Letters: Scenes of Reading and Writing in Nineteenth-Century America* (Chicago: University of Chicago Press, 1993).

88. Julie Elison, "Race and Sensibility in the Early Republic: Ann Eliza Bleeker and Sarah Wentworth Morton," in *Subjects and Citizens: Nation, Race, and Gender from Oroonoko to Anita Hill,* ed. Michael Moon and Cathy Davidson (Durham, N.C.: Duke University Press, 1995), 57–86, quotation on 60.

89. WMC, Deans Files, MCP-C4, Rachel Bodley, folder 11, 1886, Acc #291, ASCWM.

90. Agnes C. Vietor, ed., *A Woman's Quest: The Life of Marie Zakrzewska, M.D.* (New York: Appleton, 1924), 441.

91. Mark Twain and Charles Dudley Warner, *The Gilded Age: A Tale of Today,* ed. Shelley Fisher Fishkin (New York: Oxford University Press, 1996; original publication, 1873), 148.

92. *Medical and Surgical Journal* (Philadelphia), "Outrage at a Woman's Medical College," 7, no. 8 (Feb. 23, 1871): 133–34.

93. WMC, College Scrapbooks, A, 1816–48, 2, clipping from *Evening Bulletin,* Nov. 8, 1869.

94. WMC, College Scrapbooks, A, 1816–48, 25, clipping from the *Philadelphia Press,* Nov. 12, 1869.

95. WMC, College Scrapbooks, A, 1816–48, Faculty Statement, 27.

96. WMC, College Scrapbooks, A, 1816–48, Faculty Statement, 27.

97. WMC, College Scrapbooks, #3, 1868, 1869, Jan. 1870–Aug. 1871, 29.

98. Regina Markell Morantz-Sanchez, *Sympathy and Science: Women Physicians in American Medicine* (New York: Oxford University Press, 1985), chap. 3.

99. Vietor, *A Woman's Quest,* 18.

Works Cited

TWENTIETH-CENTURY SOURCES

This list includes contemporary sources and editions of works written before 1800. Works published by writers active before 1900 are included in the section "Nineteenth-Century Sources."

Abrahams, Harold J. *Extinct Medical Schools of Nineteenth-Century Philadelphia.* Philadelphia: University of Pennsylvania Press, 1966.

Abram, Ruth. *"Send Us a Lady Physician": Women Doctors in America, 1835–1920.* New York: Norton, 1985.

Alsop, Gulielma Fell. *History of the Woman's Medical College, Philadelphia, Pennsylvania (1850–1950).* Philadelphia: Lippincott, 1950.

Armstrong, D. *Political Anatomy of the Body: Medical Knowledge in Britain in the Twentieth Century.* Cambridge: Cambridge University Press, 1983.

Bacon, Margaret Hope. *Mothers of Feminism: The Story of Quaker Women in America.* New York: Harper and Row, 1986.

Balint, M. *The Doctor, His Patient and the Illness.* New York: International University Press, 1957.

Barton, Ellen. "Literacy in (Inter)Action." *College English* 59, no. 4 (Apr. 1997): 408–37.

Bates, Barbara. *Bargaining for Life: A Social History of Tuberculosis, 1876–1938.* Philadelphia: University of Pennsylvania Press, 1992.

Beer, Gillian. *Darwin's Plots: Evolutionary Narrative in Darwin, George Eliot, and Nineteenth-Century Fiction.* London: Routledge, 1983.

Belenky, Mary, and B. M. Clinchy, N. R. Goldberger, and J. M. Tarule. *Women's Ways of Knowing: The Development of Self, Voice, and Mind.* New York: Basic Books, 1986.

Benstock, Shari, ed. *The Private Self: Theory and Practice of Women's Autobiographical Writings.* Chapel Hill: University of North Carolina Press, 1988.

The Berean Manual Training and Industrial School. Philadelphia: 1907–8. Black Women Physicians Project, Anderson File. ASCWM.

The Berean Manual Training and Industrial School. Philadelphia: n.d., probably 1914. Black Women Physicians Project, Anderson File, ASCWM.

Bergman, A. B., and S. J. Stamm. "The Morbidity of Cardiac Nondisease in School Children." *New England Journal of Medicine* 276 (1967): 1008–13.

Berlin, James. *Writing Instruction in Nineteenth-Century American Colleges.* Carbondale: Southern Illinois University Press, 1984.

Biology and Gender Study Group (Athena Beldecos, Sarah Bailey, Scott Gilbert, Karen Hicks, Lori Kenschaft, Nancy Niemczyk, Rebecca Rosenberg, Stephanie Schaertel, and Andrew Wedel). "The Importance of Feminist Critique for Contemporary Cell Biology." In *Feminism and Science,* ed. Nancy Tuana, 172–87. Bloomington: Indiana University Press, 1989.

Bonner, Thomas Neville. *To the Ends of the Earth: Women's Search for Education in Medicine.* Cambridge, Mass.: Harvard University Press, 1992.

Braidotti, Rosi. *Nomadic Subjects: Embodiment and Sexual Difference in Contemporary Feminist Theory.* New York: Columbia University Press, 1994.

Braude, Ann. *Radical Spirits: Spiritualism and Women's Rights in Nineteenth Century America.* Boston: Beacon, 1989.

Brereton, John C., ed. *The Origins of Composition Studies in the American College, 1875–1925, a Documentary History.* Pittsburgh: University of Pittsburgh Press, 1995.

Brereton, Virginia. *From Sin to Salvation: Stories of Women's Conversions, 1800 to the Present.* Bloomington: Indiana University Press, 1991.

Brieger, Gert, ed. *Medical America in the Nineteenth Century: Readings from the Literature.* Baltimore: Johns Hopkins University Press, 1972.

Brinton, Howard. *Quaker Journals: Varieties of Religious Experience among Friends.* Wallingford, Pa.: Pendle Hill, 1972.

Britton, James. *The Development of Writing Abilities (11–18).* London: Macmillan Education, 1975.

Brodhead, Richard. *Cultures of Letters: Scenes of Reading and Writing in Nineteenth-Century America.* Chicago: University of Chicago Press, 1993.

Bullough, Vern, and Martha Voght. "Women, Menstruation, and Nineteenth-Century Medicine." *Bulletin of the History of Medicine* 47 (1973): 66–82.

Butler, Judith. *Bodies That Matter: On the Discursive Limits of "Sex."* New York: Routledge, 1993.

Butler, Judith. *Gender Trouble: Feminism and the Subversion of Identity.* New York: Routledge, 1990.

Bynum, W. F. *Science and the Practice of Medicine in the Nineteenth Century.* Cambridge: Cambridge University Press, 1994.

Campbell, Karlyn Kohrs. *Man Cannot Speak for Her.* Vol. 1: *A Critical Study of Early Feminist Rhetoric.* Vol. 2: *Key Texts of the Early Feminists.* New York: Praeger, 1989.

Cazort, Mimi, Monique Kornell, and K. B. Roberts. *The Ingenious Machine of Nature: Four Centuries of Art and Anatomy.* Ottawa: National Gallery of Canada, 1996.

Cervetti, Nancy. "S. Weir Mitchell: Literature and Medicine." Unpublished talk, Wood Institute for the History of Medicine, Mar. 1997. CPP.

Charlesworth, Max. "Whose Body? Feminist Views on Reproductive Technology." In

Troubled Bodies: Critical Perspectives on Postmodernism, Medical Ethics, and the Body, ed. Paul A. Komesaroff, 125–41. Durham, N.C.: Duke University Press, 1995.

Charon, Rita. "To Build a Case: Medical Histories as Traditions in Conflict." *Literature and Medicine* 11, no. 1 (spring 1992): 115–32.

Chenail, Ronald, ed. *Medical Discourse and Systemic Frames of Comprehension.* Vol. 42 of Advances in Discourse Processes. Norwood, N.J.: Ablex, 1991.

Cicourel, Aaron V. "Text and Discourse." *Annual Review of Anthropology* 14 (1985): 159–85.

Cohen, Emily Jane. "Enlightenment and the Dirty Philosopher." *Configurations* 5, no. 3 (fall 1997): 369–424.

Corbett, Mary Jean. *Representing Femininity: Middle-Class Subjectivity in Victorian and Edwardian Women's Autobiographies.* New York: Oxford University Press, 1992.

Davis, Audrey B. "Louis Thomas Jerôme Auzoux and the Papier Mâché Anatomical Model." *Estratto da atti del I congresso internazionale sulla ceroplastica nella scienza e nell'arte,* 257–79. Vol. 20 of series. Firenze: Biblioteca della "Rivista di storia della scienze mediche e naturali," 1977.

Davis, Kathy. "Paternalism under the Microscope." In *Gender and Discourse: The Power of Talk,* ed. Alexandra Dundas Todd, 19–54. Norwood, N.J.: Ablex, 1988.

Dixon, Laurinda S. *Perilous Chastity: Women and Illness in Pre-Enlightenment Art and Medicine.* Ithaca, N.Y.: Cornell University Press, 1995.

Douglas, Ann. *The Feminization of American Culture.* New York: Knopf, 1977.

Duffin, Jacalyn. "Private Practice and Public Research: The Patients of R. T. H. Laennec." In *French Medical Culture in the Nineteenth Century,* ed. A. La Berge and Mordechai Feingold, 118–49. Amsterdam and Atlanta, Ga.: Rodopi, 1994.

Elison, Julie. "Race and Sensibility in the Early Republic: Ann Eliza Bleeker and Sarah Wentworth Morton." In *Subjects and Citizens: Nation, Race, and Gender from Oroonoko to Anita Hill,* ed. Michael Moon and Cathy Davidson, 57–86. Durham, N.C.: Duke University Press, 1995.

Epps, Charles, M.D., Davis Johnson, Ph.D., and Audrey Vaughan, M.S. "Black Medical Pioneers: African-American 'Firsts' in Academic and Organized Medicine." *Journal of the National Medical Association* 85, nos. 8, 9, 10 (Aug. and Sept. 1993): 629–44, 703–20.

Epstein, Julia. "Historiography, Diagnosis, and Poetics." *Literature and Medicine* 11, no. 1 (spring 1992): 23–44.

Fausto-Sterling, Anne. *Myths of Gender: Biological Theories about Women and Men.* 2d ed. New York: Basic Books, 1992.

Fearn, Anne Walter. *My Days of Strength: An American Woman Doctor's Forty Years in China.* New York: Harper and Brothers, 1939.

Fisher, Sue, and Alexandra Dundas Todd. *The Social Organization of Doctor-Patient Communication.* 2d ed. Norwood, N.J.: Ablex, 1993.

Flexner, Abraham. *Medical Education in the United States and Canada.* New York: Carnegie Foundation for the Advancement of Teaching, 1910.

Flood, David H., and Rhonda Soricelli. "Development of the Physician's Narrative Voice in the Medical Case History." *Literature and Medicine* 11, no. 1 (spring 1992): 64–83.

Foster, Pauline Poole. *Ann Preston, M.D. (1813–1872): A Biography: The Struggle to Obtain Training and Acceptance for Women Physicians in Mid-Nineteenth Century America.* Ph.D. dissertation, University of Pennsylvania. Ann Arbor: University Microfilms, 1984.

Foucault, Michel. *The Birth of the Clinic: An Archaeology of Medical Perception.* New York: Random House, 1973.

Foucault, Michel. *Discipline and Punish: The Birth of the Prison.* Trans. Alan Sheridan. New York: Vintage, 1979.

Friedman, Susan Stanford. "Women's Autobiographical Selves." In *The Private Self: Theory and Practice of Women's Autobiographical Writings,* ed. Shari Benstock, 34–62. Chapel Hill: University of North Carolina Press, 1988.

Furst, Lilian. "Halfway up the Hill: Doctresses in Late Nineteenth-Century American Fiction." In *Women Healers and Physicians: Climbing a Long Hill,* ed. Lilian Furst, 221–38. Lexington: University Press of Kentucky, 1997.

Furst, Lilian R., ed. *Women Healers and Physicians: Climbing a Long Hill.* Lexington: University Press of Kentucky, 1997.

Galen. *On the Natural Faculties.* Trans. Arthur John Brock. Loeb Classical Library. Cambridge, Mass.: Harvard University Press, 1952.

Garber, Marjorie. *Vested Interests: Cross-Dressing and Cultural Anxiety.* New York: Harper, 1992.

Gartner, Carol. "Fussell's Folly: Academic Standards and the Case of Mary Putnam Jacobi." *Academic Medicine* 71, no. 5 (May 1996): 470–77.

Gere, Anne Ruggles. *Intimate Practices: Literacy and Cultural Work in U.S. Women's Clubs, 1880–1920.* Urbana: University of Illinois Press, 1997.

Gilder, Richard Watson. "Address." In *In Memory of Mary Putnam Jacobi,* January 4, 1907, 43–56. New York: Academy of Medicine, 1907.

Gilligan, Carol. *In a Different Voice: Psychological Theory and Women's Development.* Cambridge, Mass.: Harvard University Press, 1982.

Goldstein, Linda Lehmann. "'Without Compromising in Any Particular': The Success of Medical Coeducation in Cleveland, 1850–1856." *Caduceus* 10, no. 2 (autumn 1994): 101–15.

Gray, Chris Hables, ed. *The Cyborg Handbook.* London: Routledge, 1995.

Gross, Paul, and Norman Leavitt. *Higher Superstition: The Academic Left and Its Quarrel with Science.* Baltimore: Johns Hopkins University Press, 1994.

Hall, Diana Long. "Eakins's Agnew Clinic: The Medical World in Transition." *Transactions and Studies of the College of Physicians of Philadelphia: Medicine and History,* ser. 5, 7, no. 1 (Mar. 1985): 26–31.

Haller, John S. *Medical Protestants: The Eclectics in American Medicine, 1825–1939.* Carbondale: Southern Illinois University Press, 1994.

Halliday, M. A. K., and J. R. Martin. *Writing Science: Literacy and Discursive Power.* Pittsburgh: University of Pittsburgh Press, 1993.

Halloran, Michael. "Rhetoric in the American College Curriculum: The Decline of Public Discourse." *Pre/Text* 3 (1982): 245–69.

Haraway, Donna. "A Game of Cat's Cradle: Science Studies, Feminist Theory, Cultural Studies." *Configurations* 2, no. 1 (1993): 59–72.

Haraway, Donna. *Primate Visions: Gender, Race, and Nature in the World of Modern Science.* London: Routledge, 1989.

Haraway, Donna. *Simians, Cyborgs, and Women.* London: Routledge, 1989.

Harding, Sandra. "Rethinking Standpoint Epistemology: What Is 'Strong Objectivity'?" In *Feminist Epistemologies,* ed. Linda Alcott and Elizabeth Potter, 49–82. New York: Routledge, 1993.

Harding, Sandra. *The Science Question in Feminism.* Ithaca, N.Y.: Cornell University Press, 1986.

Harding, Sandra. *Whose Science? Whose Knowledge? Thinking from Women's Lives.* Ithaca, N.Y.: Cornell University Press, 1991.

Harvey, Joy. "Clanging Eagles: The Marriage and Collaboration between Two Nineteenth-Century Physicians, Mary Putnam Jacobi and Abraham Jacobi." In *Creative Couples in the Sciences,* ed. Helena Pycior, Nancy Slack, and Pnina Abiram, 185–95. New Brunswick, N.J.: Rutgers University Press, 1995.

Harvey, Joy. "Medicine and Politics: Dr. Mary Putnam Jacobi and the Paris Commune." *Dialectical Anthropology* 15 (1990): 107–17.

Harvey, Joy. "La Visite: Mary Putnam Jacobi and the Paris Medical Clinics." In *French Medical Culture in the Nineteenth Century,* ed. Ann La Berge and Mordechai Feingold, 350–71. Amsterdam and Atlanta, Ga.: Rodopi, 1994.

Hine, Darlene Clark. *Black Women in America: An Historical Encyclopedia.* Bloomington: Indiana University Press, 1994.

Hobbs, Catherine, ed. *Nineteenth-Century Women Learn to Write.* Charlottesville: University Press of Virginia, 1995.

Huddle, Thomas. "Competition and Reform at the Medical Department of the University of Pennsylvania, 1847–1877." *Journal of the History of Medicine and Allied Sciences* 51, no. 3 (July 1996): 251–92.

Hume, Edgar E. *Orthinologists of the US Army Medical Corps: Thirty-Six Biographies.* Baltimore: Johns Hopkins University Press, 1942.

Hunter, Kathryn Montgomery. *Doctors' Stories: The Narrative Structure of Medical Knowledge.* Princeton, N.J.: Princeton University Press, 1991.

Jelinek, Estelle. *The Tradition of Women's Autobiography: From Antiquity to the Present.* Boston: Twayne, 1986.

Jelinek, Estelle. *Women's Autobiography: Essays in Criticism.* Bloomington: Indiana University Press, 1980.

Jerrido, Margaret. "Rebecca Cole." Typed manuscript. Undated. Black Women Physicians Project, Rebecca Cole File. ASCWM.

Johnson, Nan. *Nineteenth Century Rhetoric in North America.* Carbondale: Southern Illinois University Press, 1991.

Jordanova, Ludmilla. *Sexual Visions: Images of Gender in Science and Medicine between the Eighteenth and Twentieth Centuries.* New York: Harvester, 1989.

Kaiser, Robert, Sandra L. Chaff, and Steven J. Peitzman. "A Philadelphia Medical Student of the 1890's: The Diary of Mary Theodora McGavran." *Pennsylvania Magazine of History and Biography* 108, no. 2 (Apr. 1984): 217–36.

Kass-Simon, G., and Patricia Farnes. *Women of Science: Righting the Record.* Bloomington: University of Indiana Press, 1990.

Katz, Jay. *The Silent World of Doctor and Patient.* New York: Free Press, 1984.

Keller, Evelyn Fox. *A Feeling for the Organism: The Life and Work of Barbara McClintock.* San Francisco: Freeman, 1983.

284

Keller, Evelyn Fox. "Feminism and Science." In *Feminism and Science,* ed. Evelyn Fox Keller and Helen Longino, 3–65. New York: Oxford University Press, 1996.

Keller, Evelyn Fox. *Reflections on Gender and Science.* New Haven, Conn.: Yale University Press, 1985.

Keller, Evelyn Fox, and Helen Longino, eds. *Feminism and Science.* New York: Oxford University Press, 1996.

Kitzhaber, Albert. *Rhetoric in American Colleges, 1850–1900.* Dallas: Southern Methodist University Press, 1990.

La Berge, Ann. "Medical Microscopy in Paris, 1830–65." In *French and Medical Culture in the Nineteenth Century,* ed. Ann La Berge and Mordechai Feingold, 296–326. Amsterdam and Atlanta, Ga.: Rodopi, 1994.

La Berge, Ann, and Mordechai Feingold, eds. *French Medical Culture in the Nineteenth Century.* Amsterdam and Atlanta, Ga.: Rodopi, 1994.

Lacan, Jacques. *Feminine Sexuality: Jacques Lacan and the École Freudienne.* Ed. Juliet Mitchell and Jacqueline Rose. New York: Norton, 1985.

Laclos, Pierre Choderlos de. *Les Liaisons dangereuses.* Paris: Garnier-Flammarion, 1964.

Laqueur, Thomas. *Making Sex: Body and Gender from the Greeks to Freud.* Cambridge, Mass.: Harvard University Press, 1990.

Laslett, Barbara, Sally Gregory Kohlstedt, Helen Longino, and Evelynn Hammonds, eds. *Gender and Scientific Authority.* Chicago: University of Chicago Press, 1996.

Latour, Bruno. "Socrates' and Callicles' Settlement—or, The Invention of the Impossible Body Politic." *Configurations* 5, no. 2 (spring 1997): 189–240.

Latour, Bruno, and Steve Woolgar. *Laboratory Life: The Construction of Scientific Facts.* Princeton, N.J.: Princeton University Press, 1979.

Leavitt, Judith Walzer, ed. *Women and Health Care in America: Historical Readings.* Madison: University of Wisconsin Press, 1984.

Lee, Dr. C. Bruce. Letter to the dean of the Woman's Medical College of Pennsylvania, Apr. 20, 1964. Black Women Physicians Project, Georgiana Young File. ASCWM.

Longino, Helen, and Ruth Doell. "Body, Bias, and Behavior: A Comparative Analysis of Reasoning in Two Areas of Biological Science." *Signs: Journal of Women in Culture and Society* 9, no. 2 (1983): 206–27.

Ludmerer, Kenneth. *Learning to Heal: The Development of American Medical Education.* Baltimore: Johns Hopkins University Press, 1985.

Martin, Emily. "The Egg and the Sperm: How Science Has Constructed a Romance Based on Stereotypical Male-Female Roles." *Signs: Journal of Women in Culture and Society* 16, no. 3 (spring 1991): 485–501.

Martin, Emily. *The Woman in the Body: A Cultural Analysis of Reproduction.* Boston: Beacon, 1987.

McConnell-Ginet, Sally. "Language and Gender." In *Linguistics: The Cambridge Survey,* vol. 4: *Language: The Socio-cultural Context,* ed. Frederick Newmeyer, 75–99. Cambridge: Cambridge University Press, 1988.

Miller, Susan. *Textual Carnivals: The Politics of Composition.* Carbondale: Southern Illinois University Press, 1991.

Mishler, Elliot. *The Discourse of Medicine: Dialectics of the Medical Interview.* Norwood, N.J.: Ablex, 1984.

Mishler, Elliot G., Lorna Amarsingham, Stuart Hauser, Ramsay Liem, Samuel Osherson, and Nancy Wexler. *Social Contexts of Health, Illness, and Patient Care.* Cambridge: Cambridge University Press, 1981.

Moldow, Gloria. *Women Doctors in Gilded-Age Washington: Race, Gender, and Professionalization.* Urbana: University of Illinois Press, 1987.

Monroe, William Frank, Warren Lee Holleman, and Marsha Cline Holleman. "Is There a Person in This Case?" *Literature and Medicine* 11, no. 1 (spring 1992): 45–63.

Morantz-Sanchez, Regina Markell. *Conduct Unbecoming a Woman: Medicine on Trial in Turn-of-the-Century Brooklyn.* New York: Oxford University Press, 1999.

Morantz-Sanchez, Regina Markell. "The Gendering of Empathic Expertise: How Women Physicians Became More Empathic Than Men." In *The Empathic Practitioner: Empathy, Gender, and Medicine,* ed. Ellen Singer More and Maureen Milligan, 40–58. New Brunswick, N.J.: Rutgers University Press, 1994.

Morantz-Sanchez, Regina Markell. "Making It in a Man's World: The Late-Nineteenth-Century Surgical Career of Mary Amanda Dixon Jones." *Bulletin of the History of Medicine* 69 (1995): 542–68.

Morantz-Sanchez, Regina Markell. *Sympathy and Science: Women Physicians in American Medicine.* New York: Oxford University Press, 1985.

Morantz, Regina Markell, and Sue Zschoche. "Professionalism, Feminism, and Gender Roles: A Comparative Study of Nineteenth-Century Medical Therapeutics." *Journal of American History* 67 (Dec. 1980): 568–88.

O'Hara, Leo J. *An Emerging Profession: Philadelphia Doctors, 1860–1900.* New York: Garland, 1989.

Owen, A. *The Darkened Room: Women, Power, and Spiritualism in Late Victorian England.* Philadelphia: University of Pennsylvania Press, 1990.

Parsons, Talcott. *The Social System.* Glencoe, Ill.: Free Press, 1951.

Peitzman, Steven. *A New and Untried Course: Woman's Medical College and Medical College of Pennsylvania.* New Brunswick, N.J.: Rutgers University Press, 2000.

Peterson, Linda. *Victorian Autobiography: The Tradition of Self-Interpretation.* New Haven, Conn.: Yale University Press, 1986.

Philadelphia Club of Advertising Women. "Notes of Philadelphia Friendship Dinner." Typescript, May 2, 1936. Longshore Papers. ASCWM.

Poirer, Suzanne, Lorie Rosenblum, Lioness Ayre, Daniel Brauner, Barbara Sharf, and Ann Folwell Stanford. "Charting the Chart—an Exercise in Interpretation(s)." *Literature and Medicine* 11, no. 1 (spring 1992): 1–22.

Pringle, Rosemary. *Sex and Medicine: Gender, Power, and Authority in the Medical Profession.* Cambridge: Cambridge University Press, 1998.

Raimbault, G., O. Cachin, J. Limal, C. Eliacheff, and R. Rapaport. "Aspects of Communication between Patients and Doctors: An Analysis of the Discourse in Medical Interviews." *Pediatrics* 55 (1975): 401–5.

Richardson, Ruth. *Death, Dissection, and the Destitute.* Harmondsworth: Penguin, 1989.

Rivers, Christopher. *Face Value: Physiognomical Thought and the Legible Body in Marivaux, Lavater, Balzac, Gautier, and Zola.* Madison: University of Wisconsin Press, 1994.

Roberts, K. B. "The Contexts of Anatomical Illustrations." In *The Ingenious Machine of Nature: Four Centuries of Art and Anatomy*, by Mimi Cazort, Monique Kornell, and K. B. Roberts, 71–104. Ottawa: National Gallery of Canada, 1996.

Roberts, Shirley. *Sophia Jex-Blake: A Woman Pioneer in Nineteenth Century Medical Reform*. London: Routledge, 1993.

Roman, Camille, Suzanne Juhasz, and Christanne Miller, eds. *The Women and Language Debate: A Sourcebook*. New Brunswick, N.J.: Rutgers University Press, 1994.

Rosenberg, Charles E. *The Care of Strangers: The Rise of America's Hospital System*. New York: Basic Books, 1987.

Rosenberg, Charles E. "The Therapeutic Revolution: Medicine, Meaning, and Social Change in Nineteenth Century America." In *The Therapeutic Revolution: Essays in the Social History of American Medicine*, ed. Morris J. Vogel and Charles E. Rosenberg, 3–26. Philadelphia: University of Pennsylvania Press, 1979.

Rosenberg, Charles, and Janet Golden, eds. *Framing Disease: Studies in Cultural History*. New Brunswick, N.J.: Rutgers University Press, 1992.

Rosner, Lisa. "Student Culture at the Turn of the Nineteenth Century: Edinburgh and Philadelphia." *Caduceus* 10, no. 2 (autumn 1994): 65–86.

Ross, Andrew, ed. *Science Wars*. Durham, N.C.: Duke University Press, 1996.

Rossiter, Margaret. *Women Scientists in America: Struggles and Strategies to 1940*. Baltimore: Johns Hopkins University Press, 1982.

Rothman, Sheila M. *Living in the Shadow of Death: Tuberculosis and the Social Experience of Illness in American History*. New York: Basic Books, 1994.

Ryan, Mary P. *Womanhood in America: From Colonial Times to the Present*. 3d ed. New York: Franklin Watts, 1983.

Ryan, Mary. *Women in Public: Between Banners and Ballots*. Baltimore: Johns Hopkins University Press, 1990.

Salem, Dorothy, ed. *African American Women: A Biographical Dictionary*. New York: Garland, 1993.

Sappol, Michael. "Sammy Tubbs and Dr. Hubbs: Anatomical Dissection, Minstrelsy, and the Technology of Self-Making in Postbellum America." *Configurations* 4, no. 2 (1996): 131–83.

Sappol, Michael. *A Traffic of Dead Bodies: Anatomy and Embodied Social Identity in Nineteenth-Century America*. Princeton, N.J.: Princeton University Press, 2001.

Savitt, T. L. "'A Journal of Our Own': The Medical and Surgical Observer at the Beginnings of an African-American Medical Profession in Late Nineteenth Century America," part 2. *Journal of the National Medical Association* 88, no. 2 (Feb. 1996): 115–22.

Schiebinger, Londa. *The Mind Has No Sex? Women in the Origins of Modern Science*. Cambridge, Mass.: Harvard University Press, 1989.

Schiebinger, Londa. *Nature's Body: Gender in the Making of Early Modern Science*. Boston: Beacon, 1993.

Shapin, Steven, and Simon Schaffer. *Leviathan and the Air Pump: Hobbes, Boyle, and the Experimental Life*. Princeton, N.J.: Princeton University Press, 1985.

Silverman, David. "Policing the Lying Patient: Surveillance and Self-Regulation in Consultations with Adolescent Diabetics." In *The Social Organization of Doctor-*

Patient Communication, ed. Alexandra Dundes Todd and Sue Fisher, 213–43. 2d ed. Norwood, N.J.: Ablex, 1993.

Smith, Jonathan. *Between Fact and Feeling: Baconian Science and the Nineteenth-Century Literary Imagination.* Wisconsin: University of Wisconsin Press, 1994.

Smith, Sidonie. *A Poetics of Women's Autobiography: Marginality and the Fictions of Self-Representation.* Bloomington: Indiana University Press, 1987.

Spigelman, Candace. "Dialectics of Ownership in Peer Writing Groups." Unpublished Ph.D. dissertation, Temple University, Philadelphia, 1996.

Stafford, Barbara. *Body Criticism: Imaging the Unseen in Enlightenment Art and Medicine.* Cambridge, Mass.: MIT Press, 1991.

Stanley, Liz. *The Auto/Biographical I: The Theory and Practice of Feminist Auto/Biography.* Manchester, England: Manchester University Press, 1992.

Temkin, Owei. "The Scientific Approach to Disease: Specific Entity and Individual Sickness." In *The Double Face of Janus: And Other Essays in the History of Medicine,* 441–55. Baltimore: Johns Hopkins University Press, 1977.

Theriot, Nancy. "Women's Voices in Nineteenth-Century Medical Discourse: A Step toward Deconstructing Science." In *Gender and Scientific Authority,* ed. Barbara Laslett, Sally Gregory Kohlstedt, Helen Longino, and Evelynn Hammonds, 124–54. Chicago: University of Chicago Press, 1996.

Todd, Alexandra Dundas, and Sue Fisher, eds. *The Social Organization of Doctor-Patient Communication.* 2d ed. Norwood, N.J.: Ablex, 1993; original publication, Washington, D.C.: Center for Applied Linguistics, 1983.

Tompkins, Jane. *Sensational Designs: The Cultural Work of American Fiction, 1790–1860.* New York: Oxford University Press, 1985.

Truax, Rhoda. *The Doctors Jacobi.* Boston: Little, Brown, 1952.

Tuana, Nancy. *Feminism and Science.* Bloomington: Indiana University Press, 1989.

Vietor, Agnes C., ed. *A Woman's Quest: The Life of Marie Zakrzewska, M.D.* New York: Appleton, 1924.

Viner, Russell. "Radical Medicine in Ante-Bellum New York City: Abraham Jacobi and German Social Medicine in America." Fall 1996 Workshop Series of the Department of History and Sociology of Science at the University of Pennsylvania, Philadelphia, Oct. 7, 1996.

Vogel, Morris. *The Invention of the Modern Hospital: Boston, 1870–1930.* Chicago: University of Chicago Press, 1980.

Vogel, Morris, and Charles Rosenberg, eds. *The Therapeutic Revolution: Essays in the Social History of American Medicine.* Philadelphia: University of Pennsylvania Press, 1979.

Waite, Fredrick C. "The Three Myers Sisters—Pioneer Women Physicians." *Medical Review of Reviews* (Mar. 1933): 1–7.

Waitzkin, Howard. *The Politics of Medical Encounters: How Patients and Doctors Deal with Social Problems.* New Haven, Conn.: Yale University Press, 1991.

Warner, John Harley. *Against the Spirit of System: The French Impulse in Nineteenth-Century American Medicine.* Princeton, N.J.: Princeton University Press, 1998.

Warner, John Harley. *The Therapeutic Perspective: Medical Practice, Knowledge, and Identity in America 1820–1885.* Reprint ed. Princeton, N.J.: Princeton University

Press, 1997; original publication, Cambridge, Mass.: Harvard University Press, 1986 (page references are to reprint edition).

Wegener, Frederick. "'A Line of Her Own': Henry James's 'Sturdy Little Doctress' and the Medical Woman as Literary Type in Gilded-Age America." *Texas Studies in Language and Literature* 39, no. 2 (summer 1997): 139–80.

Wells, Susan. *Sweet Reason: Rhetoric and the Discourses of Modernity.* Chicago: University of Chicago Press, 1996.

Welsh, Lilian. *Reminiscences of Thirty Years in Baltimore.* Baltimore: Norman, Remington, 1925.

West, Candace. "'Ask Me No Questions . . .': An Analysis of Queries and Replies in Physician-Patient Dialogues." In *The Social Organization of Doctor-Patient Communication,* ed. Alexandra Dundas Todd and Sue Fisher, 127–60. 2d ed. Norwood, N.J.: Ablex, 1993.

West, Candace. *Routine Complications: Troubles with Talk between Doctors and Patients.* Bloomington: Indiana University Press, 1984.

Wood, Ann Douglas. "'The Fashionable Diseases': Women's Complaints and Their Treatment in Nineteenth-Century America." *Journal of Interdisciplinary History* 4 (1973): 25–52.

NINETEENTH-CENTURY SOURCES

Note: This section includes twentieth-century editions of works by nineteenth-century writers and some articles, especially obituaries, from early in the twentieth century.

Agnew, D. Hayes, M.D. *Lecture Introductory to the One Hundred and Fifth Course of Instruction in the Medical Department of the University of Pennsylvania, Delivered Monday, October 10, 1870.* Philadelphia: Published by the class, 1870.

Agnew, D. Hayes, M.D. *Theatrical Amusements; with Some Remarks on the Rev. Henry W. Bellows' Address before the Dramatic Fund Society, N.Y.* Philadelphia: Wm. S. Young, 1857.

Alcott, Louisa May. *Hospital Sketches.* In *Alternative Alcott,* ed. E. Showalter, 1–73. New Brunswick, N.J.: Rutgers University Press, 1988; original publication, 1863.

Anderson, Matthew. *Presbyterianism: Its Relation to the Negro.* Illustrated by the Berean Presbyterian Church, Philadelphia, with Sketch of the Church and Autobiography of the Author. Philadelphia: John McGill, White, and Co., 1897.

Baker, C. Alice. Letter to Mary Putnam Jacobi. Nov. 7, 1874. Mary Putnam Jacobi Collection, Jacobi Papers, folder 10. Baker correspondence. SL.

Bartlett, H. Frances. "Report of the Entertainment Committee." In WMC, Alumnae Association, *Transactions of the Thirty-first Annual Meeting of the Alumnae Association of the Woman's Medical College of Pennsylvania,* May 24–25, 1906, 35–37. Philadelphia: Published by the association, 1906. MCP Collection. ASCWM.

Bean, Theodore W. *A History of Montgomery County, Pennsylvania.* Philadelphia: Everts and Peck, 1884. MCHS.

Beecher, Catherine. *Letters to the People on Health and Happiness.* New York: Harper and Row, 1855.

Blackwell, Elizabeth. *Essays in Medical Sociology.* New York: Arno Press, 1972; original publication, 1902.

Blackwell, Elizabeth. "The Influence of Women in the Profession of Medicine." In *Essays in Medical Sociology,* vol. 2, 1–33. New York: Arno Press, 1972; original publication, 1902.

Blackwell, Elizabeth. *The Laws of Life: With Special Reference to the Physical Education of Girls.* New York: Garland, 1986; original publication, 1852.

Blackwell, Elizabeth. *Pioneer Work in Opening the Medical Profession to Women.* New York: Schocken, 1977; original publication, 1895.

Black Women Physicians Project, 1864–1995. Files for Carolyn Still Wiley Anderson, Rebecca Cole, Eliza Grier, Rebecca Lee [Crumpler], Halle Tanner, and Georgiana Young. ASCWM.

Blankenburg, Lucretia. Notes on an interview with Mrs. Blankenburg. No date or interviewer given. Longshore Papers. ASCWM.

Boardman, Andrew. "An Essay on the Means of Improving Medical Education and Elevating Medical Character." Reprinted in Gert Brieger, ed., *Medical America in the Nineteenth Century: Readings from the Literature,* 27–28. Baltimore: Johns Hopkins University Press, 1972.

Boston Medical and Surgical Journal. "Outrage at a Woman's Medical College." 7, no. 8 (Feb. 23, 1871): 133–34.

Broomall, Anna E., M.D. Deceased Alumnae Files, MCP Collection. ASCWM.

Bruns, John Dickson. *Life, Its Relations, Animal and Mental: An Inaugural Dissertation.* Charleston, S.C.: Steam Power Press of Walker, Evans, and Co., 1857. CPP.

Campbell, Jane. "Sketch of the Life of Dr. Hannah Longshore, a Pioneer Woman Physician of Philadelphia." Manuscript, Oct. 19, 1901 (date crossed out). New York Academy of Medicine, New York City.

Carithers, Eli. Notebook of Clinical Cases, Jefferson Medical College. 1849–50. MM-014. JEFF.

Carpenter, William. *Principles of Human Physiology with the Chief Applications to Psychology, Pathology, Therapeutics, Hygiéne, and Forensic Medicine,* by William B. Carpenter, M.D., F.R.S., F.G.S., ed. with additions by Francis Gurney Smith, M.D. New American from the last London ed. Philadelphia: Blanchard and Lea, 1856.

Cass, Edward. "Letter from Ohio." *Medical and Surgical Reporter* (Philadelphia) 50, no. 22 (May 31, 1884): 685.

Clarke, Edward H. "Medical Education of Women." *Boston Medical and Surgical Journal* 4, no. 24 (Dec. 16, 1869): 346.

Clarke, Edward H. *Sex in Education: Or, A Fair Chance for Girls.* Boston: Osgood, 1873.

Cole, Rebecca. "First Meeting of the Women's Missionary Society of Philadelphia." *Woman's Era* 3, no. 4 (Oct./Nov. 1896): 4–5.

Cope, Ellen Fussell. "Bits of Background." Manuscript, undated. SC 045, Alice Fussell, Fussell-Lewis Family Papers, folder 3. FHL.

Corson, Thomas. *Physician and Patient: Address Delivered before the State Medical*

Society of New Jersey (1869), by Thos. J. Corson, M.D., President of the Society. Pamphlet, 1869. CPP.

Crumpler, Rebecca, M.D. *A Book of Medical Discourses in Two Parts.* Boston: Cashman, Keating and Co., Printers, 1883. History of Medicine Division, National Library of Medicine, Washington, D.C.

Douglass, Sarah Mapps. Letters to Hannah White Richardson. 1850–82. RG5/187: Richardson Family Papers, ser. 4. FHL.

Douglass, Sarah Mapps. Letters to Rebecca White, Philadelphia. Feb. 9, 1862, and two undated letters. QC.

Drake, Daniel. *Practical Essays on Medical Education and the Medical Profession in the United States.* Cincinnati: Roff and Young, 1832. Reprinted in Gert Brieger, ed., *Medical America in the Nineteenth Century: Readings from the Literature,* 8–24. Baltimore: Johns Hopkins University Press, 1972.

DuBois, W. E. B. *The Philadelphia Negro: A Social Study.* Philadelphia: University of Pennsylvania Press, 1996; original publication 1899.

Dunlap, J. Francis. Notebook of Clinical Cases, Jefferson Medical College. 1873–77. MM-029. JEFF.

Echo (London). Monday, Aug. 29, 1870.

Eclectic Medical Journal of Philadelphia. Ed. William Paine, M.D., and Marshall Calkin. 3, no. 6 (June 1860). CPP.

Eclectic Medical Journal of Philadelphia. "Organization of the American Eclectic Medical Association of Philadelphia." 1, no. 4 (Apr. 1858): 166.

Elliot, Rev. H. B. "Woman as Physician." In *Eminent Women of the Age; Being Narratives of the Lives and Deeds of the Most Prominent Women of the Present Generation,* by James Parton and others, chap. 2, 537–44. Hartford, Conn.: S. M. Betts and Co., 1868.

Emerson, Ralph Waldo. "Nature." *Emerson: Essays, First and Second Series,* ed. Douglas Crane, 309–26. New York: Vintage, 1990.

Fraser-Goins, Georgia. "Miss Doc." Georgia Frasier-Goins Collection. Moorland-Spingarn Research Center, Manuscript Division. Howard University Library.

Friends' Intelligencer. "Life of James Parnel and Francis Howgill." 37 (1880): 21–22, 320–24, 337–41. FHL.

Fulton, W., Dr. Case and lecture notes by Dr. W. Fulton. Bound handwritten notes on clinical cases of Prof. Ellerslie Wallace and Prof. Jacob Da Costa. Archives MM-207. JEFF.

Fussell, Edwin. "Valedictory Address to the Graduating Class of the Female Medical College of Pennsylvania at the Tenth Annual Commencement, March 13, 1861." MCP Collection, ASCWM.

Gilman, Charlotte Perkins. *The Diaries of Charlotte Perkins Gilman.* Vol. 2: *1890–1935.* Ed. Denise D. Knight. Charlottesville: University Press of Virginia, 1994.

Gilman, Charlotte Perkins. *The Living of Charlotte Perkins Gilman: An Autobiography.* New York: Appleton-Century, 1935.

Gilman, Charlotte Perkins. "The Yellow Wall-Paper." In *The Yellow Wall-Paper,* ed. E. Hedges, 9–36. Rev. 2d ed. Old Westbury, Conn.: Feminist Press, 1996; short story originally published 1892 in *New England Magazine.*

Gleason, Rachel. *Talks to My Patients: Hints on Getting Well and Keeping Well.* New ed. enlarged with the addition of nineteen "Letters to Ladies" on health, education, society, etc. New York: Holbrook, 1895.

Grier, Eliza. Letter to Susan B. Anthony. Mar. 7, 1901. Black Women Physicians Project, Grier File. ASCWM.

Grier, Eliza. Letter to the president and proprietor of the Woman's Medical College. Dec. 6, 1890. Black Women Physicians Project, Grier File. ASCWM.

Griscom, Mary, M.D. "Memorial Meeting for Dr. Anna E. Broomall." Apr. 4, 1932. Deceased Alumnae Files, Anna E. Broomall. ASCWM.

Gross, Samuel. "The Factors of Disease and Death after Injuries, Parturition, and Surgical Operations." *Reports and Papers, A.P.H.A.* 2 (1874–75): 400–14. Reprinted in Gert Brieger, ed., *Medical America in the Nineteenth Century: Readings from the Literature,* 190–200. Baltimore: Johns Hopkins University Press, 1972.

Hibbard, Sarah. Manuscript draft of lectures and sermons. Manuscripts, MS 54, Acc. #189. ASCWM.

Holmes, Oliver Wendell. "Report of the Committee on Medical Literature." *Transactions of the American Medical Association* 1 (1848): 249–88.

Hooker, Worthington. *Physician and Patient; or, a Practical View of the Mutual Duties, Relations, and Interests of the Medical Profession and the Community.* New York: Arno Press, 1972; original publication, 1849.

Hunt, Harriot Kezia. *Glances and Glimpses: Or Fifty Years Social, Including Twenty Years Professional Life.* Boston: Jewett, 1856.

Jacobi, Abraham. *Infant Diet.* A Paper Read before the Public Health Association of New York. New York: Putnam's Sons, 1873.

Jacobi, Abraham. *Infant Diet.* Revised, enlarged, and adapted to popular use by Mary Putnam Jacobi, M.D. New York: Putnam's Sons, 1874.

Jacobi, Abraham. Letter to Mary Putnam Jacobi. Mary Putnam Jacobi Collection, Jacobi Papers, a-26, folder 21. SL.

Jacobi, Mary Putnam. "Acute Fatty Degeneration of the New-born." *American Journal of Obstetrics* 2 (1878): 499. Reprinted in Mary Putnam Jacobi, *Mary Putnam Jacobi, M.D.: Pathfinder in Medicine,* ed. Women's Medical Association of New York City, 311–25. New York: Putnam's Sons, 1925.

Jacobi, Mary Putnam. "Anomalous Malformation of the Heart." *Medical Record* 7 (1872): 111.

Jacobi, Mary Putnam. "Aspiration of Dermoid Cysts Followed by Inflammation." *American Journal of Obstetrics* 16 (1883): 1160–70.

Jacobi, Mary Putnam. Autobiographical manuscript. Typescript, 1902. Mary Putnam Jacobi Collection, Jacobi Papers, a-26, folder 3. SL.

Jacobi, Mary Putnam. "Case of Absent Uterus: With Considerations of the Significance of the Hermaphrodism." *American Journal of Obstetrics* 32, no. 4 (Oct. 1895): 512.

Jacobi, Mary Putnam. "Case of Facial and Palatine Paralysis and Loss of Equilibrium Produced by a Fall on the Head." *Independent Practitioner* 2 (1881): 69.

Jacobi, Mary Putnam. "A Case of Malignant Icterus." *Medical Record* 8 (1873): 65.

Jacobi, Mary Putnam. "A Case of Probably Tumor of the Pons." *Journal of Nervous and Mental Diseases* 16 (1889): 115–25.

Jacobi, Mary Putnam. "A Case of Trephining of Sternum for Osteomyelitis." *American Journal of Obstetrics* 14 (1881): 981.

Jacobi, Mary Putnam. "Case of Uterine Fibroid Treated by Apostoli's Method: Enucleation of the Tumor." *American Journal of Obstetrics* 21 (1888): 806.

Jacobi, Mary Putnam. "The Clubs of Paris." *Scribner's Monthly* 3 (Nov. 1871): 105–8.

Jacobi, Mary Putnam. "Contribution to Sphygmography: The Influence of Pain on the Pulse Trace." *Archives of Medicine* 1 (1879): 33–35. Reprinted in Mary Putnam Jacobi, *Mary Putnam Jacobi, M.D.: Pathfinder in Medicine*, ed. Women's Medical Association of New York City, 326–28. New York: Putnam's Sons, 1925.

Jacobi, Mary Putnam. Correspondence. Mary Putnam Jacobi Collection, Jacobi Papers. SL.

Jacobi, Mary Putnam. "Croup and Diphtheria." *Medical Record* 12 (1876): 397.

Jacobi, Mary Putnam. "Curious Congenital Deformities of Upper and Lower Extremities." *Medical Record* 12 (1878): 115.

Jacobi, Mary Putnam. "Cystic Ovaries; Battey's Operation." *Medical Record* 25 (1884): 705.

Jacobi, Mary Putnam."Description of the Early Symptoms of the Meningeal Tumor Compressing the Cerebellum. From Which the Writer Died. Written by Herself." In Mary Putnam Jacobi, *Mary Putnam Jacobi, M.D.: A Pathfinder in Medicine*, ed. Women's Medical Association of New York City, 501–4. New York: Putnam's Sons, 1925. Original typescript, "Case. Description of the Early Symptoms of the Meningeal Tumor Compressing the Cerebellum. From Which the Writer Died. Written by Herself." [1903]. Mary Putnam Jacobi Collection, Jacobi Papers, folder 35. SL.

Jacobi, Mary Putnam. *Essays on Hysteria, Brain Tumor and Some Other Causes of Nervous Disease.* New York: Putnam's Sons, 1888.

Jacobi, Mary Putnam. "Foreword to the Family." Mary Putnam Jacobi Collection, Jacobi Papers, a-26, folder 3. SL.

Jacobi, Mary Putnam. "Found and Lost." In Mary Putnam Jacobi, *Stories and Sketches*, 1–49. New York: Putnam's Sons, 1907; first publication, *Atlantic Monthly*, Apr. 1860.

Jacobi, Mary Putnam. "Fragment at the thought of her twelfth birthday." Correspondence. Mary Putnam Jacobi Collection, Jacobi Papers, folder 5. SL.

Jacobi, Mary Putnam. "Inaugural Address at the Opening of the Woman's Medical College of the New York Infirmary, October 1, 1880." In Mary Putnam Jacobi, *Mary Putnam Jacobi: Pathfinder in Medicine*, ed. Women's Medical Association of New York City, 334–57. New York: Putnam's Sons, 1925.

Jacobi, Mary Putnam. "The Indication for Quinine in Pneumonia." *New York Medical Journal* 45 (1887): 589–99, 620–27. Reprinted in Mary Putnam Jacobi, *Mary Putnam Jacobi: Pathfinder in Medicine*, ed. Women's Medical Association of New York City, 419–45. New York: Putnam's Sons, 1925.

Jacobi, Mary Putnam. "Intestinal Obstruction." *Medical Record* 7 (1872): 208.

Jacobi, Mary Putnam. "Intra-Uterine Therapeutics." *American Journal of Obstetrics* 22 (1889): 449.

Jacobi, Mary Putnam. Letter to Dr. J. V. Ingham. 1900. Autograph case. CPP.

Jacobi, Mary Putnam. "Letters to the *Medical Record,* 1867–70—Medical Matters in Paris," signed P. C. M. In Mary Putnam Jacobi, *Mary Putnam Jacobi: Pathfinder in Medicine,* ed. Women's Medical Association of New York City, 1–171. New York: Putnam's Sons, 1925.

Jacobi, Mary Putnam. *Life and Letters of Mary Putnam Jacobi.* Ed. Ruth Putnam. New York: Putnam's Sons, 1925.

Jacobi, Mary Putnam. "Limitations and Dangers of Intra-Uterine Medication." *American Journal of Obstetrics* 22 (1889): 598, 697.

Jacobi, Mary Putnam. "Malignant Icterus with Great Enlargement of the Liver." *Transactions of the New York State Pathological Society* 3 (1879): 50.

Jacobi, Mary Putnam. *Mary Putnam Jacobi, M.D.: A Pathfinder in Medicine.* Ed. Women's Medical Association of New York City. New York: Putnam's Sons, 1925.

Jacobi, Mary Putnam. "Modern Female Invalidism." In Mary Putnam Jacobi, *Mary Putnam Jacobi, M. D.: Pathfinder in Medicine,* ed. Women's Medical Association of New York City, 478–82. New York: Putnam's Sons, 1925.

Jacobi, Mary Putnam. "The Nature and Dangers of Intra-uterine Medication." *Medical Record* 33 (1888): 23.

Jacobi, Mary Putnam. *New Orleans Sunday Times* columns, signed Mary Israel. Writings, 1866. Mary Putnam Jacobi Collection, Jacobi Papers, folder 28. SL.

Jacobi, Mary Putnam. "Nitrite of Amyl and Belladonna in Dysmenorrhoea." *Medical Record* 10 (1875): 11.

Jacobi, Mary Putnam. "Note on the Cause of Sudden Death during the Operation of Thoracentesis," letter to the editor. *Medical Record* 16 (1879): 139.

Jacobi, Mary Putnam. "Ovarian Tumor." *Medical Record* 8 (1873): 342.

Jacobi, Mary Putnam. "Pathogeny of Infantile Paralysis." *American Journal of Obstetrics* 8 (1874): 1–24. Reprinted in Mary Putnam Jacobi, *Mary Putnam Jacobi, M.D.: Pathfinder in Medicine,* ed. Women's Medical Association of New York City, 240–83. New York Putnam's Sons, 1925.

Jacobi, Mary Putnam. "Phenomena Attending Section of the Right Restiform Body." *Medical Record* 8 (1873): 17.

Jacobi, Mary Putnam. *Physiological Notes on Primary Education and the Study of Language.* New York: Putnam's Sons, 1889.

Jacobi, Mary Putnam. "Provisional Report on the Effect of Quinine upon the Cerebral Circulation." *Archives of Medicine* 1 (1879): 33.

Jacobi, Mary Putnam. "Puerperal Fever, Infection from Ovary through Retroperitoneal Glands." *Medical Record* 11 (1876): 307.

Jacobi, Mary Putnam. *The Question of Rest for Women during Menstruation,* Boylston Prize Essay of Harvard University, 1876. New York: Putnam's Sons, 1877.

Jacobi, Mary Putnam. "Remarks upon Empyema." *Medical News* 56 (1890): 120–21, 172–73.

Jacobi, Mary Putnam. "Remarks upon the Action of Nitrate of Silver on Epithelial and Gland Cells." *Transactions of the New York State Medical Society* (1875): 251. Reprinted in Mary Putnam Jacobi, *Mary Putnam Jacobi, M.D.: Pathfinder in Medicine,* ed. Women's Medical Association of New York City, 284–94. New York: Putnam's Sons, 1925.

Jacobi, Mary Putnam. "Reply to Prof. Munsterberg on American Women's Education." Typescript. Undated. Mary Putnam Jacobi Collection, Jacobi Papers, Writings, 1873, folder 30. SL.

Jacobi, Mary Putnam. "Salpingo-oophorectomy." *New York Medical Journal* 29 (1884): 673.

Jacobi, Mary Putnam. "Scarlatinous Nephritis." *Medical Record* 7 (1872): 354.

Jacobi, Mary Putnam. "Some Considerations on Hysteria." In Mary Putnam Jacobi, *Essays on Hysteria, Brain Tumor and Some Other Causes of Nervous Disease,* 1–80. New York: Putnam's Sons, 1888.

Jacobi, Mary Putnam. "Some Details in the Pathogeny of Pyaemia and Septicaemia." *Medical Record* 7 (1872): 73–101. Reprinted in Mary Putnam Jacobi, *Mary Putnam Jacobi, M.D.: Pathfinder in Medicine,* ed. Women's Medical Association of New York City, 171–200. New York: Putnam's Sons, 1925.

Jacobi, Mary Putnam. "Sphygmographic Experiments upon a Human Brain Exposed by an Opening in the Cranium." *American Journal of the Medical Sciences* 76 (1878): 10–21. Reprinted in Mary Putnam Jacobi, *Mary Putnam Jacobi, M.D.: Pathfinder in Medicine,* ed. Women's Medical Association of New York City, 299–310. New York: Putnam's Sons, 1925.

Jacobi, Mary Putnam. *Stories and Sketches.* New York: Putnam's Sons, 1907.

Jacobi, Mary Putnam. "Studies in Endometritis." *American Journal of Obstetrics* 18 (1885): 36–50, 113–28, 262–83, 519–37, 596–606. Continued in the same volume as "Morbid Variations in the Greater or Parturient Cycle, Subinvolution and Chronic Metritis (Studies in Endometritis)," 802–30; "Menstrual Subinvolution or Metritis of the Non-parturient Uterus (Studies in Endometritis)," 915–25; and "Theories of Menstruation: New Theory (Studies in Menstruation)," 376. Continued in a later volume as "The Ovarian Complication of Endometritis (Studies in Endometritis)," *American Journal of Obstetrics* 19 (1886): 352–67.

Jacobi, Mary Putnam. "Thrombosis of Ovarian Veins." *Medical Record* 7 (1872): 215.

Jacobi, Mary Putnam. "Urethral Irritation." *Proceedings of the Philadelphia County Medical Society* 13 (1892): 450–62.

Jacobi, Mary Putnam. "The Use of Electricity in Gynaecology." In WMC, Alumnae Association, *Report of the Proceedings of the Fourteenth Annual Meeting of the Alumnae Association of the Woman's Medical College of Pennsylvania,* Mar. 15, 1889, 60. Philadelphia: Rodgers Printing Co., 1889. MCP-D4, ASCWM.

Jacobi, Mary Putnam. *The Value of Life: A Reply to Mr. Mallock's Essay "Is Life Worth Living?"* New York: Putnam's Sons, 1879.

Jacobi, Mary Putnam. "Woman in Medicine." In *Woman's Work in America,* ed. Annie Nathan Meyer, 139–205. New York: Holt, 1891.

Jacobi, Mary Putnam, M.D., and Victoria White, M.D. *On the Use of the Cold Pack Followed by Massage in the Treatment of Anaemia.* New York: Putnam's Sons, 1880.

Jefferson Medical College. Clinical Notes (probably of the general dispensary), 1866–69. UA-JMC 014. JEFF.

Jefferson Medical College. Notebook of Clinical Cases, anonymous medical student, Oct.–Dec. 1853. MM-289. JEFF.

Jewett, Sarah Orne. *A Country Doctor.* Boston: Houghton Mifflin, 1884; reprinted, New York: Penguin, 1986.

The Journal. "Gershom M. Fitch: A Biographical Sketch." 9, no. 9 (Mar. 4, 1881): 67. FHL.

Judson, Eliza. "Address in Memory of Ann Preston, M.D., Delivered by Request of the Corporators and Faculty of the Woman's Medical College of Pennsylvania," Mar. 11, 1873. MCP Deans Files. ASCWM.

Kane, Elisha K., M.D. *Experiments on Kiesteine, with Remarks on its Application to the Diagnosis of Pregnancy.* Philadelphia: Medical Faculty of the University of Pennsylvania, 1842; reprinted from the *American Journal of the Medical Sciences* 4 (1842): 13–38. CPP.

Keller, Dr. Elizabeth C. "A Case of Laparotomy." In WMC, Alumnae Association, *Proceedings of the Twelfth Annual Meeting of the Alumnae Association of the Woman's Medical College of Pennsylvania,* Mar. 18, 1887, 61–63. Philadelphia: Rodgers Printing Co., 1887. MCP Collection, ASCWM.

Ladies' Physiological Institute of Boston and Vicinity. Secretary's Reports and Board Meetings, vol. 1, Dec. 1850, Apr. 1851. Ladies' Physiological Society Papers, MC 236. SL.

Lathrop, Ruth. Letter. Jan. 6, 1898. Black Women Physicians Project, Grier File. ASCWM.

Liston, Robert. *Elements of Surgery.* Ed. Samuel D. Gross. Philadelphia: Ed. Barrington and Geo. Haswell, 1846.

Longshore, Hannah. "Autobiography." Manuscript, in four versions, undated, unpaginated. Longshore Papers. ASCWM.

Longshore, Hannah. "A Case of Conception without Intromission." *Medical and Surgical Reporter* (Philadelphia) 50, no. 22 (May 31, 1884): 700–701.

Longshore, Joseph. *The Centennial Liberty Bell.* Philadelphia: Claxton, Remsen and Haffelfinger, 1876.

Longshore, Joseph. "History of Obstetrics." *Eclectic Medical Journal of Philadelphia* 8, no. 3 (Mar. 1865): 117–20; 8, no. 4 (Apr. 1865): 160–63; 8, no. 5 (May 1865): 1–97.

Longshore, Joseph. "Introductory Lecture, Delivered before the Class, at the Opening of the Female Medical College of Pennsylvania, Oct. 12, 1850." Philadelphia: Young, 1850. ASCWM and CPP.

Longshore, Joseph. Letter to Thomas Longshore. Jan. 24, 1834. Longshore Papers. ASCWM.

Longshore, Joseph. "The Ovular Theory of Menstruation, and Its History." *Eclectic Medical Journal of Philadelphia* 8, no. 6 (June 1865): 241–45.

Longshore, Joseph. *The Philadelphia System of Obstetrics.* Philadelphia: University Publication Society, 1868.

Longshore, Joseph. *The Principles and Practice of Nursing, or a Guide to the Inexperienced.* Philadelphia: Merrihew and Thompson, 1842.

Longshore, Joseph. "A Valedictory Address Delivered before the Graduating Class, at the First Annual Commencement of the Female Medical College of Pennsylvania, Held at the Musical Fund Hall, Dec. 30, 1851." Philadelphia: Published by the graduates, 1852. ASCWM and CPP.

Longshore, Joseph. "Woman." *Eclectic Medical Journal of Philadelphia* 8, no. 1 (Jan. 1865): 14–19.

Longshore, Joseph. *Woman and Her Maladies: The Little Book of Forbidden Knowledge.* Philadelphia: Grant, Faires, and Rodgers, 1878.

Longshore, Thomas. "Autobiography." Manuscript notebook, undated. Longshore Papers, file 11. ASCWM.

[Longshore, Thomas]. "Biography of Hannah Longshore." Manuscript notebook, bound ledger, appended pages, unsigned, undated. Longshore Papers. ASCWM.

[Longshore, Thomas]. "Biography of Joseph Skelton Longshore." Manuscript, in two versions, unsigned, undated. Longshore Papers. ASCWM.

Longshore, Thomas. *"The Christ" Interpreted.* Pamphlet, signed T. E. L. Philadelphia, July 1884.

Longshore, Thomas. *Father, Son, and Holy Ghost.* Pamphlet. N.d., n.p.

Longshore, Thomas. *George Fox Interpreted: The Religion, Revelations, Motives and Mission of George Fox Interpreted in the Light of the Nineteenth Century and Applied to the Present Condition of the Church.* Philadelphia: self-published, 1881. FHL.

Longshore, Thomas. *The Higher Criticism in Theology and Religion Contrasted with Ancient Myths and Miracles as Factors of Human Evolution and Other Essays on Reform.* New York: Somesby, 1892.

Longshore, Thomas. "History of the College." Manuscript, undated. Longshore Papers. ASCWM.

Longshore, Thomas. *Our Lord and Savior Jesus Christ.* Philadelphia, Mar. 1888, FHL.

Longshore, Thomas. "Sketch of Her Early Years." Manuscript, undated. Longshore Papers. ASCWM.

Longshore, Thomas. *The Spiritual Religion of Jesus and Salvation by Christ. Not Judaism nor Paganism; neither Greek nor Roman Mythology; Nor the Religion of Christianity as Taught by the Church in Ancient or Modern Times.* Pamphlet, signed T. E. L. Philadelphia: John Hiestand, printer, July 1884.

Longshore, Thomas, and Hannah Longshore. Letter to "you all." May 10, 1850. Longshore Papers, Family Correspondence file. ASCWM.

Longshore-Potts, Anna. *Discourses to Women on Medical Subjects.* London: self-published, 1897. ASCWM.

Longshore-Potts, Anna. *Love, Courtship, and Marriage.* Paradise Valley Sanitarium, National City, San Diego County, Calif.: self-published, 1891. ASCWM.

Marshall, Clara. *The Woman's Medical College of Pennsylvania: An Historical Outline.* Philadelphia: P. Blakiston, 1897.

McCully, S. E. "Masturbation in the Female." *American Journal of Obstetrics* 16, no. 8 (Aug. 1883): 844–45.

Medical and Surgical Reporter (Philadelphia). "The Female Students Again." 23 (Jan. 28, 1871): 85.

Medical and Surgical Reporter (Philadelphia). "Medical Lectures to Mixed Classes." 21 (Nov. 20, 1869): 325.

Medical and Surgical Reporter (Philadelphia). "The Medical Profession and the Management of Hospitals," 21 (Dec. 11, 1869): 386.

Medical and Surgical Reporter (Philadelphia). "Minutes of the Medical Society of the State of Penn'a." 22 (June 18, 1870): 529.

Medical and Surgical Reporter (Philadelphia). Obituary, Francis McCloskey. N.s. 2 (1859): 189.

Medical and Surgical Reporter (Philadelphia). "The Pennsylvania Hospital and Female Students." 22 (May 14, 1870): 420–21.

Medical and Surgical Reporter (Philadelphia). "The Pennsylvania Hospital Clinics." 23 (Aug. 26, 1871): 200–201.

Medical and Surgical Reporter (Philadelphia). "Remonstrance against Mixed Clinics." 21 (Nov. 27, 1869): 345–46.

Medical and Surgical Reporter (Philadelphia). "Report of Committee on Status of Female Physicians, Philadelphia County Medical Society." 16, no. 13 (Mar. 30, 1867): 256–62.

Medical and Surgical Reporter (Philadelphia). "The Woman Question in New York." 21 (Dec. 4, 1869): 362–63.

Medical and Surgical Reporter (Philadelphia). "The Woman's Medical College of Pennsylvania." 23 (Feb. 11, 1871): 130.

Medical and Surgical Reporter (Philadelphia). "Women Are Dirty Creatures, Anyhow!" 50, no. 1422 (May 31, 1884): 4.

Medical and Surgical Reporter (Philadelphia). "Women as Physicians." 16, no. 18 (May 4, 1867): 391–94.

Medical Gazette (New York). "Cliniques for Women." 4 (Mar. 4, 1870): 164.

Medical Gazette (New York). "The Pennsylvania Hospital Scandal." 3 (Nov. 20, 1869): 294–95.

Medical Gazette (New York). "Professional Items." 3 (Nov. 27, 1869): 307.

Meigs, Charles. *Woman; Her Diseases and Remedies.* Philadelphia: Lea and Blanchard, 1851.

Meigs, J. Forsyth, M.D. *A History of the First Quarter of the Second Century of the Pennsylvania Hospital, Read before the Board of Managers at Their Stated Meeting Held 9th Mo 25th, 1876.* Philadelphia: Board of Managers, 1877. CPP.

Men and Women Medical Students. No. 2. Anonymous pamphlet. Philadelphia, Apr. 1870. (Bound with the Minute Book of the Pennsylvania Hospital Board of Managers.) HLPH.

Meyer, Annie Nathan. *Helen Brent, M.D.: A Social Study.* New York: Cassell Publishing, 1892.

Meyer, Annie Nathan, ed. *Woman's Work in America.* New York: Holt, 1891.

Mitchell, Silas Weir. *Collected Novels.* New York: Century Co., 1915.

Mitchell, Silas Weir. *Dr. North and His Friends.* New York: Century Co., 1915.

Mitchell, Silas Weir. *Fat and Blood: And How to Make Them.* 2d ed. Philadelphia: Lippincott, 1878; original publication, 1877.

Mitchell, Silas Weir. Papers. CPP.

Mitchell, Silas Weir. *The Pearl, Rendered into Modern English Verse.* New York: Century, 1906.

Morton, Thomas, M.D. *The History of the Pennsylvania Hospital, 1751–1895.* Philadelphia: Times Printing House, 1897.

Mott, Anna. *The Ladies' Medical Oracle; or, Mrs. Mott's Advice to Young Females, Wives, and Mothers . . .* Boston: self-published, 1834.

Mott, Lucretia Coffin. *Discourse on Woman.* Delivered at the Assembly Buildings,

Dec. 17, 1849. Philadelphia: T. B. Peterson, 1850. Reprinted in Karlyn Kohrs Campbell, *Man Cannot Speak for Her,* vol. 2: *Key Texts of the Early Feminists,* 71–98. New York: Praeger, 1989.

Mumford, Mary. "Remarks at the Woman's Medical College Golden Jubilee." 1900. MCP Collection. ASCWM.

Norristown Daily Herald. Obituary for Margaret Richardson and account of her funeral. May 18, 1909. MCHS.

Osler, William. *An Alabama Student and Other Biographical Essays.* 2d impression. New York: Oxford University Press, 1909.

Packard, Francis R., M.D. "The Pennsylvania Hospital." In *Founders' Week Memorial Volume,* ed. Frederick P. Penry, A.M., M.D., 595–612. Published by the City of Philadelphia in Commemoration of the Two Hundred and Twenty-fifth Anniversary of Its Founding. Philadelphia, 1909.

Pennsylvania Hospital. Minute Book of the Pennsylvania Hospital Board of Managers. 1855–70. R11D12. HLPH.

Phelps, Elizabeth Stuart. *Doctor Zay.* New York: Feminist Press, 1987; original publication, 1882.

Phelps, Elizabeth Stuart. Correspondence with S. Weir Mitchell. Jan. 25, 1884. Mitchell files. CPP.

Philadelphia Club of Advertising Women. "Notes of Philadelphia Friendship Dinner." Typescript. May 2, 1936. Longshore Papers. ASCWM.

Philadelphia Inquirer. "Reunion, University of Pennsylvania." Clipping dated Dec. 20, 1875. William Pepper Papers. PA.

Preston, Ann. *Cousin Ann's Stories for Children.* Philadelphia: McKim, 1849.

Preston, Ann. "Introductory Lecture to the Class of the Female Medical College of Pennsylvania, Delivered at the Opening of the Tenth Annual Session, Oct. 19, 1859," by Ann Preston, M.D., Professor of Physiology and Hygiene. CSHN.

Preston, Ann. "Introductory Lecture to the Course of Instruction in the Female Medical College of Pennsylvania for the Session 1855–56," by Ann Preston, M.D., Professor of Physiology. MCP Deans Files, Preston Papers. ASCWM.

Preston, Ann. Letter to Hannah Monaghan Darlington. May 26, 1833. MCP Deans Files, Preston Papers. ASCWM.

Preston, Ann. Letter to Hannah Monaghan Darlington. Jan. 4, 1851, Philadelphia. Deceased Alumnae Files, Preston Papers. ASCWM.

Preston, Ann. Letter to Lavinia Passmore. Oct. 8, 1843. Letter Collection. Chester County Historical Society, West Chester, Pa.

Preston, Ann. "Nursing the Sick and the Training of Nurses," an Address Delivered at the Request of the Board of Managers of the Woman's Hospital, at Philadelphia, by Ann Preston, M.D. 1863. Typed transcript. CSHN.

Preston, Ann. "Valedictory Address to the Graduating Class of the Female Medical College of Pennsylvania at the Twelfth Annual Commencement, March 16, 1864," by Ann Preston, M.D., Professor of Physiology and Hygiene, with Announcement of the Fifteenth Annual Session. MCP Deans Files, Preston Papers. ASCWM.

Preston, Ann. "Valedictory Address to the Graduating Class of the Female Medical College of Pennsylvania for the Session of 1857–58," by Ann Preston, M.D., Professor of Physiology and Hygiene. MCP Deans Files, Preston Papers. ASCWM.

Preston, Ann. "Valedictory Address to the Graduating Class of the Woman's Medical College of Pennsylvania at the Eighteenth Annual Commencement, March 12th, 1870," by Ann Preston, M.D., Professor of Physiology and Hygiene. CSHN.

Preston, Ann. "Women as Physicians." [1875]. CSHN. Originally published as a letter, "Women as Physicians," *Medical and Surgical Reporter* (Philadelphia) 16, no. 18 (May 4, 1867): 391–94.

Preston, Ann, and Emeline Cleveland. "Statement of the Woman's Medical College of Pennsylvania." Reprinted in Clara Marshall, *The Woman's Medical College: An Historical Outline,* 24–27. Philadelphia: Lea and Blanchard, 1897.

Preston, Ann, T. Morris Perot, Joseph Jeanes, and Emeline Cleveland. Letter to Pennsylvania State Medical Society. June 8, 1866. Reprinted in Clara Marshall, *The Woman's Medical College: An Historical Outline,* 40–41. Philadelphia: Lea and Blanchard, 1897.

Reade, Charles. *The Woman-Hater.* 3 vols. Paris and Boston: Grolier Society, n.d.; original publication, 1877.

Reber, John W. H. Surgical Clinic Notebook, Jefferson Medical College, Philadelphia. 1866. MM-25. JEFF. (Notebook contains materials for 1863–65.)

Scarlett, M. J. "Valedictory Address of Prof. M. J. Scarlett, before the Graduating Class of the Female Medical College of Pennsylvania, March 16, 1867." Additional Holdings, Publications, MCP Collection, ASCWM.

Scott, Sir Walter. *Waverly.* New York: Penguin, 1972; original publication, 1814.

Smith, Stephen, M.D. "The Medical Co-education of Women." Appendix to Elizabeth Blackwell, *Pioneer Work in Opening the Medical Profession to Women,* 255–59. New York: Schocken, 1977; original publication, 1895.

Stewart, F. Campbell. "The Actual Condition of the Medical Profession in This Country; with a Brief Account of Some of the Causes Which Tend to Impede Its Progress, and Interfere with Its Honors and Interests." *New York Journal of Medicine* 6 (1846): 151–71. Reprinted in Gert Brieger, ed., *Medical America in the Nineteenth Century: Readings from the Literature,* 62–74. Baltimore: Johns Hopkins University Press, 1972.

Thomas, Kersey. Notebook, "Female Medical College of Pennsylvania, N 229 Arch Street, Philadelphia." 1854–55. ASCWM.

Transactions of the Medical Society of New Jersey. Thomas Corson obituary. P. 209. Newark, N.J.: Hardham, 1979.

Twain, Mark, and Charles Dudley Warner. *The Gilded Age: A Tale of Today.* Ed. Shelley Fisher Fishkin. New York: Oxford University Press, 1996; original publication, 1873.

University of Pennsylvania Medical Faculty. "Report on the Medical Department of the University of Pennsylvania," for the Session of 1851–52, to the Alumni of the School by the Medical Faculty. Unpaginated. (Bound with University of Pennsylvania School of Medicine pamphlets, M378.748 PZME.8). PA.

Upham, Ella. "Women in Medicine." *North American Journal of Homeopathy* reprint, no date.

Varney-Brownell, Emily A., M.D. "A Case of Hemoptysis." In WMC, Alumnae Association, *Report of the Proceedings of the Fourteenth Annual Meeting of the Alum-*

nae Association of the Woman's Medical College of Pennsylvania, Mar. 15, 1889, 89–90. Philadelphia: Rodgers Printing Co., 1889. MCP Collection. ASCWM.

Velpeau, Alf., A.L.M. *New Elements of Operative Surgery.* First American from the last Paris ed. New York: Langley, 1845. CPP.

Wharton, Anna L. Letter to her husband, Joseph Wharton. Mar. 12, 1856. RG5/162: Joseph Wharton Papers, ser. 4. 2. FHL.

Wheeler, Edith Flower. "She Saunters into Her Past." Typescript. 1946. Wheeler Collection, Deceased Alumnae Files, MCP Collection, ASCWM.

White, J. William, M.D. "Memoir of D. Hayes Agnew, M.D., LL.D." *Transactions of the College of Physicians,* 3d ser., 15 (Jan. 4, 1893): xxix–lxv.

Wiley-Anderson, Caroline V. "Popliteal Aneurism." In WMC, Alumnae Association, *Report of the Proceedings of the Thirteenth Annual Meeting of the Alumnae Association of the Woman's Medical College of Pennsylvania,* Mar. 16, 1888, 33–35. Philadelphia: Rodgers Printing Co., 1888. MCP Collection. ASCWM.

Wilson, Erasmus, M.D. *A System of Human Anatomy, General and Special.* Ed. Paul Goddard. Fourth American from the last London ed. Philadelphia: Lea and Blanchard, 1850.

Woman's Hospital of Pennsylvania. Board of Managers Minutes. 1864. Hospitals, MCP-G3a. ASCWM.

Woman's Hospital of Pennsylvania. Patient Records. 1868–76. CSHN.

Woman's Medical College of Pennsylvania (WMC). Alumnae Association. "Addresses at the Unveiling of a Memorial Tablet in Honor of Mary Putnam-Jacobi." In *Transactions of the Thirty-second Annual Meeting of the Alumnae Association of the Woman's Medical College of Pennsylvania.* May 23–24, 1907, 56–71. Philadelphia: Published by the association, 1907. MCP Collection. ASCWM.

Woman's Medical College of Pennsylvania (WMC). Alumnae Association. *Report of the Proceedings of the Fourteenth Annual Meeting of the Alumnae Association of the Woman's Medical College of Pennsylvania.* Mar. 15, 1889. Philadelphia: Rodgers Printing Co., 1889. MCP Collection. ASCWM.

Woman's Medical College of Pennsylvania (WMC). Alumnae Association. *Report of the Proceedings of the Nineteenth Annual Meeting of the Alumnae Association of the Woman's Medical College of Pennsylvania.* May 9–10, 1894. Philadelphia: Buchanan, 1894. MCP Collection, ASCWM.

Woman's Medical College of Pennsylvania (WMC). Alumnae Association. *Report of Proceedings of the Seventeenth Annual Meeting of the Alumnae Association of the Woman's College of Pennsylvania.* May 6–7, 1892. Philadelphia: Smith and Salmon, 1892. MCP Collection. ASCWM.

Woman's Medical College of Pennsylvania (WMC). Alumnae Association. *Report of the Proceedings of the Thirteenth Annual Meeting of the Alumnae Association of the Woman's Medical College of Pennsylvania.* Mar. 16, 1888. Philadelphia: Rodgers Printing Co., 1888. MCP Collection, ASCWM.

Woman's Medical College of Pennsylvania (WMC). Alumnae Association. *Report of Proceedings of the Twelfth Annual Meeting of the Alumnae Association of the Woman's Medical College of Pennsylvania.* Mar. 18, 1887. Philadelphia: Rodgers Printing Co., 1887.

Woman's Medical College of Pennsylvania (WMC). Alumnae Association. *Transactions of the Thirty-eighth Annual Meeting of the Alumnae Association of the Woman's Medical College of Pennsylvania.* June 5–6, 1913. Philadelphia: Published by the association, 1913. MCP Collection. ASCWM.

Woman's Medical College of Pennsylvania (WMC). Alumnae Association. *Transactions of the Thirty-first Annual Meeting of the Alumnae Association of the Woman's Medical College of Pennsylvania.* May 24–25, 1906. Philadelphia: Published by the association, 1906. MCP Collection. ASCWM.

Woman's Medical College of Pennsylvania (WMC). Alumnae Association. *Transactions of the Thirty-fourth Annual Meeting of the Alumnae Association of the Woman's Medical College of Pennsylvania.* May 27–28, 1909. Philadelphia: Published by the association, 1909. MCP Collection. ASCWM.

Woman's Medical College of Pennsylvania (WMC). Alumnae Association. *Transactions of the Twenty-seventh Annual Meeting of the Alumnae Association of the Woman's Medical College of Pennsylvania.* May 22–23, 1902. Philadelphia: Published by the association, 1902. MCP Collection. ASCWM.

Woman's Medical College of Pennsylvania (WMC). College Scrapbooks. MCP-C7, Acc. #133. Scrapbook A, 1816–48; Scrapbook 3, 1868, 1869, Jan. 1870–Aug. 1871. ASCWM.

Woman's Medical College of Pennsylvania (WMC). Deans Files, MCP-C4, Ann Preston Papers. ASCWM.

Woman's Medical College of Pennsylvania (WMC). Deans Files, MCP-C4, Rachel Bodley Papers, folder 11, 1886, Acc. #291. ASCWM.

Woman's Medical College of Pennsylvania (WMC). Deceased Alumnae Files. ASCWM.

Woman's Medical College of Pennsylvania. "Eighteenth Annual Announcement of the Woman's Medical College of Pennsylvania . . . for the Session of 1867–68." MCP Collection. ASCWM.

Woman's Medical College of Pennsylvania (WMC). "Eleventh Annual Announcement of the Female Medical College of Pennsylvania . . . for the Session 1860–61." MCP Collection. ASCWM.

Woman's Medical College of Pennsylvania (WMC). Faculty Minutes, 1850–64. MCP Collection. ASCWM.

Woman's Medical College of Pennsylvania (WMC). "First Annual Announcement of the Female Medical College of Pennsylvania for the Session of 1850–51. . . ." MCP Collection. ASCWM.

Woman's Medical College of Pennsylvania (WMC). "Fourteenth Annual Announcement of the Female Medical College of Pennsylvania . . . for the Session of 1863–64." MCP Collection. ASCWM.

Woman's Medical College of Pennsylvania (WMC). "Fourth Annual Announcement of the Female Medical College of Pennsylvania . . . for the Session 1853–54." MCP Collection. ASCWM.

Woman's Medical College of Pennsylvania (WMC). "Nineteenth Annual Announcement of the Woman's College of Pennsylvania . . . for the Session of 1868–69." MCP Collection. ASCWM.

Woman's Medical College of Pennsylvania (WMC). "Second Annual Announcement, of the Female Medical College of Pennsylvania for the Session of 1851–52, Situ-ated in Philadelphia." MCP Collection. ASCWM.

Woman's Medical College of Pennsylvania (WMC). "Seventeenth Annual Announce-ment of the Female Medical College of Pennsylvania . . . for the Session of 1866–67." MCP Collection. ASCWM.

Woman's Medical College of Pennsylvania (WMC). "Sixth Annual Announcement of the Female Medical College of Pennsylvania . . . for the Session of 1855–56." MCP Collection. ASCWM.

Woman's Medical College of Pennsylvania (WMC). "Tenth Annual Announcement of the Female Medical College of Pennsylvania . . . for the Session of 1859–60." MCP Collection. ASCWM.

Woman's Medical College of Pennsylvania (WMC). "Third Annual Announcement, of the Female Medical College of Pennsylvania for the Session of 1852–53, Situ-ated in Philadelphia." MCP Collection. ASCWM.

Woman's Medical College of Pennsylvania (WMC). "Twentieth Annual Announce-ment of the Woman's Medical College of Pennsylvania . . . for the Session of 1869–70." MCP Collection. ASCWM.

Woman's Medical College of Pennsylvania (WMC). "Twenty-first Annual Announce-ment of the Woman's Medical College of Pennsylvania . . . for the Session of 1870–71." MCP Collection. ASCWM.

Woman's Medical College of Pennsylvania (WMC). "Twenty-second Annual An-nouncement of the Woman's Medical College of Pennsylvania . . . for the Session of 1871–72." MCP Collection. ASCWM.

Woman's Medical College of Pennsylvania (WMC). "Twenty-third Annual An-nouncement of the Woman's College of Pennsylvania . . . for the Session of 1872–73." MCP Collection. ASCWM.

Wood, George, M.D., et al. *To the Contributors of the Pennsylvania Hospital.* Phila-delphia, spring 1870. HLPH.

Wood-Armitage, Eliza, M.D. Scrapbook. Deceased Alumnae Files, MCP Collec-tion. ASCWM.

UNPUBLISHED THESES BY NINETEENTH-CENTURY
MEDICAL STUDENTS

Note: In thesis titles, I have reproduced the orthography of the title page as closely as possible, adding quotation marks to designate the main title.

UNIVERSITY OF PENNSYLVANIA MEDICAL DEPARTMENT

Allen, Joshua. "An Essay on Organic Life Force" for the Degree of Doctor of Medi-cine, by Joshua G. Allen, County of Delaware, State of Pennsylvania. Preceptor Dr. Charles J. Morton of Pa. Duration of studies three years. Presented 2nd mo. 15th, 1850. PA.

Cook, John S. "An Essay on Diabetes" for the Degree of Doctor of Medicine, by

John S. Cook, Easton, Northampton County, Penna. Preceptor Lewis C. Cook, M.D., 1850. PA.

Corson, Thomas. "An Essay on Health versus Fashion" for the Degree of Doctor of Medicine, in the University of Pennsylvania. By Thomas J. Corson, of New Hope, Bucks county, State of Pennsylvania. Residence in city, 293 Race Stre., Preceptor, Chas. Foulke, M.D., Duration of studies, three and a half years. Presented, Jany 18th, 1851. PA.

Crawford, S. Wylie. "An Essay on Hypertrophy and Atrophy" for the Degree of Doctor of Medicine in the University of Pennsylvania. by S. Wylie Crawford of Philad., State of Pennsylvania. Residence—Philadelphia, Arch St. above. Preceptor, Wm. E. Horner, M.D. Duration of Studies, three years; Presented, February 4th, 1850. PA.

Richardson, John P. "Enteric or Typhoid Fever," Department of Medicine, University of Pennsylvania. Preceptor H. D. W. Pawling, Department of Medicine. Feb 17, 1863. PA.

Rivins, Jesse. "An Essay on Auscultation in the Diagnosis of Pulmonary Disease." For the Degree of Doctor of Medicine in the University of Pennsylvania by Jesse A. Rivins of Rutherford County, Tennessee. Preceptors. Watson and Wendel. Duration of studies 3 years and 4 months. Presented Jan 22nd, 1850. PA.

Sale, John W. "An Essay on Haemoptysis" For the Degree of Doctor of Medicine in the University of Pennsylvania, by John W. Sale, of Bedford County, State of Virginia. Residence in the City No 13th Filbert St. Preceptor R. A. Sale, M.D. Duration of Studies 3 years. Presented on the 15th of Jany, 1850. PA.

Smith, Abram. "An Essay on the Moral and Physical Education of Females" For the Degree of Doctor of Medicine in the University of Pennsylvania by Abram Smith of Easton, Northampton County, State of Pennsylvania, Residence No. 91 South Eighth Street, Philada. Preceptor S. Morton Zulich M.D. Duration of Studies 3 years. Presented Feby 1850. PA.

WOMAN'S MEDICAL COLLEGE OF PENNSYLVANIA: CLASS OF 1852

Ellis, Susanna H. "A Disquisition on the Influence of the Nervous System on the Functions of Respiration and Digestion." Respectfully submitted to the Faculty of the Female M. College of Pennsylvania as an inaugural thesis; for the Degree of M.D. By Susanna H. Ellis of Philadelphia. Preceptor J. W. Comfort, M.D. Period of study 3 years, 1851. ASCWM.

Hunt, Angenette. "A Disquisition on the True Physician." Respectfully submitted to the Faculty of the Medical College of Pennsylvania, as inaugural Thesis for the degree of M.D. by Angenette Hunt of Hamilton, N.Y. Term of study 3 years. Preceptor Dr. H. N. Hunt. Philadelphia, Nov. 26th, 1851. ASCWM.

Longshore, Anna M. [Anna Longshore-Potts]. "A Disquisition on Electricity." Respectfully submitted to the Faculty of the Female Medical College of Pennsylvania As an Inaugural Thesis For the Degree of M.D. By Anna M. Longshore of Bucks County Pa. Period of Study three years. Preceptor J. S. Longshore, M.D. November 1851. ASCWM.

Longshore, Hannah. "A Disquisition on Neuralgia, its Treatments," respectfully submitted to the Faculty of the Female Medical College of Pennsylvania as an Inaugural Thesis for the Degree of M.D. by Hannah E. Longshore of Philadelphia. Period of Study, Three Years. Preceptor Dr. Joseph S. Longshore, M.D., November 1851. ASCWM.

Mitchell, Frances. "A Disquisition on Chlorosis." Respectfully submitted to the Faculty of the Female Medical College of Pennsylvania as an Inaugural Thesis for the degree of the Doctorate in the Female Medical College of Pennsylvania. By Frances G. Mitchell of England. Period of Study three years. Preceptor J. F. X. McCloskey, M.D., Philadelphia, Dec 1st 1851. ASCWM.

Preston, Ann. "A Disquicition on General Diagnosis," Respectfully submitted to the Faculty of the Female Medical College of Pennsylvania as an Inaugural Thesis for the Degree of M.D. by Ann Preston of West Grove, Penna, term of study 3 years, preceptor, N. R. Moseley, M.D., Phila, Nov. 26th, 1851. ASCWM.

Sawin, Martha. "A Disquisition on Anaemia." Respectfully Submitted to the Faculty of the Female Medical College of Pennsylvania as an Inaugural Thesis For the Degree of M.D. by Martha A. Sawin of Boston Mass. Period of Study 3 years. Preceptors E. C. Rolfe, M.D., W. M. Cornell, M.D. ASCWM.

Way, Phebe. "A Disquisition on Wounds." Respectfully submitted to the Faculty of the Female Medical College of Pennsylvania. As an Inaugural Thesis for the Degree of M.D. by Phebe M. Way of Chester County, Pennsylvania. Preceptor, J. W. Comfort. ASCWM.

WOMAN'S MEDICAL COLLEGE OF PENNSYLVANIA: CLASS OF 1853

Adams, Charlotte. "Disquisitio De Physiologus Effectis Nutricum A Lactatione Nimia." Verecundie Submittitur ad Professores Feminae Medicinalis Collegii Pennsylvaniae, Quasi Inauguratum Propositum Pro Grado Doctoris Medicinae. Per Charlotte G. Adams, Bostonae. Praeceptores Guilielmus M. Cornell M.D., Enochus C. Rolfe, M.D., Tempus Studii—Tres Annos. Philadelphia, Januaris Primo Die. Annodomini MDCCCLII. ASCWM.

Anderson, Annah N. S. "A Disquisition on General Physiology," Respectfully Submitted to the Faculty of the Female Medical College of Pennsylvania as an Inaugural *thesis*, for the Degree of *Doctorate of Medicine*. By Annah N. S. Anderson of Bristol, Bucks County Pennsylvania. Period of study 3 years. Preceptor *Dr. Benjamin Malone* Philadelphia. January 1853. ASCWM.

Beverly, Julia A. "A disquistion on Iron," Respectfully Submitted to the Faculty of the Female Medical College of Pennsylvania As an Inaugural Thesis for the Degree of Doctor in Medicine, January 7th, 1853 by Julia A. Beverly of Prov. Rhode Island. Preceptors, W. M. Cornell, M.D. and E. C. Rolfe, M.D. Period of study three years. ASCWM.

Ellis, Hannah W. "A Disquisition on Labor." Respectfully submitted to the Faculty of the Female Medical College of Pennsylvania as an Inaugural Thesis for the Degree of Doctorate of Medicine by Hannah W. Ellis of Pennsylvania. Period of study 3 years. Preceptor [   ] Philadelphia, 1853. ASCWM.

Johnson, Henrietta W. "A disquisition on the Skin and its Functions": Respectfully Submitted to the Faculty of the Female Medical College of Pennsylvania as an

Inaugural thesis For the degree of M.D. by Henrietta W. Johnson of New Jersey. Preceptor I. W. Redfield M.D., Term of Study Three Years. ASCWM.

Minnis, Maria. "Disquisition on Medical Jurisprudence" Respectfully Submitted to the Faculty of the Female Medical College of Pennsylvania as an Inaugural Thesis for the Degree of the Doctorate in Medicine, by Maria Minnis of Phelps, New York. Period of study, four years. Preceptors, Caleb Bannister, M.D. and G. F. Horton. Philadelphia, January 10th, 1853. ASCWM.

Montgomery, Augusta. "A Disquisition on the Medical Education of Woman" Respectfully Submitted to the Faculty of the Female Medical College of Pennsylvania as an Inaugural Thesis for the Degree of Doctor of Medicine. By Augusta R. Montgomery. Residence: Attica, New York. Term of Study. Three years. Preceptors: Drs. Hayes and Hadley. Philadelphia, January 1st, 1853. ASCWM.

Richardson, Margaret. "A Disquisition on Phthisis Pulmonalis," respectfully Submitted to the Faculty of the Female Medical College of Pennsylvania as an Inaugural Theses for the Degree of the Doctorate in Medicine. By Margaret Richardson of Pennsylvania. Period of Study, three years, Preceptor, J. S. Longshore, M.D., Philadelphia, December 30th, 1852. ASCWM.

WOMAN'S MEDICAL COLLEGE OF PENNSYLVANIA: CLASS OF 1864

Putnam, Mary. "Theorae ad Lienis officium." Thesis Medicinae Collegii Foeminis Pennsylvaniae Facultati submissa ad gradum obtinendum Medicinae Doctoris. Maria C. Putname scripta. New York, 1864. ASCWM.

WOMAN'S MEDICAL COLLEGE OF PENNSYLVANIA: CLASS OF 1870

Hall, Sarah. "A Thesis on The Physical and Moral Effects of Abortion." Presented to the Faculty of the Woman's Medical College of Pennsylvania by Sarah C. Hall, Philadelphia Session of 1869–70. ASCWM.

WOMAN'S MEDICAL COLLEGE OF PENNSYLVANIA: CLASS OF 1878

Wiley, Caroline V. "A Thesis on Fibromata," Presented to the Faculty of the Woman's Medical College of Pennsylvania for Degree of Doctor of Medicine by Caroline Wiley, Philadelphia, Session of 1877–78. ASCWM.

Young, Georgiana. "A Thesis on Opium," Presented to the Faculty of the Woman's Medical College of Pennsylvania, for degree of Doctor of Medicine by Georgie E. Young, Philadelphia, Session of 1877–8. ASCWM.

WOMAN'S MEDICAL COLLEGE OF PENNSYLVANIA: CLASS OF 1888

Bennett, Juan F. "Sanitary Chemistry." Submitted to the Faculty and Corporators of the Woman's Medical College for the Degree of Doctor of Medicine. Juan F. Bennett, 1888. ASCWM.

Index

307

DATE DUE

MAR 0 5 2003		
APR 2 2 2003		
NOV 0 7 2003 LL		
JAN 0 7 2004		
MAY 0 4 2005		
MAY 1 0 2005		
GAYLORD		PRINTED IN U.S.A.